PREFACE

This Instructor's Manual, prepared in conjunction with *Family-Centered Nursing Care of Children*, 2nd edition, by Cecily Lynn Betz, Mabel Hunsberger, and Stephanie Wright, is intended to facilitate the effective use of the comprehensive information in the textbook. The manual offers the instructor of pediatric nursing a variety of ideas and approaches to both classroom and clinical teaching of nursing care of children and families.

The first part of the Instructor's Manual is organized chapter by chapter to correlate with the textbook. Each chapter contains discussion questions, student learning activities, and audiovisual resources. Selected chapters contain case studies, pretests, and student worksheets designed to ascertain the students' knowledge and ability to apply previously learned and newly acquired information on the nursing care of children and families. Following the last chapter is an Audiovisual Resource Guide (see below) and a short section on Strategies for Clinical Instruction, which includes a Clinical Preparation Worksheet, a Weekly Care Plan, and a Clinical Student Self-Evaluation form. The Test Items form the second half of the manual and include multiple choice questions that are directly related to chapter content. Its description is given below following a brief description of each section within the chapters.

DISCUSSION QUESTIONS

These questions closely follow chapter content and reflect important concepts found in the textbook. The discussion questions can be used as classroom discussion topics, essay test questions, individual student presentation assignments, or review questions.

STUDENT LEARNING ACTIVITIES

This part includes a variety of teaching strategies for the classroom or clinical setting. Each activity reflects chapter content and is designed to promote the students' application of theoretical concepts to actual situations in pediatric nursing. The activities include guidelines for written analysis projects, clinical assignments, observational experiences, group participation activities, and group discussions.

AUDIOVISUAL RESOURCES

This section of each chapter includes an annotated summary of audiovisual programs that relate to the content of that chapter. Suggestions for classroom, clinical, or independent use of these resources as alternate or supplementary teaching modalities are provided for the programs that were previewed in the first edition of the Instructor's Manual. An Audiovisual Resource Guide (pages 195–196) is provided following the last chapter, which contains addresses and telephone numbers for program distributors.

CASE STUDIES

The case studies are brief descriptions of a particular child and family interacting with the health care system. The presentations include questions designed to promote application of knowledge to actual situations. These case studies can be used to stimulate discussion, to illustrate conceptual or problem-solving modalities, as essay test questions, or as part of a written analysis exercise.

STUDENT WORKSHEETS AND ASSESSMENT FORMS

The student worksheet and assessment forms are for enhancement of student understanding and application of knowledge gained through classroom instruction or independent study. These forms may be reproduced and used in a variety of ways, including written projects, interviewing and assessment practice, and patient teaching plan development.

PRETESTS

These tests are designed to assist the instructor in identifying the knowledge level of the student in areas basic to nursing practice, such as growth and development, nutrition, fluid and electrolyte balance, and structure and function of each body function. Use of these pretests will help in planning appropriate review and individual study activities by assessing student learning needs. Answers to the pretest questions are on the page immediately preceding each test.

TEST ITEMS

The test items that make up in the second half of this manual include nearly 400 multiple choice questions that are derived from the chapter content. Each question is accompanied by the correct answer and its rationale, as well as its cognitive type: knowledge (K), interpretation (I), or application (A). These questions are also available in computerized software form by contacting your local W. B. Saunders representative.

ACKNOWLEDGMENTS

This revision was based on the first edition of the Instructor's Manual, which was written by Lynn Kelly and Susan Saltstein. We thank them for their work.

We also acknowledge with great appreciation the test item contributors to the first edition:

Lynn Kelly	Carol A. Flaugher
Susan Saltstein	Agatha M. Gallo
Ann Barlett	Terea Giannetta
Rosalie Benchot	Carole Kenner
Joan E. Bowers	Charlotte R. Patrick
Beth M. Donaher	Ruth R. Voignier
Peggy J. Drapo	Marilyn L. Winkelstein

INSTRUCTOR'S MANUAL AND TEST QUESTIONS TO ACCOMPANY

BETZ, HUNSBERGER, AND WRIGHT

N F

1994
W. B. SAUNDERS COMPANY
A Division of Harcourt Brace & Company
Philadelphia • London • Toronto • Montreal • Sydney • Tokyo

W. B. Saunders Company
A Division of Harcourt Brace & Company

The Curtis Center
Independence Square West
Philadelphia, Pennsylvania 19106

Design, layout, and editing; Kathy Walker
Editorial Technologies
Renton, Washington

Instructor's Manual and Test Questions to Accompany
Family-Centered Nursing Care of Children ISBN 0-7216-4573-9

Printed in the United States of America.

Last digit is the print number: 9 8 7 6 5 4 3 2 1

Instructor's Manual and Test Questions to Accompany

Betz, Hunsberger, and Wright

FAMILY-CENTERED NURSING CARE OF CHILDREN

Table of Contents

UNIT I

PERSPECTIVES ON NURSING CARE OF CHILDREN AND ADOLESCENTS

CHAPTER 1

CHILD HEALTH ISSUES, ETHICS, AND NURSING PROCESS

DISCUSSION QUESTIONS

1. Discuss the meaning of the terms *morbidity* and *mortality*. What are the major causes of morbidity in the pediatric population?
2. Describe poverty in the United States and how this affects children. Discuss the implications for nursing care.
3. What are the health care needs for children in the twenty-first century?
4. Discuss the historical evolution of health care provided to children. What is the current status of child health care?
5. List functions of the pediatric nurse as patient advocate and teacher.
6. Describe the steps of the Thomasma model for ethical decision making.
7. Describe the five phases of the nursing process in relation to planning care of the child.

CLASSROOM EXERCISES

1. In group discussion, have students identify areas of nursing practice that might result in ethical dilemmas. Begin by having students define the terms *ethics*, *values*, and *beliefs* and the relationship among them. Ask students their feelings regarding withholding treatment from an infant with a profound neurological deficit or physical disorder. What rights do parents have in determining the type of treatment that their children receive?
2. Examine the United Nations Declaration of the Rights of Children. What are some instances when it would be difficult to maintain a particular principle?
3. Collaborate with the nursing research course. Ask students to identify areas of research within pediatric nursing. Develop mini-research proposals, including identification of the research question, procedure for collecting the data, and expectation of the findings based on current scientific data.

CASE STUDY

Apply the steps of the ethical decision-making model (Thomasma, 1978) to one of the case studies presented in the ethic boxes throughout the text.

STUDENT LEARNING ACTIVITIES

1. Ask students to contact local and state departments of public health to identify the major causes of morbidity and mortality for children in various age groups. Are there differences related to socioeconomic status? What resources are available in the community to deal with childhood morbidity and mortality? Ask students to make a list of measures that would help communities and families begin to reduce childhood morbidity and mortality.

2. Divide the students into small groups and ask each group to observe nurses practicing in various pediatric settings, including well child clinics, inpatient general floor, emergency room, specialty clinics, and intensive care. Ask the students to develop a list of nursing practices common to all of the settings and a list of practices unique to a particular setting. Ask the students to give examples of how the observed nurses functioned in the role of patient advocate, teacher, and care giver.

3. Obtain copies of hospital policies on (a) cardiopulmonary resuscitation, (b) determination of brain death, and (c) informed consent. What rights do these policies provide children and families? What responsibilities do nurses have for maintaining these policies?

AUDIOVISUAL RESOURCES

1. **The Pediatric Nurse as Teacher**
   This program is valuable for demonstrating the teaching role in pediatric nursing. It reviews basic childhood growth and development and presents appropriate teaching strategies for use with children. Individual developmental assessments and educational strategies to foster a child's understanding of unfamiliar hospital surroundings and procedures are presented.

Videocassette: 20 minutes

Distributor: Altschul Group Corporation

2. **Critical Choice**
   This videotape dramatizes a hospital director's struggle to decide whether to allocate scarce resources to one child in need of an emergency liver transplant or to fund a new program that could save the lives of many infants over the next year. Since this program is an open-ended presentation, it can be used to stimulate discussion of ethical, legal, and economic issues associated with the nursing care of children.

Videotape: 15 minutes

Distributor: Pyramid Film and Video

3. **Who Should Decide?**
   A woman with spina bifida learns her unborn child has the same condition. She and her husband must make a decision about whether to terminate the pregnancy. This drama is one in a bioethics series designed to stimulate discussion about ethical issues raised by advances in modern science and technology.

Videocassette: 13 minutes

Distributor: Pyramid Film and Video

4. **I'm Just Your Mother—Ethical Dilemmas in the NICU: The Parent's Perspective**
   This program portrays the story of one family faced with the birth of a premature infant. It is designed to help nurses understand how parents perceive the decision-making process and lead to further discussion of the issues involved.

Videocassette: 23 minutes

Distributor: Health Sciences Consortium

CHAPTER 2

FAMILY THEORIES AND ASSESSMENT

DISCUSSION QUESTIONS

1. How is the family defined?
2. Why is the view of the nuclear family not representative of contemporary families?
3. Describe the historical growth process of the family.
4. How is the family conceptualized in various nursing theoretical frameworks?
5. How is the family conceptualized in the following frameworks: (a) systems theory, (b) structural-functional, (c) social exchange, (d) interactional, and (e) developmental. Identify the strengths and limitations of each framework.
6. Discuss the components of the nursing process from a family-centered approach. What constitutes a family health problem? What important factors should be considered in establishing priorities for identified problems?
7. Identify the basic assumptions of family assessment and family nursing.
8. Describe the following family assessment tools in relation to content and priority focus: (a) family APGAR, (b) Otto's 13 assessment criteria, (c) family genogram, and (d) family ecomap.
9. Why is it important for the nurse working with families to be aware of her own values?
10. Describe four models of family health according to Loveland-Cherry.
11. What is meant by the term *vulnerable families*?
12. What is meant by the term *families at risk*? Identify factors that put a family at risk.
13. What are the advantages and disadvantages of a multidisciplinary approach to working with families at risk?
14. What are the primary nursing roles in working with families at risk?

CASE STUDY

Jody Williams, 8 years old, is brought to the clinic by his mother who tells the nurse that Jody was not allowed to attend school because his immunization schedule is not up to date. Jody has not had a medical evaluation in two years. On exam, Jody is at the 50th percentile for height and just below the 5th percentile for weight. Her mother, Christine, is a single mother who works as a housekeeper in a hospital. She often works overtime and gets home after midnight. Jody's older sister, who is 13 years old, baby-sits for Jody. The family lives close to a fast food restaurant and they often eat dinner there. Jody likes school and received good marks in first grade. Christine reports that Jody is not interested in playing outside with other children and spends much of his time at home watching TV.

On physical exam, Jody's right ear shows signs of chronic infection. Christine says that Jody often complains of pain on the right side of his face, but she attributes it to growing pains. During the exam, Jody maintains close contact with his mother, and she holds his hand during the immunization injection and hugs him after the injection is given.

What actual and potential difficulties in family functioning are present in the Williams family? What strengths can be identified in the family?

What are the actual and potential nursing diagnoses for this family? What interventions can the nurse initiate for these diagnoses?

STUDENT LEARNING ACTIVITIES

1. Select one of the tools provided for family assessment and use the tool to assess the family of the child to whom they are assigned on the hospital unit. Ask the student to critique the tool with respect to biases relating to the following: (a) the picture of an ideal family, (b) ethnic or cultural biases, and (c) utility and content.
2. Ask students to construct a family genogram for the family of the child to whom they are assigned. Ask students to write a paragraph describing the information obtained from the genogram.
3. Assign to each student a child hospitalized with chronic health problems. Ask students to assess the family functioning using the family ecomap.

AUDIOVISUAL RESOURCES

1. Patterns of Family Interaction
This program is designed to help viewers think about how families communicate and what causes them to function poorly. The program consists of eight different vignettes of a family portraying a spectrum of family structures.

Videocassette: 25 minutes

Distributor: Health Sciences Consortium

2. Family and Survival
This program, hosted by Phil Donahue, provides insight into the changing role of the American family—changes brought about by unprecedented stress and changing societal needs and pressures. It points out that less than 5% of American households still fall into the "traditional" family mold. The program looks at the effects of broken homes, battered wives, estranged children, and corporate nomads on the children growing up in these environments.

Videocassette: 52 minutes

Distributor: Indiana University Audio-Visual Center

3. The Single Parent Family
This program dramatizes the problems, frustrations, and anxieties of being a single parent. One single mother and her three children share their experiences.

Videocassette or 16-mm film: 15 minutes

Distributor: Indiana University Audio-Visual Center

4. Suffer The Children
Five families who live in urban poverty are profiled. The effect of poverty on the children is discussed. This program looks at the circumstances that perpetuate poverty and the hostility, anger, and despair caused by limited opportunity.

Videocassette: 86 minutes

Distributor: Indiana University Audio-Visual Center

5. Teenage Parents
This program explains the problems that arise and the adjustments that are necessary when teenagers become parents. Interviews with two teenage couples are included. The program addresses differences in the lifestyles of these two teenage couples.

16-mm film: 13 minutes

Distributor: Indiana University Audio-Visual Center

6. Cultural Assessment
Nursing experts share experiences with patients from various cultures with real-life vignettes in this program. Included are a nurse using pictures to communicate with a patient who speaks very little English, offering a visit from the hospital priest to help a patient, and integrating the patient's dietary preferences into her total care. An assessment tool that includes ethnic/racial identity, language, healing beliefs and practices, and religious beliefs is discussed. Although this program is not tailored to children, it offers the student valuable information about cultural assessment.

Videocassette: 28 minutes

Distributor: American Journal of Nursing Company

7. Family Assessment
This program begins with an overview of the family assessment process. Health-related questioning, particularly relevant to the family's cultural background, is presented. Pertinent observations and assessment strategies such as a genogram are emphasized.

Videotransfer: 16 minutes

Distributor: Concept Media

CHAPTER 3

DEVELOPMENT OF CHILDREN

DISCUSSION QUESTIONS

1. Why is a thorough understanding of all facets of growth and development important for nurses working with children?
2. Distinguish between the terms *physical, intellectual,* and *emotional-social competency.*
3. Describe the interrelationships between growth and development.
4. Outline the characteristics of the child in each of Piaget's stages of cognitive development.
5. Compare and contrast the innate theory, social reinforcement theory, and social learning theory of language development.
6. Identify the task for each of the eight stages of Erikson's theory of psychosocial development.
7. Describe the characteristics of each stage of faith development according to Fowler.
8. Describe the characteristics of each of the stages of moral development according to Kohlberg. What are the criticisms of Kohlberg's theory?
9. What is temperament? How is temperament manifested? What aspects of behavior are influenced by temperament? How does Thomas categorize temperament?
10. Compare and contrast the terms *growth, development,* and *maturation.*
11. Give examples of each of the following developmental progressions: (a) simple to complex, (b) general to specific, (c) cephalocaudally, and (d) proximodistally.
12. Discuss the factors that can either facilitate or deter a child from achieving an optimum level of development.
13. What does research suggest about the influence of television on children?

STUDENT LEARNING ACTIVITIES

1. At the beginning of the course, give students the Pretest for Growth and Development (following this chapter). Review and discuss their answers in class.
2. Ask students to evaluate the developmental status of both a well child and a sick child. Students should evaluate the child's psychosocial, cognitive, and moral development using the Developmental Assessment Form. In a clinical conference, ask students if levels of development are always consistent for children of the same chronological age. Are differences in development observed for children with chronic illnesses?

AUDIOVISUAL RESOURCES

1. **The Growing Child: Infancy through Adolescence**
   This series addresses growth and development in each age group as well as health needs of children in each age group. Nursing assessments and interventions for children and adolescents experiencing potential disruptions in development are included.

Videocassette: 30 minutes each

Distributor: J.B. Lippencott Company

2. **Baby Talk**
   This program examines modern research in language development. Specifically, fetal and infant responses to speech, the relationship between language and cognitive development, and the processes by which infants and children interpret adult speech to build grammar are addressed.

Videocassette: 49 minutes

Distributor: Indiana University Audio-Visual Center

3. **Out of the Mouths of Babes**
   This program offers a chronology of language acquisition from birth to 6 years of age. Researchers in language acquisition Peter and Jill de Villiers describe linguistic development and discuss the games and tests they have devised for their research.

Videocassette or 16-mm film: 28 minutes

Distributor: Filmakers Library

4. **Everybody Rides the Carousel, Parts I & II**
   These programs address Erikson's theory of personality development from infancy through young adulthood. Vignettes of typical life situations are presented.

Videocassette: 24 minutes each part

Distributor: Pyramid Film and Video

5. **The Impact of Media on Children**
   This program features a consultant to a state department of public instruction discussing the impact of media on children and adolescents. Interviews with children, parents, and educators are included. Parental responsibilities are outlined.

Videocassette: 28 minutes

Distributor: Indiana University Audio-Visual Center

6. **Infancy through Adolescence**
   This five-part series depicts growth and development from infancy through adolescence. Health issues for each age group are addressed.

Videocassette: 38–44 minutes

Distributor: American Journal of Nursing

ANSWERS TO PRETEST

1. a
2. c
3. a
4. b
5. c
6. a
7. b
8. b
9. c
10. b
11. b
12. a
13.
14. c
15. d
16. b

PRETEST: GROWTH AND DEVELOPMENT

Circle the letter that corresponds to the correct answer.

1. At the conclusion of Piaget's sensorimotor stage, which of the following skills has the child acquired?

a. object permanence

b. ability to use symbols

c. reversibility

d. conservation

2. According to Erikson, the major task of infancy is to establish

a. autonomy

b. intimacy

c. trust

d. initiative

3. During the pre-operational period, the child exhibits all of the following *except*

a. primitive responses to stimuli

b. magical thinking

c. transductive reasoning

d. concentration

4. According to Freud, what are the most important activities for infant development?

a. rocking and holding

b. eating and sucking

c. contact with many people

d. long periods of sleep

5. What factor(s) is consistent in influencing the normal physical development of most infants?

a. timing

b. order

c. level of ability

d all of the above

6. Which if the following is an example of cephalocaudal development?

a. sitting before standing

b. babbling before saying words

c. scribbling before printing letters

d. running before skipping

7. Which of Piaget's stages is characterized by "thought influenced by egocentricism and exhibiting *centration* and *irreversibility*"?

a. sensorimotor stage

b. pre-operational stage

c. concrete operational stage

d. formal operational stage

8. According to Erikson, which of the following is the task that children develop between the ages of 3 and 6 years?

a. intimacy

b. initiative

c. industry

d. identity

9. According to Freud, which child would most likely exhibit castration complex?

a. 18-month-old David

b. 24-month-old Sarah

c. 3-year-old Steven

d. 4-year-old Monica

10. Which of the following age groups usually demonstrates fears and concerns regarding the genital areas?

a. toddlers

b. preschool children

c. school age children

d. adolescents

11. Moral reasoning that effects behavior during the pre-operational period is most influenced by

a. intention

b. consequences

c. sex of the child

d. parental reaction

12. The adolescent exhibiting formal operational thought is able to do which of the following?

a. think hypothetically

b. consider single alternatives to problems

c. deal only with problems in the present

d. understand objects only in relation to function

13. According to Erikson, which of the following is the major developmental task the adolescent should achieve?

a. identity

b. industry

c. autonomy

d. intimacy

14. Piaget postulated that in *animistic thinking*, the child

a. connects sleep with death

b. views all behavior under her control

c. believes inanimate objects possess living attributes

d. fears all animals

15. Which of the following is most typical of the school-age child?

a. more interested in peers than family activities

b. appears self sufficient in most activities

c. busy trying out his skills within peer group

d. all of the above

16. According to Piaget, a major cognitive task of the school-age child is to develop the ability to conserve. Which of the following is a good example of "the ability to conserve" for the school-age child?

a. realizing the importance of preserving natural resources

b. two balls of different shapes can be made out of the same amount of clay

c. ice returns to water when thawed

d. the speed of a swinging object is determined by its weight

STUDENT WORKSHEET: DEVELOPMENTAL ASSESSMENT

	Normal Behavior/Stage (textbook picture)	Child's Observed Behavior/Stage	Evaluation (Is child at expected level?)
Gross motor skills			
Fine motor skills			
Psychosocial			
Cognitive			
Moral/Faith			

(continued)

Student Worksheet (continued)

	Normal Behavior/Stage (textbook picture)	Child's Observed Behavior/Stage	Evaluation (Is child at expected level?)
Sexuality			
Language			
Play			
Effects of Illness or Hospitalization			

UNIT TWO

GROWTH AND DEVELOPMENT OF CHILDREN WITHIN FAMILIES

CHAPTER 4

FAMILIES WITH NEONATES

DISCUSSION QUESTIONS

1. What is the difference between the terms *attachment* and *bonding*? What measures can nurses apply that help facilitate bonding between parents and their newborn?
2. Define the term *maternicity* and describe behaviors that indicate the development of maternicity in mothers.
3. Describe the four elements included in an assessment of father-infant bonding.
4. Describe the five components of the Apgar score and the procedure for arriving at an infant's score.
5. How does the nurse evaluate a neonate's gestational age?
6. What is the normal physical appearance of the neonate? What are normal findings for each body system?
7. Name each of the infantile reflexes and describe how to elicit each. What are the normal and abnormal responses for each reflex?
8. Identify nursing interventions related to newborn screening.
9. What information would be included when teaching parents about newborn bathing and temperature regulation?
10. What safety concerns should be addressed with parents before the neonate is discharged from the hospital or birthing center?

CASE STUDY

Baby Adam Fletcher is born at 40 weeks gestation and weighs 7 pounds 8 ounces. His Apgar scores are 8/9. He is the first child of Judy and James Fletcher. Judy is planning to breastfeed. When would Adam receive his first feeding?

The next day, Judy tells the nurse, "I'm very nervous about giving Adam a bath. What should I do about his umbilical cord?" What would the nurse teach Judy about bathing and cord care?

The nurse informs Judy and Steve that Adam received the first dose of the hepatitis B vaccine. What is the nurse's response to their question, "Why did Adam need to have that?"

The Fletchers have decided to have their son circumcised. What are some of the issues surrounding routine circumcision? What nursing assessments and interventions are appropriate following circumcision?

STUDENT LEARNING ACTIVITIES

1. Complete the teaching sheet for normal newborn care.
2. Ask the students to prepare a nursing care plan for the neonate immediately after birth and identify at least three nursing diagnoses applicable to the needs of neonates immediately after birth.

AUDIOVISUAL RESOURCES

1. **Appraisal of the Newborn**
This film demonstrates the physical examination of the normal newborn infant. The importance of observation and documentation as a basis for assessing changes is discussed. This program is concise yet comprehensive for demonstrating newborn assessment

Videocassette: 26 minutes

Distributor: American Journal of Nursing Company

2. **Physical Assessment of the Neonate, Part2: Gestational Age Assessment**
This program demonstrates the Dubowitz method for determining the gestational age of the newborn. Also identified are common hazards for the neonate who is pre- or post-term or small or large for gestational age.

Videocassette: 17 minutes

Distributor: Concept Media

3. **Thermal Environment of the Neonate**
This program presents the causes and modalities of heat exchange in the newborn and interventions for minimizing thermal stress for newborns. Common hospital situations that cause thermal stress and factors that increase infant vulnerability to heat exchange are identified. Self-instructional materials accompany this program, thus it can be used as an independent learning activity for students.

Slide and tape: 11 minutes

Distributor: University of Michigan, Medical Center Media Library

4. **Breast Feeding: A Practical Guide**
This is a two-part program that clearly illustrates the how-to's of breast feeding. Part I includes a brief overview of breast milk production, maternal preparation, breast feeding positions, and how to attach and release the baby from the breast. Part II discusses the let-down reflex, common problems and interventions, methods of expressing and storing milk, nursing in public, attitudes, and parental roles.This is a comprehensive program to familiarize the student with the practical aspects of breast feeding.

Videocassette: 30 minutes

Distributor: American Journal of Nursing Company

5. **Assessment and Care of the Newborn**
This program focuses on assessment and nursing interventions for the first 24 hours of a newborn's life. Immediate care to facilitate the newborn's adjustment to extrauterine life is identified. Physical assessment of the newborn and guidelines for feeding and bathing are presented.

Videocassette: 15 minutes

Distributor: Health Sciences Consortium

6. **Physical Examination of the Newborn**
A complete physical examination of a newborn is demonstrated by a nurse in this program.

Videocassette: 18 minutes

Distributor: Health Sciences Consortium

STUDENT WORKSHEET: NORMAL NEWBORN CARE

1. **Bathing and Skin Care**

2. **Cord Care**

3. **Circumcision Care**

4. **Nutrition and Feeding**

5. **Elimination**

6. **Safety**

Chapter 5

Families with Infants

DISCUSSION QUESTIONS

1. Identify potential stressors for families adjusting to an infant.
2. Describe the nurse's role in promoting family adjustment for families with infants.
3. What changes in height, weight, and head circumference occur during the first year of life?
4. Identify the sequence of gross and fine motor development during the first year.
5. Describe the four substages of the sensorimotor period that occur during infancy.
6. Define *object permanence.* How does object permanence relate to cognitive development?
7. What anticipatory guidance should be provided to parents of infants to encourage cognitive and language development?
8. Describe psychosexual development of the infant according to Freud.
9. What is the psychosocial task of the infancy period according to Erikson? How can the nurse facilitate parent-infant attachment?
10. Discuss the current nursing research on the mother's and the infant's temperament.
11. Identify health concerns for the infancy period.
12. What is the recommended schedule for immunizations during the first year?
13. Identify anticipatory guidance related to tooth eruption and dental care for the parents of an infant.
14. What are the developmental characteristics of the infant's sleep? Describe strategies to promote healthy sleep.
15. How does an infant's nutritional needs vary from 0 to 3 months, from 4 to 6 months, and from 6 to 12 months?
16. What are the issues surrounding a parent's choice to use cloth or disposable diapers?
17. What are safety concerns for families with infants? How can families prevent injury to their infants?

CASE STUDY

Maria Juarez brings her 4-month-old daughter Alicia into the well-child clinic for a routine checkup. Alicia was a full-term infant. Her birth weight was 8 pounds 2 ounces, and her length at birth was 21 inches. Alicia's well-child visit at 2 months was normal, and she received immunizations at that time.

Her present weight is 15 pounds 8 ounces and her length is 27 3/4 inches. Do these measurements indicate adequate growth?

Maria is breastfeeding Alicia. She asks the nurse about adding juice and cereal to her diet. What would the nurse tell the mother about the introduction of solid foods? The water in the Juarez home is not fluoridated. What type of fluoride supplement should Alicia receive?

Maria asks the nurse when Alicia will roll over and be able to sit by herself. What anticipatory guidance would the nurse give her about gross motor development? What kinds of toys are appropriate for the 4- to 6-month-old infant?

What immunizations would Alicia receive at this well-child visit? Maria is concerned about complications associated with immunizations. What information would the nurse give her?

STUDENT LEARNING ACTIVITIES

1. Complete the Teaching Sheet for Normal Infant Care (next two pages).
2. Assign students to care for infants 0–6 months old and 6–12 months old. Have students evaluate development using the Developmental Assessment Form (Chapter 3).
3. Make an assignment for the students to visit a pediatrician's office or a well-child clinic to observe routine visits for infants. Ask the students to compile a list of questions that are asked by parents. Compare concerns expressed by parents of young infants 0–6 months old and 6–12 months old.

AUDIOVISUAL RESOURCES

1. Infancy
This program addresses the developmental changes that occur during infancy. The theories of Erikson, Piaget, and Freud as they relate to infancy are compared. Growth and nutritional needs are included as well as anticipatory guidance for parents.

Videocassette: 30 minutes

Distributor: J. B. Lippincott Company

2. Human Development: The First 2 1/2 Years
This four-part series includes physical growth and motor development, cognitive development, language development, and emotional/social development. Strategies for promoting development are provided in each video.

Videocassette: 19–25 minutes

Distributor: Concept Media

3. Infant
This program depicts the growth process from 1 month to 1 year of age. The importance of immunizations is emphasized.

Videocassette: 38 minutes

Distributor: American Journal of Nursing Company

STUDENT WORKSHEET: NORMAL INFANT CARE

1. **Nutrition**
   a. **Introduction to solid foods**

   b. **Weaning**

   c. **Using cup**

2. **Teething**

3. **Sleep patterns**

4. **Elimination**

(continued)

5. Promoting development

a. Motor skills

b. Social skills

c. Language

6. Toys

7. Safety

8. Health promotion: Immunizations

CHAPTER 6

FAMILIES WITH TODDLERS

DISCUSSION QUESTIONS

1. What characteristics of the toddler stage can cause difficulty with family relationships? What measures can families institute that facilitate healthy adaptation to the toddler?
2. What suggestions would you offer expectant parents for preparing their toddler for the arrival of a new baby?
3. Describe the physical growth of a toddler. How does the child's physical appearance change from 1 year of age to 3 years?
4. What gross motor and fine motor skills are acquired during toddlerhood? Identify the age at which these skills are achieved.
5. Describe the advances in cognitive development that occur during the toddler period.
6. Describe the characteristics of toddler speech. How can parents facilitate language development?
7. Why is toddlerhood identified as the anal stage of psychosexual development according to Freud?
8. What suggestions can nurses offer parents to promote healthy toddler sexual development?
9. Identify nursing interventions to alleviate a hospitalized toddler's separation anxiety.
10. Describe the development of autonomy during the toddler period.
11. Why do toddlers most often express anger by hitting and having temper tantrums?
12. Identify measures to help parents deal with the toddler's negativism and dawdling.
13. What stages of moral and faith development apply to the toddler?
14. What health screening would be included in a well-child visit between 1 and 3 years of age?
15. What immunizations should the toddler receive and when?
16. What are typical sleep behaviors exhibited by toddlers? How are these behaviors related to toddler development? What suggestions can nurses offer parents regarding management of toddler behaviors at bedtime?
17. What anticipatory guidance would the nurse offer to parents about dental care and nutrition?
18. What developmental prerequisites are necessary prior to the onset of toilet training?
19. Describe the play of toddlers.
20. Identify safety concerns and prevention strategies for families with toddlers.

CASE STUDY

William, age 18 months, is brought to the pediatrician for a well-child visit. He is the first child of the Prestons and is well nourished and in good health. His behavior indicates that he is at the expected developmental level. William is carrying a bottle containing milk. His mother, Kay Preston, states that he still takes a bottle to bed with him. What information related to William's use of a bottle should the nurse give to Kay?

What motor milestones generally occur at 18 months? What anticipatory guidance is appropriate regarding these new motor skills? What eating and self-care activities should William be able to perform?

William's mother states that although William is a poor eater, he always drinks plenty of milk. What should the nurse's response be?

When William is weighed, Kay mentions that she is worried that he has been gaining so little weight between visits lately. When he was an infant, each visit showed a large weight gain. What explanation should the nurse offer her regarding William's slow weight gain?

Kay states that William talks constantly even when alone, but refuses to speak in sentences and almost all of his statements begin with "me." What information can the nurse offer about the characteristics of toddler speech?

Kay relates that recently William says "no" to everything and refuses to come when called. She is worried that he is developing a behavior problem. What information can the nurse provide her that would be helpful?

STUDENT LEARNING ACTIVITIES

1. Develop a teaching plan for parents of a toddler focused on this nursing diagnosis: Knowledge deficit related to normal toddler development.
2. Compile a list of toys and play activities that promote toddler motor, language, social, and cognitive development. For each toy or activity, explain how it influences development.
3. Ask students to talk with the parents of toddlers to find out which aspects of toddler behavior parents find most positive and those which are most difficult to deal with. Students should ask these questions: How are temper tantrums and other forms of negative behavior handled? How does the toddler spend a typical day?
4. Visit a local day care facility to observe normal toddler development and group behavior.
5. Visit toy stores and review catalogs of infant and children merchandise for safety products that parents of toddlers can use to child-proof their homes.
6. Make clinical assignments to toddlers. Ask students to compile a list of safety hazards on the hospital unit and develop measures for child-proofing the unit for the toddler age group.
7. Evaluate a toddler's development using the developmental assessment form in Chapter 3. Have the students compare their findings.

AUDIOVISUAL RESOURCES

1. **Toddlerhood**
   Physical, cognitive, and psychosocial development from 1 year through 3 years of age is the focus of this program. Also included are nurse's responsibilities for documenting and reporting child abuse.

Videocassette: 30 minutes

Distributor: J. B. Lippincott Company

CHAPTER 7

FAMILIES WITH PRESCHOOLERS

DISCUSSION QUESTIONS

1. Identify potential stressors for families with preschoolers.
2. What is the average height and weight for the 3-year-old, 4-year-old, and 5-year-old preschooler? Describe the preschooler's general appearance.
3. Describe gross and fine motor development of the 3 year old, 4 year old, and 5 year old.
4. What are the characteristics of the preoperational period of cognitive development? What is meant by the terms *centration, animism,* and *transductive thinking*?
5. What are the characteristics of preschooler speech?
6. What behaviors of the preschool child are consistent with Erikson's stage of initiative versus guilt?
7. Discuss sex role identification for the preschool age child.
8. What anticipatory guidance can be offered to parents in dealing with preschooler fears?
9. What is the preschooler's stage of moral or faith development?
10. What is included in an assessment of cardiovascular risks in the preschool period?
11. Why are vision and hearing screening an important part of the preschooler's health promotion?
12. Develop a teaching plan for parents of preschoolers covering dental care, sleep behaviors, nutrition, and sex education.
13. Differentiate between nightmares and night terrors.
14. Describe the characteristics of preschooler play.
15. What options are available to working parents for child care? What questions should parents ask when selecting child care?
16. Identify behaviors that indicate a child's readiness for school.
17. Develop a teaching plan for preschoolers and their families about safety .

CASE STUDY

Tommy Santos is brought to the clinic by his mother for a routine visit. Tommy is 4 years old and in good health. He is within the normal parameters for height and weight. What health screening would be done at a 4-year visit?

Anna Santos, Tommy's mother, states that he is very active and often sustains minor injuries. She is concerned that Tommy has recently begun to masturbate and often touches his genitals in front of people. What areas concerning safety would be appropriate for the nurse to review with Anna? What is the best way for Anna to deal with Tommy's episodes of masturbation?

Anna Santos tells the nurse that she is very concerned about Tommy's poor appetite, and she feels that he is much too thin. How can the nurse demonstrate to the mother that Tommy is nutritionally healthy and a normal size for his age? What suggestions might Anna use that will help Tommy develop good eating habits?

Anna relates that Tommy has recently begun to resist going to bed and that he says that "monsters are under his bed." What can the nurse tell the mother about the basis of Tommy's fears? How can Tommy's parents help to minimize his fears regarding bedtime?

STUDENT LEARNING ACTIVITIES

1. Assign students to care for preschool-age children. Evaluate a preschooler's development using the Developmental Assessment Form (Chapter 3). Have students compare their findings.
2. Contact the local poison control center and make a list of the most common agents found in childhood poisonings. Ask the students to identify measures that reduce the chances of accidental poisoning among children.
3. Ask students to spend a day in the local daycare center and preform a written evaluation (following the guidelines in the textbook) of the program's structure, personnel, facilities, health and safety, and special services.
4. Ask students to talk to parents of preschoolers to discover what aspects of preschooler behavior they find most positive and those they find most negative or irritating.

AUDIOVISUAL RESOURCES

1. **Preschool Child**
   This film demonstrates the growth and development of the normal preschool child through play activities. The emergence of the preschooler as a thinking, social being and a member of the family is discussed.

Videocassette: 41 minutes

Distributor: American Journal of Nursing Company

2. **Human Development: 2 1/2 to 6 Years**
   This four-part series is a comprehensive look at preschool development, including physical growth and motor development, language and cognitive development, sex differences, socialization, and the role of play.

Videocassette: 21–28 minutes

Distributor: Concept Media

3. **Physical Examination of the Preschool Child**
   This program demonstrates physical assessment techniques for use in the examination of the preschool child. It is useful for students in both acute and primary care practice settings.

Videocassette: 32 minutes

Distributor: Altschul Group Corporation

4. **Cockaboody**
   This animated program shows the nature of children's play and examines the child's make-believe world as two sisters, age 3 and 5 years old, explore their parent's bedroom, bathroom, and closet.

16-mm film: 9 minutes

Distributor: Indiana University Audio-Visual Center

5. **Child, Part 5: 4 Years–6 Years**
   The nature of children between 4 and 6 years of age is the focus of this program. The similarities and differences of children in this age group are described.

16-mm film: 27 minutes

Distributor: Indiana University Audio-Visual Center

6. **Preschooler**
   This program addresses preschooler characteristics and stages, health needs, and disruptions in development. Developmental assessment tools are also covered.

Videocassette: 30 minutes

Distributor: J. B. Lippincott Company

7. **The Preschool Years**
   This program offers an overview of physical, emotional, and cognitive development and aspects of family relationships for the preschool period.

Videocassette: 18 minutes

Distributor: Medcom/Trainex

CHAPTER 8

FAMILIES WITH SCHOOL-AGE CHILDREN

DISCUSSION QUESTIONS

1. Which aspects of change confront the family and child during the school-age years?
2. Discuss the physical growth and maturation of the school-age child.
3. Describe the progressive refinement in motor skill development during the school-age years.
4. What information should parents be given regarding the interpretation of intelligence tests that are given to their children?
5. What is the definition of *intuitive thought*? What types of thinking are characteristic of children who are in the stage of intuitive thought?
6. Describe Piaget's *concrete operational stage*. What types of thinking are characteristic of this stage?
7. What changes in language development occur during the school-age years? What social function does language have for the school-age child?
8. Discuss the psychosexual development of school-age children.
9. What behaviors of the school-age child are consistent with Erikson's stage of *industry versus inferiority*?
10. Explain how temperament style may effect school adjustment and performance.
11. How does emotional development progress during the school-age years? What is the major task for the child in relation to emotional expression?
12. How can parents help their school-age child learn to deal with anger constructively?
13. Describe the coping mechanisms school-age children use to deal with stressors.
14. What are the characteristics of the school-age child's moral or faith development?
15. Describe the school-age child's peer group relationships.
16. What health screening is appropriate for school-age children?
17. Identify dental health concerns for the school-age population.
18. Develop a teaching plan for parents of school-age children regarding sleep, nutrition, play and sports activities, and safety.
19. The school nurse takes the height and weight of a 10-year-old boy and finds that his height is at the 50th percentile for his age but his weight is above the 95th percentile. What implications do these findings have for health teaching for the school nurse?
20. Why do sleepwalking and sleeptalking occur?
21. What guidelines should the nurse consider for sex education with school-age children and their parents?

CASE STUDY

Rebecca is 10 years old and has come to the school nurse several times in the past two months complaining of stomach pain and asking to be sent home. Rebecca has not had a fever, vomiting, or diarrhea with these episodes. In talking with Rebecca's teacher, the school nurse learns that Rebecca has recently begun to have difficulty with her studies and has done poorly on several exams.

Based on the knowledge of the developmental characteristics of the school-age child, what could we assume might be the basis of Rebecca's physical complaints and school problems? What suggestions could the nurse offer Rebecca's parents that would help her adjust to school?

STUDENT LEARNING ACTIVITIES

1. Make assignments to the students to observe for a day in a grade school classroom and record the teacher's role in promoting intellectual, emotional, and social growth for the children. Ask each student to observe one child in particular and compare that child's fine and gross motor development and social and language skills to those expected for that age.

2. After the students have observed the children in the grade school class during play activities (see assignment above), ask the students to answer the following questions:

   a. How would you describe the characteristics of play of the school-age child?

   b. Is the play cooperative? Are there rules? Do boys and girls play together or do play groups consist of same-sex playmates?

   c. During the play activities, are there indications of Erikson's stage of industry versus inferiority? If so, what are some examples?

AUDIOVISUAL RESOURCES

1. **School-Age Child**
   This program addresses refinement of motor skills, socialization through play, cognitive development, and impact of school for children 6 to 12 years of age.

Videocassette: 41 minutes

Distributor: American Journal of Nursing Company

2. **School Age**
   The theories of Piaget, Erikson, Kohlburg, and Freud are reviewed for school-age stages, as well as health needs and health screening for this age group.

Videocassette: 30 minutes

Distributor: J. B. Lippincott Company

3. **The School Age Years**
   This program offers an overview of physical, emotional, and cognitive development for children 6 to 9 years of age.

Videocassette: 17 minutes

Distributor: Medcom/Trainex

CHAPTER 9

FAMILIES WITH ADOLESCENTS

DISCUSSION QUESTIONS

1. What characteristics of adolescence may result in communication problems with parents and other adults? What methods can parents use to help keep communication open with their adolescent?
2. Adolescent development results in behaviors that are potentially stressing to the family system. What areas of potential stress can result from both the cognitive change and the psychosocial change that occur in adolescence?
3. Identify the major physical development characteristics for the adolescent period.
4. Describe the sexual maturation process for males and females.
5. According to the theory of Piaget, what are the characteristics of adolescent cognitive development?
6. What is adolescent egocentricism? How does it relate to cognitive development?
7. Describe sexual development during adolescence. What are the behavioral consequences of sexual development, and what role does the nurse play in promoting healthy sexual development?
8. Describe the process of developing an identity as a gay or lesbian individual.
9. What adolescent behaviors are consistent with Erikson's stage of identity versus role confusion?
10. The adolescent who is striving to develop a sense of identity is subject to many types of stresses and influences. What are these, and what can nurses and parents do to assist the adolescent in adopting a healthy identity?
11. Describe the characteristics of adolescent moral or faith development.
12. What health screening is recommended for the adolescent period? What is the nurse's role in adolescent health promotion?
13. What information should the adolescent and his parents receive on balancing rest and activity, nutrition, recreation, and safety?
14. What types of accidents are commonly associated with adolescent injury and death? How could these accidents be prevented?
15. What would the nurse include in a teaching session with adolescents about sexually transmitted diseases?
16. Identify health concerns related to adolescent use of anabolic steroids.
17. Discuss the health and social consequences of adolescent pregnancy.

CASE STUDY

Mindy, a 14-year-old teenager, visits the physician for a routine checkup. She is doing well in school and wears glasses for seeing the board and watching television. She has a favorite boyfriend, but is not yet allowed to go out on dates. Her only reported concern is that she is taller than all the boys in her class.

Mindy has been wearing a bra for a year and has some pubic and axillary hair, but has not yet begun to menstruate. What information can the nurse provide regarding the timing for the onset of menarche?

During the physical assessment, what important aspects of development should the nurse discuss with Mindy? What can the nurse tell Mindy about the rate of growth for males and females during adolescence? What aspects of anticipatory guidance would be pertinent for the nurse to discuss with Mindy and her mother?

STUDENT LEARNING ACTIVITIES

1. Assign students to care for adolescents. Evaluate development using the Developmental Assessment Form (Chapter 3).
2. Ask students to interview two different age groups of adolescents: 14–15 year olds and 17–18 year olds. Record their attitudes regarding the following issues: relationships with their parents, attitudes toward school, future plans for education, current political issues, and employment. Ask adolescents to describe a typical weekday and how they usually spend their weekends. Ask students to compare and contrast the responses of the two age groups. What might explain the differences?
3. As a group project, ask the students to develop a teaching session focused on adolescent sexuality. The information could be developed into a packet or a loose leaf booklet to be used in the adolescent clinic or inpatient unit. Areas to include are normal anatomy and physiology for males and females, contraception, sexually transmitted diseases, and guidelines for making healthy decisions regarding sexual activity. Instruct students to include ample diagrams to facilitate learning and interest.

AUDIOVISUAL RESOURCES

1. The Adolescent
This program describes theoretical concepts and the growth and development of adolescents. Content includes rapid growth patterns leading to sexual maturation, identity conflicts associated with wide mood swings, and problems important to the teenager. Substance abuse, pregnancy, and sexually transmitted diseases are discussed with emphasis on health promotion and protection during adolescence. This film is a good general overview of the teenage period.

Videocassette: 44 minutes

Distributor: American Journal of Nursing Company

2. Sex and the American Teenager
This film dramatizes adolescent and parental feelings about sexuality and love. It is intended to challenge teenagers to examine their values and to consider consequences of sexual activity. It also emphasizes to parents the need for open communication with their teenager. The film is nonthreatening to teenagers and/or parents and would be valuable to stimulate interaction in families with adolescents.

Videocassette: 32 minutes

Distributor: Pyramid Film and Video

3. All the Kids Do It
This film dramatizes the danger of drinking alcohol and driving and identifies statistical information related to teenagers and alcohol-related vehicular accidents. The film is narrated by a popular young actor and emphasizes the teenager's responsibility for safe driving practices.

Videocassette: 30 minutes

Distributor: Pyramid Film and Video

4. **Sex Education: Too Little, Too Late**
The pressures faced by teenagers and issues surrounding school sex education programs are examined. Teens, teachers, and policy makers evaluate sex education in the schools.

Videocassette: 26 minutes

Distributor: Films for the Humanities and Sciences

5. **What If I'm Gay?: A Search for Understanding**
As an adolescent realizes he is gay, he considers how his sexuality will affect relationships with family and friends and shape the course of his future. This program should provoke thoughtful discussion about stereotyping and assumptions about sexual orientation.

Videocassette: 30 minutes

Distributor: Coronet/MTI Film & Video

6. **Adolescent Health: Nursing Implications Series**
This eight-part series includes adolescent physical and psychosocial changes, nutritional needs and obesity, adolescent anorexia, adolescent sexuality, the pregnant adolescent, nursing needs of the adolescent during the intrapartum period, adolescent parenting, and the adolescent with a long-term health problem. Programs are also available individually.

Videocassette: 30 minutes each part

Distributor: Health Sciences Consortium

7. **Adolescence—The Winds of Change**
Physical, sexual, and cognitive changes are discussed through interviews with adolescents and child development authorities. Parental impact on adolescent development is also addressed.

16-mm film: 31 minutes

Distributor: Indiana University Audio-Visual Center

8. **Adolescence**
This program reviews adolescent development and is intended to help nurses identify health needs and provide interventions for this age group. Specifically addressed are peer groups, relationships with the opposite sex, and establishing a personal identity.

Videocassette: 30 minutes

Distributor: J. B. Lippincott Company

9. **The Adolescent Years**
This program discusses adolescent physical, emotional, and cognitive development.

Videocassette: 17 minutes

Distributor: Medcom/Trainex

UNIT III

PROMOTING HEALTH

CHAPTER **10**

HEALTH CONCEPTS: CHILDREN'S PERCEPTIONS AND BEHAVIORS

DISCUSSION QUESTIONS

1. How would you describe a healthy individual? What constitutes healthy behavior in the areas of (a) adaptation and stability, (b) actualization, (c) effectiveness, and (d) assuming responsibility for one's own health? How can the nurse promote optimal functioning in each of these areas?
2. Explain how each of the following describes the child's concept of health: (a) cognitive-developmental model and (b) expectancy theory?
3. How does the psychological concept of locus of control relate to health behaviors?
4. What is the meaning of the following terms: (a) *prevention*, (b) *health maintenance*, and (c) *health promotion?* What causes people problems in trying to differentiate among these terms?
5. What are some examples of services provided to children and their families in (a) primary prevention, (b) secondary prevention, and (c) tertiary prevention?
6. Discuss the nurse's role in health promotion of children.
7. Suggest topics for future research on family and children's health.
8. What are the components of a nursing assessment of child health?
9. What processes are involved in the acquisition of healthy behavior by children? How can the nurse help children to assume more responsibility for their health?
10. What is meant by the following terms: (a) *natural immunity*, (b) *natural active immunity*, (c) *natural passive*, and (d) *natural passive immunity?*
11. Discuss current issues regarding childhood immunizations.
12. What is the immunization schedule for DPT, MMR, polio, HIB, and hepatitis B vaccines?
13. What types of reactions can occur after administration of DPT?
14. What are contraindications to further pertussis vaccination?
15. What is the current status of the pneumococcal polysaccharide, meningococcal polysaccharide, and varicella vaccines?
16. What are the American Academy of Pediatrics (AAP) recommendations for tuberculin testing?
17. If a mother brought her 4-year-old child into the clinic and the child had not received any previous immunizations, what immunizations should be received on this visit? What would be the schedule of immunizations to the age of 12 years?
18. What assessments should the nurse make prior to the administration of immunizations?
19. What information should the parents receive before their child receives an immunization? What information would the nurse record when administering immunizations?

CASE STUDY #1

Mark, age 6 years, is admitted to the hospital after falling off his bike and fracturing his arm. The fracture is reduced in the operating room under general anesthesia. The following day, Mark complains of some discomfort but is walking around the unit and interacting with other children. Discharge is planned for later in the afternoon. Mark will wear a cast for eight weeks.

In planning Mark's discharge, what responsibilities for care can the nurse teach Mark? What difficulties can Mark be expected to experience in understanding the need for the cast, restriction of his activity, and prevention of damage to the cast?

Mark's mother tells the nurse that she has difficulty getting Mark to brush his teeth. What suggestions can the nurse offer that will help Mark's parents promote good health behaviors?

CASE STUDY #2

Julia Little brings 8-month-old Gretchen to the pediatrician's office because she is concerned about the runny nose and cough her daughter has had for the past three days. In reviewing Gretchen's record, the nurse notes that she missed her 6-month well-child visit and is behind in her immunizations.

Describe how the nurse would explain to Julia the importance of regular well-child care for Gretchen. Develop a teaching plan for the mother that focuses on anticipatory guidance.

No problems were identified during Gretchen's physical examination. What immunizations should she receive? What information would the nurse give to Julia before the immunizations are administered?

Julia tells the nurse that she is not sure about when to call the physician when Gretchen is sick. How would the nurse advise her?

STUDENT LEARNING ACTIVITIES

1. Assign students to spend a day in a well-child clinic or pediatrician's office. Ask them to develop teaching sheets on immunizations for parents. Make sure the students include the rationale for the immunization, the common side effects, and the treatment for side effects.
2. Interview hospitalized children of different developmental levels. What explanations do they provide for their illness? How do they perceive the reasons for medical and nursing procedures? How do they describe a healthy or ill person? Compare responses to the norms presented in the cognitive developmental model for children's health concepts.

AUDIOVISUAL RESOURCES

1. **Immunization: Your Child's Protection**
This program explains the immunizations against diphtheria, pertussis, tetanus, polio, measles, mumps, and rubella, along with the recommended ages for administration. Risks associated with DPT are discussed. Information about the Haemophilus B conjugate vaccine is included. This program may be useful for parent education.

Videocassette: 10 minutes

Distributor: Milner-Fenwick

CHAPTER 11

COMMUNICATING WITH CHILDREN AND FAMILIES

DISCUSSION QUESTIONS

1. Developing a positive relationship with the child and family is important for the nurse to be an effective teacher and caregiver. What are the skills and attitudes that a nurse should have to develop good relationships with children and families?
2. Differentiate between the two types of communication.
3. Describe the various components of the Social Model of Intercultural Communication.
4. What advances in cognitive development influence communication during the concrete operational period? During the formal operational period?
5. What forms of communication are characteristic of children during the pre-operational stage of cognitive development?
6. Communicating effectively with children requires the application of certain principles by the nurse. What are these principles? How would a nurse apply each principle to the care of a preschooler and the care of an adolescent?
7. Explain the direct and indirect communication techniques that can be used with children to encourage conversation.

CASE STUDY

Brian, age 4 years, was diagnosed with acute lymphocytic leukemia at age 2. He has recently relapsed and is now admitted to the hospital for chemotherapy. Brian frequently requires venipunctures and intravenous insertions.

How can the nurse use communication techniques to reduce some of Brian's anxiety related to future painful procedures?

How best can the nurse explain to Brian his need for painful procedures and tests?

What are some examples of ways the nurse can help Brian to express his fears and questions regarding his illness and hospitalization?

STUDENT LEARNING ACTIVITIES

1. Assign students to interview a preschool child, a school-age child, and an adolescent in relation to their school activities, hobbies and interests, and families. What special interview techniques worked best with each age group? What difficulties were encountered in gaining the information from the children?
2. Have students observe nurses involved in interviewing children and families. Ask the students to identify and give examples of particular approaches used by the nurses that demonstrated good communication skills.
3. Develop a nursing care plan for preparing a preschool child for surgery using techniques of art, play, and story telling.

AUDIOVISUAL RESOURCES

1. **Interviewing Children: The Initial Assessment**
   This program focuses on the special skills involved in interviewing children. The purposes of an initial assessment interview are discussed and delineated into four phases with elements of each phase being demonstrated through videotapes of interactions between a nurse and a child in different settings.

Videocassette: 34 minutes

Distributor: University of Michigan

2. **Pediatrics: Psychosocial Implications, Part I—The Nursing Challenge**
   This program emphasizes the developmental knowledge and observational skills necessary for communication with children and monitoring their physical and emotional condition. The nurse's relationship with the family is stressed as a means of involving parents in the child's care.

Filmstrip or videotransfer: 18 minutes

Distributor: Concept Media

3. **Interviewing Techniques for Pediatric Nurses**
   This program discusses appropriate interviewing techniques and ways of providing information to the young patient.

Videocassette: 29 minutes

Distributor: Altschul Group Corporation

CHAPTER 12

PROMOTING HEALTHY PARENTING

DISCUSSION QUESTIONS

1. What are the major goals of parenting? What factors influence the degree of emphasis parents place on each of these goals?
2. What are the essential elements of parenting, and how do these elements promote healthy socialization of the child?
3. What is the most effective way that parents can teach rules to children? What guidance can the nurse use to assess parental use of rules in parenting behavior?
4. What is *negative reinforcement?* What types of negative reinforcement could a parent use to discipline a child?
5. What would a nurse include in an assessment of a parent's use of negative reinforcement?
6. Why would a nurse discourage the use of physical punishment as a method of negative reinforcement?
7. What is *positive reinforcement?* What criteria must be met for positive reinforcement?
8. What measures help parents assess whether positive or negative reinforcement is appropriate for a given situation?
9. What ways can parents use a child's imagination to teach healthy behaviors?
10. What guidance can the nurse offer parents about the child's temperament and parenting style?
11. How does the parenting role change throughout childhood?
12. When both parents are working in a family, what effect does this have on (a) the mother, (b) the father, and (c) the children?
13. What is meant by the term *home-alone children?* Discuss the findings that reflect the effects of this experience on those children?
14. What issues should the nurse discuss with a parent who is considering leaving a school-age child home alone after school?
15. Describe measures to facilitate family functioning within blended families.

CASE STUDY

Melissa, age 5, and Sean, age 9, are brought to the pediatrician for routine well-child visits. Their mother, Cathy Lee, tells the nurse that she has been having difficulty disciplining the children. They often respond to the mother's requests with smart remarks, they resist participating in family duties such as cleaning their rooms, and react to any form of discipline with anger and crying. Cathy has been divorced for two years and has recently begun to date again. She plans to marry again in the future.

What advice can the nurse offer Cathy regarding effective parenting? When applying any method of parenting, what important considerations are necessary?

The Lee children exhibit temperament styles characteristic of the slow-to-warm child. What parenting approaches work best with this personality type?

What suggestions can the nurse offer Cathy that would assist the children in adjusting to a new father?

STUDENT LEARNING ACTIVITIES

1. Ask students to observe children of various ages in the hospital unit. Ask them to note how nurses control the children's behavior. Are their methods effective? What principles of reinforcement do the nurses use most often? How do approaches to control behavior differ among children of various developmental levels?

AUDIOVISUAL RESOURCES

1. **Parents and Children**
The parent-child relationship is examined as a special learning experience in this program. The purposeful use of rewards can play a crucial role in the relationship. The program uses behavioral methods to demonstrate the proper use of time-out and ignoring inappropriate behavior.

16-mm film: 23 minutes

Distributor: Indiana University Audio-Visual Center

2. **Psychology of Parenting**
This program explores some of the problems of being a parent. It includes scenes from a parenting workshop where parents share positive and negative experiences and solutions are offered for improved communication between parents and teenagers.

Videocassette: 19 minutes

Distributor: Films for the Humanities and Sciences

3. **Latch-Key Families**
This program offers guidance to working parents whose children are on their own after school, now termed *home-alone children*. Educational and law enforcement specialists explain how parents can provide for the physical safety and emotional needs of their children and how rules for conduct can be set so that the experience will help teach children maturity and independence. This program could be useful for students involved in child and parent teaching.

Videocassette: 23 minutes

Distributor: Films for the Humanities and Sciences

4. **Stepparenting Issues**
This program illustrates common experiences and problems for stepfamilies, such as testing of authority and sibling rivalry, using vignettes. This program, designed to help viewers identify and cope with predictable emotional patterns, could be useful for student discussion or family teaching programs.

Videocassette: 20 minutes

Distributor: Coronet/MTI Film & Video

5. **Child's Game**
This program describes specific skills to be used to control the behavior of children ages 2 through 8 years. The film demonstrates ways to encourage desirable behavior and how to discourage undesirable behaviors such as tantrums, whining, and other attention-seeking acts. This film could be used to illustrate effective parenting skills for students or for family teaching programs.

Videocassette: 24 minutes

Distributor: Health Sciences Consortium

CHAPTER 13

ASSESSING CHILD HEALTH

DISCUSSION QUESTIONS

1. What are the two types of interviews that a nurse conducts with families and children? What is the purpose of each?
2. Identify principles of interviewing.
3. What are developmental considerations when interviewing preschool children, school-age children, and adolescents?
4. From the pairs of questions listed below, select the one that best facilitates the gathering of information during a health history. Provide a rationale for your selection.

   a. Is Jessica walking yet?
   b. What new things has Jessica done since her last visit?

   a. Do you find it difficult to discipline Steven?
   b. It is sometimes difficult to discipline toddlers, but you must have a method. What is it?

   a. Has Justin been in good health since his last visit?
   b. Tell me how Justin has been doing since his last visit.
5. Describe the steps in the health history. What information is gathered on the (a) present illness, (b) family profile, (c) past history, (d) developmental history, and (e) review of systems?
6. How would the nurse obtain the height and weight of an 8-month-old infant?
7. In what order would the nurse obtain vital signs for an 18-month-old child? Why?
8. Describe the four assessment techniques.
9. How is *visual acuity* defined? What are important considerations for reliable testing of visual acuity?
10. Describe how to perform a screening test for strabismus.
11. Describe the components of assessment of the (a) skin, (b) head and neck, (c) heart and lungs, and (d) abdomen.
12. Discuss developmental approaches to hearing testing.
13. What areas are included in a neurological assessment?
14. What is the purpose of the Denver II in child assessment? How is the Denver II different from the Denver Development Screening Test (DDST)?
15. What routine laboratory screening is part of the health visit?

CASE STUDY

Erin is brought to the clinic for her 5-year-old well-child visit by her mother who reports no serious problems. Erin's height and weight are measured to be 42 inches and 30 pounds, respectively. Erin's mother is curious about her daughter's percentiles on the growth chart. Plot Erin's height and weight on the appropriate growth chart. At her last well-child visit, Erin was 39 inches and 34 pounds. How have her percentiles changed?

How would the nurse assess Erin's visual acuity and hearing?

As part of the visit the nurse performs a Denver II. Erin's birth date was May 16, 1988. Today's date is March 31, 1993. What would the nurse tell Erin's mother regarding the purpose of the Denver II? Describe the four sections of the Denver II. Which items cross Erin's age line?

Erin's performance in all categories falls between the 50th and 70th percentiles. What does this finding indicate about Erin's developmental status?

STUDENT LEARNING ACTIVITIES

1. Observe a nurse in a well-child clinic who is obtaining a health history. Describe the procedure she follows. How does she organize her data and identify real and potential problems? How does the nurse establish rapport with the child and the family? What type of questioning does he nurse use? Is her approach effective in obtaining a clear picture of the child?
2. Perform a physical assessment on a toddler, a young school-age child, and an adolescent. What aspects of the exam produced anxiety or resistance for each age group? Relate these reactions to the cognitive and emotional development of that age.

AUDIOVISUAL RESOURCES

1. **Physical Assessment of a Child**
   This film demonstrates and explains how to perform a physical examination on a young child. The four basic techniques of inspection, palpation, percussion, and auscultation are covered. Detailed examination of the head and neck, the respiratory system, the cardiovascular system, and the nervous system are included. Techniques for establishing trust and positive rapport with a child during the physical examination are also demonstrated. This straightforward, comprehensive program is an excellent resource for nursing students in pediatric settings.

Videocassette: 33 minutes

Distributor: American Journal of Nursing Company

2. **Pediatrics: Physical Care, Program I—Physical Differences**
   This program describes important physical differences between children and adults. It focuses on anatomical and physiological differences in the pulmonary, cardiovascular, and central nervous systems. Implications for nursing care unique to children are emphasized. This program is useful for comparing and contrasting normal physical findings in children versus adults.

Videocassette: 20 minutes

Distributor: Concept Media

3. **Pediatrics: Physical Care, Program 6—Using an Otoscope**
This program describes the anatomy of the outer and middle ear and illustrates the procedure for viewing these structures with the otoscope. Normal and abnormal findings are described. The program is designed for parents as well as health care professionals and could be used for parent teaching activities as well as student practice instruction.

Videocassette: 18 minutes

Distributor: Concept Media

4. **Modification of Examination Techniques: The Difficult-to-Handle Child**
This program describes and illustrates specific ways to handle a child who is especially fearful or uncooperative during a physical examination. Included are methods to involve the child, ways to reassure the child and mother, various methods of restraint, sequencing procedures, and ways to promote rapport.

Videocassette: 33 minutes

Distributor: Altschul Group Corporation

5. **Physical Examination of the Preschool Child**
This program presents observations that should be made during the physical examination of the preschool child. Methods to facilitate the physical assessment are discussed.

Videocassette: 32 minutes

Distributor: Altschul Group Corporation

ANSWERS TO THE PRETEST

1. inspection, palpation, percussion, and auscultation
2. decreases
3. brachial, radial
4. pearly gray
5. rales
6. vagus
7. dorsal surface of the foot
8. pinching the skin between the finger and thumb and noting the reaction of the skin when released
9. head and neck, axilla, and inguinal area
10. two
11. c
12. b
13. a and b
14. b
15. b
16. a
17. a
18. d

PRETEST: PHYSICAL ASSESSMENT

Fill in the blanks.

1. The four basic physical assessment techniques are ______________________, ______________________, ______________________, and ______________________.

2. The normal heart rate ______________________ as children get older.

3. The two major palpable arteries of the arm are the ______________________ and the ______________________.

4. The normal appearance of the tympanic membrane is ______________________ ______________________.

5. When auscultating breath sounds, fine, crackling sounds are termed ______________________.

6. The cranial nerve responsible for the gag reflex is the ______________________.

7. The major pedal pulse is located on the ______________________ ______________________.

8. Skin turgor is usually evaluated by ______________________ ______________________ ______________________ ______________________.

9. Complete physical assessment includes the examination of lymph nodes in what three major areas?

   ______________________.

   ______________________.

   ______________________.

10. In normal children, an examiner can most commonly hear how many heart sounds? ______________________

Matching

Match the following organs with their location(s) in the abdomen (a–d).

11. appendix ________
12. stomach ________
13. pancreas ________
14. left kidney ________
15. spleen ________
16. gallbladder ________
17. liver ________
18. sigmoid colon ________

a. right upper quadrant

b. left upper quadrant

c. right lower quadrant

d. left lower quadrant

CHAPTER 14

FOSTERING SELF-ESTEEM

DISCUSSION QUESTIONS

1. What constitutes a child's self-concept?
2. How do the following factors influence the development of the self-system: (a) developmental psychosocial crises, (b) significant other's expectations, (c) social role expectations and cultural factors, (d) physical health status, and (e) temperamental coping style?
3. Describe the influence that each of the following parenting styles has on a child's developing self-concept: (a) permissive (b) autocratic, and (c) democratic.
4. What methods are available to assess a child's self-concept? Identify the strengths and weaknesses of these measures.
5. Certain conditions tend to foster the development of positive self-systems. What are some examples of the ways parents and nurses can help a child develop a sense of (a) security, (b) identity, (c) belonging, (d) purpose, and (e) personal competence?
6. What measures assist children in enhancing their own self-concept?

STUDENT LEARNING ACTIVITIES

1. Ask your students to describe the children for whom they care during their weekly clinical experience. Also ask them to answer the following questions: Why were they hospitalized? What aspects of their home environment, culture, socioeconomic status, illness, and hospitalization may have positive or negative influences on their self-concept development? Each student can develop a care plan for the child using the following nursing diagnosis: *Potential for disturbances in self-concept.* The care plan should include ways to foster self-concept during hospitalization and a teaching plan for providing parents with measures to help facilitate their child's self-concept.

AUDIOVISUAL RESOURCES

1. **How to Develop Self-Confidence When You're Not the Fastest, the Smartest, the Prettiest, or the Funniest**
   This film shows four scenarios depicting pre-adolescent children in situations that illustrate the importance and difficulties of developing independence and self-confidence. Issues raised include pleasing others, living up to parental expectations, and unhealthy dependence on others. Also included are suggestions for handling disappointment, making responsible decisions, establishing and realizing personal goals, and how to feel good about oneself. This program would be useful for stimulating student discussion and ideas for promoting self-esteem or for well-child teaching projects.

Videocassette

Distributor: The Center for Humanities

2. **Proud To Be Me: Developing Self-Esteem**
This four-part program uses interviews and scenarios to illustrate the problems of identity and self-esteem in adolescence. The discussion focuses on ways to explore what makes one feel good, how parents and peers hinder or help attempts to build self-esteem, why strengths and weaknesses should be identified and accepted, and strategies for dealing with problem times. This program is designed for adolescent viewing and could be used to heighten student understanding of adolescent self-system or as a teaching tool for teenage health promotion projects.

Videocassette

Distributor: The Center for Humanities

3. **Pediatrics: Psychosocial Implications, Part 5—Alterations in Body Image**
This film addresses changes in body image that result from childhood disease or injury. It discusses how body image perception is affected by the child's developmental stage and the responses of significant others. Cues that indicate body image concerns and problems are described. Suggestions for professional intervention during each stage of body image reintegration are identified. This program could be used to assist students in developing care plans to promote positive self-concept in children who are a risk for or are experiencing alterations in body image.

Filmstrip or videocassette: 20 minutes

Distributor: Concept Media

4. **My Self-Esteem**
This program tells the story of an 11-year-old girl who receives a low grade in spelling. The girl is embarrassed and her self-esteem is at a low point. She learns techniques for raising her self-esteem from her alter ego. While directed to a school-age audience, this program offers nursing students practical suggestions for helping children with an alteration in self-esteem.

Videocassette: 18 minutes

Distributor: Pyramid Film and Video

CHAPTER 15

PROMOTING SAFETY

DISCUSSION QUESTIONS

1. Identify the five leading causes of injury resulting in death of children.
2. The three factors contributing to the incidence of accidents among children are (a) host characteristics, (b) agent characteristics, and (c) the environment. Discuss each of these factors and how each effects the incidence of accidents among children.
3. Give an example of an active and a passive approach to injury prevention.
4. What is the major intervention responsible for the reduction in incidence of accidents among children?
5. Automobile accidents are the leading cause of death in children older than 1 year of age. What changes in legislation have made an impact upon the incidence of automobile injuries and deaths?
6. Develop a nursing care plan for parents that focuses on prevention of injuries to children related to automobiles.
7. What is the incidence of childhood homicide? What patterns have been identified in childhood homicide?
8. What is the incidence of drowning accidents? Which populations are most at risk for drowning?
9. Identify strategies to prevent childhood drowning.
10. What are the typical burn injuries that occur in children under 5 years of age? Over 5 years of age? What developmental characteristics help explain the types of burns found in these two age groups?
11. What is the peak age of accidental poisonings in children? Why are poisonings so prevalent during this period?
12. Why is suffocation a threat to infants under 1 year of age? What actions can parents take to prevent infant suffocation?
13. What guidance would the nurse give to parents of infants to prevent foreign body aspiration? How does this information change for the toddler?
14. What would the nurse teach parents to do if a child aspirates a foreign body?
15. Why are infants placed in infant walkers at risk for injury?
16. What would the nurse teach a 5-year-old child about bicycle safety? A 10-year old child?
17. What is *street-proofing?* List the areas important to cover when street-proofing the young school-age child.
18. The nurse that provides anticipatory guidance to parents on accident prevention may encounter parental attitudes that reduce the effectiveness of her teaching. What are these attitudinal stances and how can the nurse overcome these barriers to safety education?

CASE STUDY

Clara, age 7 months, is brought to the clinic for a routine checkup. She is healthy and on schedule in her development. Clara still uses a pacifier, and her mother had put it on a ribbon around the infant's neck so that she can easily reach it. Clara has an older brother, Mark, who has just turned 2 years old.

What areas of anticipatory guidance would the nurse review with Clara's mother regarding safety? What should the nurse explain to the mother about the pacifier?

What information should the nurse give to the mother regarding food and the danger of aspiration for Mark's age group? Describe the information the mother should receive on the correct action to take if one of her children accidentally aspirated a foreign object.

STUDENT LEARNING ACTIVITIES

1. Assign the students to visit one of the following: (a) urban, (b) suburban, or (c) rural hospital emergency room. Ask students to review the records and interview nurses regarding the common types of accidents experienced by the children living in that area. Are there differences in the incidence of accidents among the three environments? What characteristics of the children and their environment contribute to the common accidents that occur? What teaching methods or written materials are used by the emergency room staff in accident prevention? If none are used, what suggestions do the students have for such teaching?

AUDIOVISUAL RESOURCES

1. **Preventing Injuries**
   This program addresses the most common areas of danger and makes some basic points about common sense and risk taking. Injury prevention is divided into five major categories: wearing seatbelts, using safe toys, care in sports on land and in the water, and winter hazards. The program discusses safety helmets, floatation devices, hypothermia, accidental poisoning, and the effects of alcohol.

Videocassette: 26 minutes

Distributor: Films for the Humanities and Sciences

2. **The Heimlich Maneuver**
   This program identifies the signs of choking and actions to take to remove foreign matter from a victim's airway. Thorough step-by-step demonstrations are offered for performing the maneuver on the adult, child, and infant.

Videocassette: 14 minutes

Distributor: Films for the Humanities and Sciences

3. **Choking Emergency**
   Clear, easy-to-follow steps to follow during a choking emergency are offered in this program. Information includes how to open the airway, perform rescue breathing, recognize a choking victim, apply the Heimlich maneuver to conscious and unconscious victims, and what to do when a conscious victim becomes unconscious. Special techniques to use with infants and children are included. This program could be useful for safety education.

Videocassette: 12 minutes

Distributor: Pyramid Film and Video

4. **Water: Friend or Foe**
   In a series of dramatic episodes, this program addresses accident prevention in and around water as well as how to save yourself and others when accidents occur. It includes step-by-step instructions for common water emergencies involving swimming, boating, fishing, scuba diving, and being near a pond or swimming pool.

Videocassette: 23 minutes

Distributor: Pyramid Film and Video

5. **Bicycle Safety: How To Prevent an Accident**
   This program is intended for a primary to intermediate level audience and includes facts about bicycle laws and equipment, crash and theft prevention, repair and maintenance, emergency precautions, and defensive driving. It could be useful for health and safety education.

Videocassette: 19 minutes

Distributor: Pyramid Film and Video

6. **Smart, Safe, and Sure: Preventing Child's Abduction**
This program offers practical and essential advice to parents, suggests how children can protect themselves, and reviews the responsibility of health care professionals in educating the public to identify and avoid high-risk situations.

Videocassette: 28 minutes

Distributor: American Journal of Nursing Company

7. **Pediatrics: Physical Care, Part 2—Safety**
This program describes factors in growth and development that make infants, toddlers, and preschool children prone to accidents and discusses interventions to protect them. Emphasis is placed on prevention of strangulation, aspiration, and falls. This program could be used to heighten student awareness of the safety risks associated with developmental levels of children.

Videotransfer: 13 minutes

Distributor: Concept Media

CHAPTER 16

HEALTHY DIETARY PRACTICES

DISCUSSION QUESTIONS

1. Give the findings of various surveys of the nutritional status of children in the United States that were discussed in the text. What are the difficulties in establishing the incidence and prevalence of nutritional problems in children?
2. What influence does the eating experience have on the development of children?
3. Describe the influence that the woman's nutritional status has on the growing fetus and the newborn infant.
4. What are the findings on the relationship of an infant's nutritional status to later intellectual development and immune competence?
5. When are the energy requirements greatest? Why?
6. What factors influence a child's dietary practices?
7. What information is gathered in the nutritional history?
8. What would a nurse tell parents regarding the nutritional quality of meals consumed in fast food restaurants?
9. What can parents do to help their child develop positive eating behaviors?
10. Explain the etiology and management of the following diseases: (a) marasmus, (b) kwashiorkor, and (c) rickets.
11. Explain how infant obesity can be prevented.
12. What are the potential nutritional problems for children on vegetarian diets? How can these nutritional problems be prevented?
13. What are the criteria for an infant to be diagnosed as *failure to thrive* (FTT)?
14. Describe the characteristics of the following types of FTT: (a) organic FTT, (b) nonorganic FTT, and (c) mixed FTT.
15. What are the common characteristics of parents having an infant with FTT?
16. What is the current view regarding the etiology of FTT?
17. Infants with what personality types are more likely to experience FTT?
18. What are the physical manifestations exhibited by infants with FTT?
19. What assessments would the nurse make about the infant who is diagnosed with FTT?
20. What is the nursing care for the infant hospitalized with FTT?
21. What are the components that make up parenteral nutrition and fat emulsions?
22. What are the indications for parenteral nutrition?
23. Describe the nursing responsibilities related to the administration of parenteral nutrition, and provide the rationale for each.
24. How are enteral formulas classified?
25. What are the various methods of administering enteral tube feedings?

CASE STUDY

John Campbell brings his daughter Katie, 14 months old, to the well-child clinic. He reports that Katie has a poor appetite for solids, but drinks plenty of whole milk. John reports that Katie goes to bed with a bottle. Katie has been well since her last visit except that she is often cranky and takes two long naps per day. On physical examination, Katie is found to be at the 25th percentile for height and above the 95th percentile for weight. An analysis of her blood indicates a hemoglobin of 7.6 grams.

What is the most likely reason for her weight status and anemia? Why might Katie be cranky?

What information should the nurse tell the father regarding putting Katie to bed with her bottle? What guidelines can the nurse offer John regarding eating behaviors and acceptance of new foods?

AUDIOVISUAL RESOURCES

1. **Unfinished Child**
This film, narrated by Patricia Neal, discusses the impact of maternal, fetal, and infant nutrition on physical and mental development. Poor nutrition is identified as a factor in the perpetuation of the poverty cycle. Also discussed are ways to provide every child with a better start through a healthy diet.

Videocassette: 30 minutes

Distributor: March of Dimes Birth Defects Foundation

2. **Burning Questions: America's Children—Diet in Danger**
Interviews with dieticians and health experts reveal that as many as 50% of the next generation of Americans will die of heart attack if the dietary and exercise patterns of children today continue. The program discusses myths about school nutrition and exercise programs as well as the impact of the media on nutrition.

Videocassette: 48 minutes

Distributor: Coronet/MTI Film and Video

3. **Being a Fat Child**
This program examines the stigma of being an overweight child. Interviews with several teenagers and their families at a camp specializing in weight reduction illustrate how childhood obesity can be controlled through proper nutrition, exercise, and behavior modification.

16-mm film: 15 minutes

Distributor: Coronet/MTI Film and Video

4. **Home Enteral Nutrition**
The focus of this program is to educate health professionals about the technology involved in enteral nutrition and learn how to monitor the procedure in the home setting. Indications for enteral feeding, contraindications, cost, and technology are addressed. The discussion includes designing a plan that consider's the patient's lifestyle, physical environment of the home, and support systems. A study guide is available. While the program is not directed to pediatrics, it may be useful for independent student viewing.

Videocassette: 28 minutes

Distributor: American Journal of Nursing Company

5. **Enteral Therapy: Nursing Implications**
All aspects of enteral therapy, including nasogastric tube, gastrostomy, and jejunostomy, are detailed in this program showing actual patients. Tube feeding procedures are detailed step-by-step. Formula preparation, care of the tube, and the delivery system are addressed. This program does not focus specifically on children.

Videocassette: 25 minutes

Distributor: American Journal of Nursing Company

6. **Total Parenteral Nutrition**
   This two-part program provides an introduction and overview of total parenteral nutrition (TRN) for adult patients. Nutritional requirements during disease, indications for TPN therapy, catheter insertion and care, and specific information regarding TPN solutions are discussed. Part II focuses on the technical, metabolic, and septic complications of TPN. It should be noted that these programs are directed to the medical student or physician audience.

Videocassette: 21 and 29 minutes

Distributor: University of Michigan Medical Center, Media Library

7. **Home Gastrostomy for Infants and Young Children**
   This program is designed to familiarize students with the principles and techniques of caring for infants and young children who have a gastrostomy. It covers two types of surgical procedures, different tubes used in feeding, steps in the feeding process, administering medications, safety precautions, and signs of problems.

Videocassette: 25 minutes

Distributor: Pyramid Film and Video

8. **Nutritional Needs and Obesity of the Adolescent**
   This program explains the usual nutritional requirements during each phase of adolescence and factors influencing an adolescent's food intake. Nutrients most likely to be deficient during adolescence are identified. Coping mechanisms used by an adolescent who is obese and the nurse's role in improving adolescent nutrition are discussed.

Videocassette: 30 minutes

Distributor: Health Sciences Consortium

ANSWERS TO PRETEST

1. carbohydrates
2. calories
3. metabolic rate
4. building body tissue
5. simple sugars, glycogen
6. liver, muscles
7. hemorrhage, poor healing, susceptibility to infection, scurvy
8. vitamin A
9. milk
10. calcium, phosphorus
11. vitamin K
12. lactose
13. vitamins A, D, E, and K
14. an amino acid that the body cannot synthesize

PRETEST: NUTRITION

Fill in the blanks.

1. The greatest source of energy for cells is ______________________________.
2. The energy content of food is expressed as ______________________________.
3. The speed at which the body uses energy is the ______________________________ ______________________________.
4. The primary function that protein serves is ______________________________ ______________________________.
5. Carbohydrates are broken down into ______________________________ and then stored as ______________________________.
6. The break-down products of carbohydrates are stored in the ______________________________ ______________________________ and ______________________________.
7. Two results of inadequate intake of vitamin C include ______________________________ ______________________________ and ______________________________.
8. The vitamin required for night vision is ______________________________.
9. The minimum requirement of riboflavin is difficult to maintain without a diet that includes ______________________________.
10. Vitamin D is required for utilization of ______________________________ and ______________________________.
11. The vitamin necessary for normal blood clotting is ______________________________.
12. The primary source of carbohydrates in young infants is ______________________________ ______________________________.
13. The four fat-soluble vitamins are ______________________________, ______________________________, ______________________________, and ______________________________.
14. An *essential amino acid* is defined as ______________________________ ______________________________ ______________________________.

CHAPTER 17

PROMOTING HEALTHY PLAY

DISCUSSION QUESTIONS

1. What are the similarities of and the differences between the definitions of *play*?
2. Describe the eight characteristics of play.
3. Describe the characteristics of the following forms of play: (a) unoccupied, (b) onlooker, (c) solitary independent, (d) parallel, (e) associative, and (f) cooperative.
4. Describe the play of infants and toddlers.
5. What are typical play activities of the preschool child?
6. Describe the play activities of the school-age child.
7. How does play facilitate physical development and motor skills?
8. Why is play critical to a child's cognitive development?
9. How is play related to language development?
10. Discuss how play contributes to a child's social and moral development.
11. How can the nurse guide parents regarding play and development?
12. How is play useful in an assessment of a child with problematic human responses?
13. What is therapeutic play?
14. Under what circumstances is play therapy indicated?
15. What are the four characteristics of medical play?
16. How would the nurse incorporate play into the preparation of a 4-year-old child for placement of a hip spica cast?

CASE STUDY #1

Juanita Sanchez brings Tina, age 3 months, to the clinic for a routine visit. The nurse taking a history asks Juanita about the types of toys she has for Tina and what play activities she engages in with Tina. Juanita says that Tina is too young to play and she keeps the home quiet so that Tina can sleep.

What aspects of development might be adversely affected by Tina's lack of play experiences?

Develop a teaching plan for the mother that is directed at the following nursing diagnosis: *Potential for altered growth and development related to lack of appropriate play opportunities.*

CASE STUDY #2

Four-year-old Marvin is admitted to the hospital for surgical repair of a hernia. He appears very frightened and cries when the nurse comes into the room. He tells her that he doesn't want an operation.

How can the nurse use play to reduce Marvin's anxiety and prepare him for surgery?

What developmental characteristics will the nurse need to consider when planning play activities for Marvin?

STUDENT LEARNING ACTIVITIES

1. Spend a day in the playroom in the hospital unit or at a local nursery school or daycare center. Observe several children. Keep a log of the characteristics of their play. How do these activities relate to the child's developmental level? What types of learning result from the play experience? For the hospitalized child, how do the play activities assist adaptation to the hospital experience?

AUDIOVISUAL RESOURCES

1. **Parents and Children Series, Play Subseries: Part I—How To Play with a Child**
   This videotape teaches how to interact with children in play through the use of vignette demonstrations of both appropriate and inappropriate interactions. This program identifies ways to recognize children's capabilities and needs, provide positive support for play, help children develop imaginative and creative play, build self-esteem and self-concept, handle boredom, avoid power struggles, and understand the importance of adult attention. This film is comprehensive and well illustrated. It is valuable as an instructional tool for students in all pediatric settings and for developing parent teaching projects that center on promoting healthy play and interaction.

Videocassette: 36 minutes

Distributor: Health Sciences Consortium

2. **Inpatient Play Assessment and Therapy**
   This program presents examples of directive and non-directive play therapy for young children. Also discussed is the assessment and management of the pediatric patient.

Videocassette: 30 minutes

Distributor: Altschul Group Corporation

3. **Children's Play and the Real World**
   The relevance of play in developing the child's self-awareness, thinking, and learning is discussed in this program. Examples are provided of Piaget's three forms of play—sensorimotor, aymbolic, and games with rules. The program offers suggestions for ways adults can support children's play. Also included are standards for evaluating the quality of play.

16-mm film: 16 minutes

Distributor: Indiana University Audio-Visual Center

UNIT IV

CONCEPTS RELATED TO ILLNESS

CHAPTER 18

STRESS, CRISIS, AND COPING

DISCUSSION QUESTIONS

1. Describe how the body responds to stressful situations.
2. What are some criticisms of the research that has been done on children and stress?
3. Describe the three models that explain why some children do not respond negatively to stress.
4. Explain what is meant by *maturational crisis*, *situational crisis*, and *unanticipated crisis*.
5. What are the steps in crisis intervention? What is the nurse's role at each of the steps?
6. What function do coping strategies play in response to stress?
7. What are examples of stressors to children that originate in the (a) microsystem, (b) exosystem, and (c) macrosystem?
8. What explanations for illness are given by children who display the following reasoning processes: (a) prelogical, (b) concrete logical, and (c) formal logical?
9. Describe the requirements of parents experiencing each of the following forms of stress: (a) intellectual, (b) instrumental, (c) interpersonal, (d) emotional, and (e) existential.

STUDENT LEARNING ACTIVITIES

1. Ask students to describe their assigned patients and families. What stresses are experienced by the child and the family members as a result of the illness and hospitalization? What other sources of stress exist for the family? Have the child and the family members developed healthy behaviors for dealing with stressful experiences?

AUDIOVISUAL RESOURCES

1. **Stress**
   This series of programs discusses stress as an expected component of life changes. Specifically identified are sources of stress, the body's response, stress and disease, managing stress, and stress as a nursing concern. This program is not pediatrically oriented, but it is comprehensive in conceptual content. It could be used for students as independent review or to stimulate discussion about the similarities and differences in childhood and adult responses to stress.

Videotransfers: 19–28 minutes each part

Distributor: Concept Media

2. **Knowing, Feeling, Growing**
   This program uses puppetry do demonstrate how to use coping techniques to solve problems and decrease anxiety. The approach is simple and is designed to teach young children. It could be used in health promotion activities for preschool and young school-age children.

Videocassette

Distributor: University of Minnesota

Chapter 19

Chronic Illness

DISCUSSION QUESTIONS

1. What are the characteristics of a disorder that is considered chronic?
2. What are the different ways that chronic illnesses are divided into categories?
3. Why do children have difficulty understanding the concept of health?
4. What factors influence the development of wellness behaviors by children?
5. Why is it dysfunctional for the child with chronic illness to assume the sick role?
6. Describe the factors that will influence how the child and family respond to and manage the consequences of the child's chronic disorder.
7. Describe the factors that place the child at risk for illness. What is the major task related to risk for the child with chronic illness?
8. Discuss the health practices of Native Americans, African Americans, Mexican Americans, and Chinese Americans. What are the nursing implications in each case for caring for a child and their families?
9. The text discusses seven factors that influence a child's response to a chronic illness. What are these factors?
10. What are the three stages of children's reactions to separation?
11. The family of a child with a chronic illness experiences many stresses. What are these stresses, and what are some means by which the stresses can be reduced?
12. What effect does chronic illness have on the development of the infant or toddler?
13. How does the preschool child typically perceive the basis of his or her illness?
14. What effect does chronic illness have on the psychosocial development of the school-age child?
15. What responses to chronic illness are typical of adolescents? What characteristics of adolescent development explain these responses?
16. Siblings of a child with a chronic illness can experience difficulties coping with the effects that the ill child has on family life. What factors will influence the types of responses siblings experience?
17. How are maternal and paternal roles and marital relationship affected when a child has a chronic illness?
18. Summarize the findings of theorists regarding family coping behaviors. What constitutes healthy family coping responses to the child with a chronic disorder?
19. What are the nursing goals of caring for the child with a chronic disorder? Describe the nursing interventions for each of these goals for the (a) infant, (b) toddler, (c) preschool child, (d) school-age child, and (f) adolescent.
20. Discuss methods children use to cope with their chronic illnesses.
21. How can the nurse facilitate the family's utilization of community resources?

CASE STUDY #1

Calvin is a 6-month-old infant who has been hospitalized since birth with tracheoesophageal fistula and bronchopulmonary dysplasia. He has been on a respirator since shortly after birth and has experienced numerous complications of this disorder. Calvin has received all nutrition first parenterally and recently via a gastrostomy tube. Calvin's parents visit twice weekly and take an active role in his care.

Explain why chronic illness during the infancy period may interfere with the following: (a) parental attachment, (b) physical development, (c) cognitive development, and (d) social-emotional development.

What are some of the effects that Calvin's illness may have on the following people: (a) his mother, (b) his father, (c) the parent's marital relationship, and (d) his 5-year-old sister Adrian?

CASE STUDY #2

Carole, age 28 months, was diagnosed with cystic fibrosis shortly after birth. She is now admitted with pneumonia. Because she is experiencing some degree of hypoxia, Carole is placed on complete bed rest and must remain in a mist tent with oxygen. Carole's mother has just given birth to her second child and is only able to visit Carole in the evenings.

What developmental characteristics of the toddler will influence Carol's response to hospitalization?

When the nurse attempts to administer an oral medication to Carole, she resists and becomes frightened. What is the best way for the nurse to gain Carole's cooperation and reduce her fear? Why would it probably not be helpful for the nurse to tell Carole that the medicine will help her to feel better?

According to Erikson, the major task of the toddler period is to establish autonomy. What problems does Carole's hospitalization present for her need to develop autonomy? Why is the absence of Carole's mother so stressful for the toddler?

STUDENT LEARNING ACTIVITIES

1. Ask students to discuss the children that they cared for during the week's clinical experience. What types of coping strategies did the children use to deal with the stresses of illness and hospitalization? Were there differences in strategies used by children with chronic versus acute illnesses? How did the child's developmental level influence coping strategies? Were the coping strategies used by the children helpful in facilitating healthy adaptation to the illness and hospitalization?

   Have students develop a care plan with the goal to promote effective coping behaviors for their assigned patient. They should include rationales for interventions based on developmental level and the child's physical status.

2. Interview parents of children with chronic illnesses. What resources do they find helpful in assisting them to care for or adjust to the demands of the child? How did they find out about these resources? What methods are used by the hospital to connect parents to the types of resources that they need?

AUDIOVISUAL RESOURCES

1. **Living with Chronic Illness: Reaching for Hope . . . Learning to Cope**
   This film discusses the changes in daily living patterns experienced by the chronically ill child and family. Vignettes provide the focal point for identifying feelings and fears of the children and families portrayed. The film focuses on preparation of the health professional in helping children cope effectively and in guiding families toward acceptance and behavior that reinforces a chronically ill child's self-concept and development. This program is a dramatic representation of the problems associated with chronic illness in children and is valuable to heighten student awareness and the ability to participate in supportive care strategies.

Videocassette: 33 minutes

Distributor: Health Sciences Consortium

2. **The Same Inside**
   In this film, four children with special needs share their feelings about their birth defects. These children discuss fears and dreams that are similar to all children. The intent is to help the viewer understand that children who are disabled or those that look different have the same emotional and psychosocial needs as "normal" children. This is a film for anyone who is unfamiliar with children who have chronic illnesses or birth defects. An educator's guide accompanies the film to facilitate use with parent or child teaching projects.

Videocassette or 16-mm film: 13 minutes

Distributor: March of Dimes Birth Defects Foundation

CHAPTER 20

DEATH AND DYING

DISCUSSION QUESTIONS

1. Explain how the terms *grief* and *mourning* differ?
2. What are the five stages outlined by Kubler-Ross in the individual's response to terminal illness? For each stage, identify the role that the nurse can assume in assisting the terminally ill child?
3. How is the process of grief explained by (a) Freud, (b) Lindemann, and (c) Engel?
4. What purposes does anticipatory grief serve?
5. How do children in the following age groups typically view the experience of death: (a) 3 to 5 year olds, (b) 5 to 9 year olds, (c) 10 to 12 year olds, and (d) adolescents?
6. How does the response to loss differ among (a) younger, (b) middle, and (c) older adolescents?
7. What nursing interventions are helpful to parents when their child is diagnosed with a disease having a poor prognosis?
8. What common emotions are expressed by parents of terminally ill children? How do these emotions influence behaviors directed toward the child and other family members?
9. What is the major death-related fear for a child of the following ages: (a) less than 5 years old, (b) 5 to 10 years, and (c) over 10 years old?
10. How can parents provide experiences that help children understand and develop healthy reactions to death?
11. Discuss ways that nurses can identify and cope with their own feelings and expressions of grief in response to dying children and death.

CASE STUDY #1

Jason, age 2 years, is admitted to the hospital with a relapse of leukemia. He is terminal, and medical and nursing interventions are focused on keeping him comfortable and providing family support. Jason has two older siblings. His parents are with Jason most of the time, but leave daily to be with their other children.

What perceptions regarding dying does Jason most likely have? What are the best means by which Jason could be comforted? What types of interventions by the nurse would be most helpful to Jason and his parents?

Jason continues to linger near death for three weeks. How can the nurse help the parents to experience the process of grieving constructively?

Jason's parents express a wish to provide a means for Jason's body to contribute to the perpetuation of another child's life. What information can the nurse give the parents regarding the possible use of Jason's organs after his death?

Because Jason's parents are unable to remain with him constantly, it is important for the nurse to be alert for signs of Jason's impending death so that the parents can be summoned in time if they are away from the hospital. Describe the signs that indicate that such a child is near death.

Jason dies with both of his parents present. Also present is the nurse who has cared for Jason during much of his illness. In what ways would it be appropriate for the nurse to express her sorrow over Jason's death?

CASE STUDY #2

Lilly, who is 8 years old, is hospitalized for liver failure. She has been hospitalized many times in the past and has undergone two liver transplants, both unsuccessful. Lilly is in the terminal stage of her disease. Both of her parents work, but they visit her nightly. She has a teenage brother, age 15 years, and a younger sister who is 5 years old. Lilly is familiar with the hospital routine and understands about her disease. She has been told that this hospitalization is to try the effectiveness of a new drug.

What influence may Lilly's previous hospital experiences have on her perception of death? What type of associations with death consistent with her developmental level would she be expected to have?

Lilly asks the nurse if she is going to die. After consulting with Lilly's parents, what response would be most appropriate for the nurse to give?

How best can Lilly's parents and the nurse provide comfort to Lilly during the terminal stage of her illness? What methods can the parents use to begin to prepare Lilly's younger sibling for her death?

Lilly's parents decide that they wish to take her home to die. What criteria should be met to make home care appropriate for Lilly?

What problems related to nutrition would Lilly be likely to experience? Why do these problems exist in terminally ill children? Develop a care plan with measures to help alleviate nutritional problems for these children.

Lilly dies after being home for two weeks. Her sister is at the grandparents' house at the time. The parents ask the visiting nurse how best to explain to Lilly's sister that Lilly has died and if they should allow her to attend the funeral. What information should the nurse provide to the parents that would help her sister adjust to Lilly's death? What are the findings on children who attend funerals?

STUDENT LEARNING ACTIVITIES

1. Ask students to interview nurses in the hospital unit about their experiences with dying children. What are their coping strategies for dealing with the loss? How do they feel dealing with the family before and after the child's death? Do they go to the funeral or keep in touch with families of children they are close to?
2. Tell students to collect books for children about death. Read them to (or with) children of different ages. Then ask the children to talk about their perceptions and feelings about the book's material.
3. Interview young children regarding their experiences with the death of a relative or pet. How do the children explain death? Is it consistent with the behaviors described for their age?
4. Assign the students to attend a community support group such as Candlelighters, Compassionate Friends, or SIDS Support Group. What methods do the groups use to provide support to parents?

AUDIOVISUAL RESOURCES

1. **Children and the Grief Process**
   This program presents the child's perspective of death through discussions between Rabbi Earl Grollmann and a group of children. The program illustrates ways to help children deal with their feelings about death and separation in a positive manner.

Videocassette: 21 minutes

Distributor: Coronet/MTI Film & Video

2. **A Child Dies**
   Two nurse clinicians share their experiences of working with families who have lost a child. This informative program is designed to fortify nurses to meet the challenges of supporting the family after the death of a child.

Videocassette: 28 minutes

Distributor: American Journal of Nursing Company

3. The Grieving Family
Interventions to help the family grieving the death of a child are discussed. The program provides a checklist of actions for nurses. The need for nurses to be aware of their own feelings is also addressed.

Videocassette: 28 minutes

Distributor: American Journal of Nursing Company

4. Death of a High Risk Infant
This program outlines the stages of parents' grief and includes an actual parents' support meeting. Practical pointers are offered to help parents cope with their loss. May also be useful for patient education.

Videocassette: 30 minutes

Distributor: American Journal of Nursing

UNIT V

MANAGING ILLNESS

CHAPTER 21

NURSING CARE DURING HOSPITALIZATION

DISCUSSION QUESTIONS

1. What are the conclusions from research on the child's response to the hospitalization experience?
2. For each of the following stressors of hospitalization, identify which children are most at risk and list the interventions the nurse can use to reduce the child's stress: (a) separation, (b) harm and injury, (c) unknown events and environment, and (d) unclear limits and loss of control.
3. Robertson has identified stages in a child's adjustment to hospitalization. What are these three stages and what behaviors are characteristic of each stage?
4. How does hospitalization affect the development and coping of the (a) infant and toddler, (b) preschool child, (c) school-age child, and (d) adolescent?
5. What factors influence a child's response to the stress of hospitalization?
6. Discuss guidelines for conducting hospital tours with young school-age children.
7. How can parents prepare a child for hospitalization?
8. Describe how the physical environment, social environment, and admission procedures can affect a child and parents during the hospital admission process.
9. Identify nursing interventions to help children cope with hospital procedures. How would nursing actions differ for the (a) infant and toddler, (b) preschool child, (c) school-age child, and (d) adolescent?
10. Hospitalization causes an interruption in the child's normal pattern of life. What interventions by the nurse are helpful in promoting (a) rest and sleep, (b) nutrition, (c) elimination, (d) activity patterns, (e) self-care, (f) development, and (g) body image?
11. How can the nurse promote positive parental competence during the child's hospitalization?
12. What types of support do parents need who have a hospitalized child at each of the following stages: (a) infant, (b) toddler, (c) preschool child, (d) school age, and (e) adolescent?
13. What measures help the siblings of the hospitalized child to adjust to the experience?
14. The nurse is about to perform the first post-operative dressing change on David's surgical incision. David is 5 years old. Outline how the nurse should prepare David for the procedure. What explanations should she provide? What typical reactions will David most likely exhibit?
15. What are the components included in the discharge instructions provided to the child and family?

CASE STUDY #1

Wendy, age 22 months, is admitted to the hospital with orbital cellulitis. She will require 10 days of intravenous antibiotics. This is Wendy's first admission to the hospital. Wendy's parents both work but will visit her each evening. When her parents leave the first day, Wendy cries violently, calls for her mother, and tries to climb out of the crib. Wendy is in which of Robertson's stages? What interventions by the nurse at this time would be most helpful to Wendy and her parents?

What major stressors will Wendy most likely experience? Develop a care plan to minimize these stressors.

The nurse is assisting the physician in inserting an intravenous line for the administration of the antibiotics. How best can the nurse prepare and support Wendy during this procedure?

After three days in the hospital, Wendy's mother tells the nurse that she is concerned because Wendy has begun to ask for a bottle again and wet her pants. Wendy had been toilet trained prior to coming into the hospital. What explanation for these behaviors can the nurse give the mother and how should the parents react to these behaviors?

CASE STUDY #2

Phillip, age 10 years, is admitted to the hospital after being hit by a car while riding his bike. He has a fractured skull and a fractured left femur. He is placed in a spica cast shortly after admission. On arrival to the floor, he is awake and alert, anxious, and crying for his parents. Why is it likely that Phillip will adjust more readily to the hospital experience than a toddler or preschooler?

What stressors is Phillip most likely to experience? Develop a nursing care plan to minimize these stressors.

What problems related to elimination will Phillip most likely experience? What can the nurse do to minimize these problems?

Phillip will be hospitalized for three weeks and will remain in a cast for a total of three months. What characteristics of school-age thought will guide the nurse in explaining to Phillip his injuries and needed medical and nursing management? Develop a nursing care plan for Phillip.

STUDENT LEARNING ACTIVITIES

1. Have students observe the meals presented to hospitalized children. Are they prepared in a manner that promotes the child's interest and desire to eat? Do hospitals consider the developmental characteristics of children when preparing meals? Is there a special place where children who are allowed out of bed can eat?
2. Provide each student with the opportunity to admit a child to the hospital. Ask another student to observe the process and offer feedback regarding skills of taking the history, ability to minimize the child's and family's fear and anxiety, and ability to provide a clear orientation to the unit's physical environment and routines.
3. Ask students to describe the reactions to hospitalization for their assigned patients. Were the reactions consistent with those typical of their developmental level? Were there differences between the reactions of those children who were being hospitalized for the first time and those who have been hospitalized before? What measures did students use to minimize the stressors of hospitalization? Were parents effective in providing emotional support and comfort to their children?
4. Ask each student to complete a nursing process plan following the outline in Table 21-2 (in the textbook) for the child they care for.
5. Provide experiences for students to discharge children. What information did they provide to the families? What questions did families have regarding home care? What assessment criteria were used to determine the adequacy of this preparation for discharge?

AUDIOVISUAL RESOURCES

1. **Young Children's Reactions to Hospitalization**
   This film presents interviews with parents and children portraying behavioral changes that may occur during hospitalization. The effects of separation are discussed with suggestions for dealing honestly with the young child. The film is intended to inform and assist parents in dealing with reactions such as regression in toilet skills, increased demands from the child, or withdrawal. This program is useful in illustrating the impact of hospitalization on children and in providing the student with guidelines for parent education.

Videocassette: 14 minutes

Distributor: American Journal of Nursing Company

2. **Promoting Normal Growth in the Hospitalized Child**
   This video details developmental stages and describes strategies for promoting the normal progression of growth and development in the hospitalized child. Specific topics include nutrition, comfort, and stimulation needs of infants; safe opportunities to encourage the toddler's developing autonomy; creative play and problem-solving experiences for the preschooler; strategies for maintaining the school-age child's sense of industry while immobilized; and provision for peer interactions for the adolescent. This is an excellent film that is useful in orienting students to clinical and caring for hospitalized children.

Videocassette: 12 minutes

Distributor: American Journal of Nursing Company

3. **The Hospitalized Adolescent**
   This program offers creative approaches for promoting independence and self-esteem of hospitalized adolescent patients.

Videocassette: 29 minutes

Distributor: Altschul Group Corporation

4. **A Hospital Adventure: Starring Boris the Bear**
   This program for children portrays what goes on in a hospital in a warm and understandable way. Boris the Bear narrates his experiences from the emergency room to his hospital room. This program is recommended for use by pediatric staffs. Also included is a package of camera-ready art to develop a Boris coloring book or other Boris items.

Videocassette: 11 minutes

Distributor: American Journal of Nursing Company

5. **Initial Nursing Assessment of a Hospitalized Child: Basis for Developing a Nursing Care Plan**
   This video dramatizes the admission of a 3 1/2-year-old child to the hospital for chemotherapy. The nurse is shown assessing the physical, psychological, cognitive, and language development of the child. Using the data obtained, she goes on to develop a care plan for the child. This is a good film that illustrates the parameters of comprehensive assessment and planning strategies for the hospitalized child.

Videocassette: 36 minutes

Distributor: Health Sciences Consortium

6. **Play Experiences During Hospitalization**
   This film demonstrates several play sessions for hospitalized children of all ages, including a diagnostic play experience in which a child is encouraged to act out how she deals with the hospital, a therapeutic session for a group of pre-operative children to learn about the procedures they will undergo, a school activity session, and a picnic outside the hospital for children who are able to leave for short periods. This program would be useful in illustrating to students how play sessions allow children to express and master fears, release tension, and learn while hospitalized.

Videocassette: 15 minutes

Distributor: University of Michigan

7. **Going to the Hospital**
   This program with Mr. Rogers offers viewers a general introduction to the sights and sounds of the hospital and some feelings children may experience there. This program could be useful to students involved in planning hospital tours for young children. Also available in Spanish.

Videocassette: 20 minutes

Distributor: Family Communications

8. **Having an Operation**
   This Mr. Rogers program presents a preschool child's experiences during a tonsillectomy. The child is admitted to the hospital the day before surgery and her parents leave in the evening. The next morning the child is followed through pre-operative medications, going to the operating room, receiving anesthesia, moving into the recovery room, and returning to her room. Later the child is discharged from the hospital with her parents. The distributor recommends this program only for children scheduled for simple surgery. It could be useful to students doing pre-operative teaching. Also available in Spanish.

Videocassette: 17 minutes

Distributor: Family Communications

9. **Child Development Series: Assessment and Planning**
   This program focuses on factors that influence the needs of the hospitalized child. Specific nursing actions designed to meet the physical and emotional needs of hospitalized children are discussed.

Videocassette: 23 minutes

Distributor: Medcom/Trainex

CHAPTER 22

COMMUNITY AND HOME CARE

DISCUSSION QUESTIONS

1. Differentiate between the three major areas of pediatric home care: (a) physician-directed intermittent skilled care, (b) physician-directed hourly skilled care, and (c) hourly support services.
2. How did the concept of home care for children develop?
3. How has the work of Ida Martinson influenced pediatric home care?
4. How have the following social factors influenced the use of pediatric home care: (a) cost containment, (b) quality of care, and (c) technology?
5. Outline the steps of the nursing process applied to preparing a child for home care.
6. What family factors indicate that the family is ready to assume the care of an ill child at home?
7. Describe the nursing interventions applicable during the following periods of home care: (a) engagement, (b) assessment, (c) intervention, and (d) termination.
8. What characteristics must a nurse possess in order to provide care to children in their home?
9. How does the nurse's role differ for intervention in the home versus the acute care institution?
10. What are the three types of home care available to children and the objectives of each?
11. Describe the types of agencies that deliver home care services.
12. Identify four differences between adult and pediatric home care.
13. What is the future outlook for home care for children, and what are the implications for nursing practice?

CASE STUDY

Jesse Wells, age 18 months, has been hospitalized since birth with complications related to prematurity. He has a tracheostomy tube and a gastrostomy tube for feedings. Jesse's parents are preparing to take him home in two weeks. Due to his illness, Jesse is developmentally delayed and demonstrates the motor skills of a 12 month old. He is not able to speak, but has learned a few basic words in sign language. He will need frequent suctioning, percussion, and postural drainage, as well as constant respiratory and cardiac monitoring. A program has been put together to facilitate language, motor, and cognitive development. The Wells will care for Jesse both day and evening shifts and will have a nurse for the night shift.

List areas of assessment that Jesse's nurse will perform to evaluate the parent's readiness for caring for Jesse at home.

What skills will be necessary for the parents to learn? What measures by the nurse will help the parents learning how to care for Jesse?

What types of support services should be made available to the Wells?

The nurse who will provide care for Jesse during the night shift is planning a meeting with the Wells. What are the major objectives of this meeting? What approach by the nurse will assist in meeting these objectives?

STUDENT LEARNING ACTIVITIES

1. Assign students to children with chronic illnesses that will require continuation of care at home. Ask the students to develop a nursing process plan for home care using Table 22-1 (in the textbook) as a guide.
2. Assign students to make a home visit with a nurse providing care in the home to a child. The students should report on the following: (a) the role of the family in providing care, (b) changes in family roles related to the presence of the ill child in the home, and (c) adaptation of family members to the experience.

AUDIOVISUAL RESOURCES

1. **Discharge Planning in Pediatric Catastrophic Illness**
This two-part program emphasizes the unique qualifications of the nurse in managing the process of planning for care of children at home. The importance of keeping children's hospital stay to a minimum to promote optimal growth and development is stressed. Part I focuses on the discharge planning process while a child is still in the hospital and is illustrated by a clinical case. Part II describes the nurse's role in pediatric home care with regards to planning, coordinating health support services, and maintaining contact with hospital-based professionals. This comprehensive program could be used with students in both acute and community health care practice settings.

Videocassette: 28 minutes each part

Distributor: American Journal of Nursing Company

2. **Only a Breath**
This program depicts the lives of five families with children who are ventilator-assisted and living at home. The children and their families describe their experiences in learning to live with the technology, problems with support systems, and how these problems affect each family member. By contrast, the health professionals responsible for primary care, management and support of these children and their families discuss their issues of concern. This program helps students identify special health needs of families caring for sick children at home who often require a complex array of services. It also illustrates the future of pediatric home care.

Videocassette: 30 minutes

Distributor: Altschul Group Corporation

3. **Parents and Nurses: Separate Roles, Common Goals**
In this program, family members and nurses discuss the problems, limitations, and benefits of home care for technologically assisted children.

Videocassette: 21 minutes

Distributor: Altschul Group Corporation

4. **Educational Planning for the Child with Special Health Care Needs**
Parents and educators address the issues involved in planning education for families with children having special health care needs.

Videocassette: 30 minutes

Distributor: Altschul Group Corporation

CHAPTER 23

PRINCIPLES AND SKILLS ADAPTED TO THE CARE OF CHILDREN

DISCUSSION QUESTIONS

1. Bobby O'Hare, 14 years old, arrives at the emergency room with a neighbor. He has fallen and lacerated his forehead and will require sutures. What procedures must the nurse follow to obtain parental consent before Bobby can be treated?
2. What do the terms *mature* and *emancipated minor* mean in regards to consent for treatment?
3. Explain the procedures that must be followed before a child can be a subject in a research project.
4. The nurse is planning a teaching session with Cindy and her parents. Cindy has had surgery and will be discharged home soon. She will need daily dressing changes and management of a surgical drain. Before the nurse begins teaching, what factors should she assess that could influence the learning process?
5. Describe the safety risks to the hospitalized child. How can the nurse minimize each of these risks?
6. The risk of a fall is a special threat to the hospitalized child. What types of common nursing practices place children at risk for falls? Describe the principles of safety that should be applied to all children to prevent the danger of falls.
7. The nurse is taking Megan, age 2 years, to the X-ray department. Megan's mother asks the nurse if she can carry her. What would the nurse's response be?
8. Describe the procedures for providing the hygienic needs of the child during hospitalization.
9. Discuss research related to the impact of parental presence during procedures.
10. What factors influence the route selected for obtaining a child's temperature?
11. Describe the correct procedure for obtaining temperature, pulse, respiration, and blood pressure in infants and children.
12. The nurse needs to collect a urine specimen from Anna, who is 13 months old. Describe the correct procedure for the nurse to follow.
13. Identify situations when the use of restraints would be indicated.
14. What are nursing diagnoses and interventions for the child with restraints?
15. When does the nurse use universal precautions? What does this involve?
16. What physiological processes produce fever? Explain the beneficial effects of fever.
17. What factors are considered when evaluating the seriousness of a fever?
18. Describe the reactions to stressful experiences and the typical coping abilities of the (a) infant, (b) toddler, (c) preschooler, (d) school-age child, and (e) adolescent. What nursing strategies for reducing stress are most effective for each of these age groups?

CASE STUDY #1

Carl, age 4 years, is scheduled to enter the hospital in a week for repair of a hernia and undescended testicles. When should Carl's parents begin to prepare him for the hospitalization?

After Carl is admitted to the hospital, how can the nurse help him to verbalize his fears regarding hospitalization and surgery?

Carl is to have blood drawn. How best can the nurse prepare him for this experience? What kinds of fears would Carl be most likely to experience that are typical of his developmental level? Carl's mother requests to stay with her son during the venipuncture. What would be the nurse's response?

Outline the nursing responsibilities related to Carl's pre-operative and immediate post-operative periods.

CASE STUDY #2

Tegan is brought to the pediatrician's office by her mother, Joann Peterson, complaining of sore throat and fever. She is 3 years old and in good health. After the exam, strep throat is diagnosed. Tegan is placed on penicillin, and her mother is instructed to give her Tylenol every four hours if she has fever at or above 101°F.

Tegan weighs 17 kg. How many milligrams of Tylenol should she receive? If Joann has the Tylenol preparation of 160 mg/5 ml, how many milliliters should Tegan receive?

Construct a teaching sheet on fever management for the mother.

How does sponging reduce fevers? Outline the proper procedure for sponging. Why should the nurse not advise Joann to place alcohol in the water used to sponge Tegan?

STUDENT LEARNING ACTIVITIES

1. Review the procedure manual in the pediatric unit regarding common procedures performed, such as giving oral and parenteral medications, obtaining urine specimens, insertion of nasogastric tubes, and nasogastric feeding. Have the students explain how these procedures differ from those followed with adults and identify the rationale for why these differences are necessary.
2. Tour the pediatric unit with the students. Ask them to identify potential safety problems and ways that would reduce the risk of injury. What measures related to maintaining child safety are practiced on the unit?
3. Assign students to follow a child through the pre-operative period, surgical procedure, and post-operative period. What preparation did the child and family receive prior to surgery? What was their reaction to the information? Did the student feel preparation was adequate? What suggestions does the student have to improve the preparation?

AUDIOVISUAL RESOURCES

1. **Restraints: The Difficult Decision, Part 5—Restraining Infants and Children**
   This program illustrates commonly used restraining procedures and devices for children, including assessment of need and appropriate documentation. This program could be used for students in the learning laboratory to demonstrate restraint procedures and to stimulate discussion of nursing strategies to prevent associated problems.

Filmstrip and videocassette: 16 minutes

Distributor: J. B. Lippincott Company

2. **Preparing Children for the Hospital Experience**
   This program includes a review of child cognitive developmental levels with specific recommendations for keying explanations to the level of understanding of each child. The use of books, diagrams, dolls, and hospital equipment for patient teaching is demonstrated. Also emphasized is the importance of preparing children and their parents to assist and cooperate in care during a hospital experience.

Videocassette: 28 minutes

Distributor: American Journal of Nursing Company

3. **Let's Talk about the Hospital . . . with Mr. Rogers**
This four-part series, narrated by Fred Rogers, is designed to familiarize young children with hospitalization and medical procedures. The four programs are entitled "Going to the Hospital," "Having an Operation," "Wearing a Cast," and "A Visit to the Emergency Department." They present actual and detailed illustrations of the events and experiences a child would encounter in each of these situations. These programs could be used by students involved in pre-operative or anticipatory guidance teaching projects.

Videotape: 16–18 minutes each part

Distributor: Family Communications

4. **Pediatrics: Psychosocial Implications, Part 9—I Went to the Hospital**
This program is designed to acquaint children with the hospital surgical experience and to alleviate associated fears. A 5-year-old girl, hospitalized for minor surgery, describes for the viewer the medical personnel, equipment, procedures, and possible discomfort they may encounter in a similar situation. The supportive and caring attention of the hospital staff is emphasized.

Filmstrip or videotransfer: 13 minutes

Distributor: Concept Media

5. **Infection Control**
This five-part program reflects updated guidelines from the Centers for Disease Control (CDC) and Occupational Safety and Health Association (OSHA). The five parts included are "Basic Principles of Infection Control," Preventing Nosocomial Infections," "Universal Precautions" "Specific Infectional Control Techniques," and "Patient Education Program of Infection Control." A study guide is also included.

Slide-tape: 12–15 minutes each part

Distributor: American Journal of Nursing Company

6. **Current Infection Control Guidelines for Healthcare Professionals**
This program emphasizes the most current preventive measures and infection control guidelines. Procedures for practicing universal precautions are addressed.

Videocassette: 22 minutes

Distributor: Medcom/Trainex

Chapter 24

Pharmacologic Principles Applied to the Care of Children

DISCUSSION QUESTIONS

1. What actions occur at the cellular level to produce the desired effects of drugs?
2. What is meant by a drug's *therapeutic index?*
3. What is meant by *bioavailability?* What route of drug administration results in optimal bioavailability?
4. Give an example of the clinical effects that result when drugs interact with (a) the same receptor, (b) identical receptors located in different tissues, and (c) different types of receptors.
5. Describe how the age of a child influences the (a) absorption of drugs, (b) distribution of drugs, (c) metabolism, and (d) elimination of drugs.
6. What questions should the nurse ask parents when collecting a medication history?
7. What guidelines should the nurse follow for using EMLA cream to prevent discomfort for an intramuscular injection?
8. What are the two methods for calculating the safe dose range of a medication ordered for a child?
9. Describe nursing actions related to the safe administration of medications to children. What is the rationale for each action?
10. How would the nurse administer an oral medication to the (a) infant, (b) toddler, (c) preschooler, (d) school-age child, and (e) adolescent?
11. What is the correct procedure for the administration of eye drops, nose drops, and ear drops to children?
12. For each of the following age groups, what is the procedure followed for giving intramuscular injections? How does the nurse prepare the parents and child? What injection sites are used and why are these sites preferred? (a) infant, (b) toddler and preschooler, (c) school-age child, and (d) adolescent

CASE STUDY

Shawna, age 5 years, has elevated blood lead levels and is being admitted to the hospital for chelation therapy. This is her first hospitalization. What information about medications would the nurse ascertain from Shawna's mother during the admission history?

The physician orders Shawna to receive $CaNa_2$ EDTA intravenously and BAL intramuscularly every 4 hours for 5 days. Formulate a plan for preparing Shawna for the frequent injections that is consistent with her developmental level. What strategies would the nurse use to prevent injury when administering the intramuscular injections?

STUDENT LEARNING ACTIVITIES

1. Require that students calculate safe dosages for all children to whom they administer medications.
2. Assign students to make "hero badges" for the younger patients who are anxious about receiving medications or treatments. After the children receive the medication or procedure, they get a badge that says "I was brave today." Children receive the badge even if they did not fully cooperate.

3. Require students to complete drug cards on all medications that are given to the patients they care for. The cards should include the following information:

   a. Name of drug

   b. Drug action

   c. Reason child is receiving drug (Note: many drugs serve numerous functions. Stress to students that the information on the card should relate directly to the use of the drug for their particular patient.)

   d. Recommended safe dose and their own safe dose calculation to ensure that medication is within the safe range

   e. Common side effects

   f. Nursing implications related to drug action, administration, and side effects

   g. Learning needs of the child and family related to the medication

AUDIOVISUAL RESOURCES

1. **Medicating Children**
   This program presents general considerations and details of the administration of medications to children of various ages. Included are all routes of administration, safety factors in calculation and administration of comfort measure. Developmental, psychosocial, and communication skills are illustrated. This is an excellent program for students.

Videocassette: 23 minutes

Distributor: American Journal of Nursing Company

2. **With Care and Caring: Pediatric Medication Administration**
   This program illustrates specific physical techniques, practical considerations, and developmental approaches for medicating children. Safety measures are identified. This film could be used for student instruction with guidance from an experienced professional.

Videocassette: 30 minutes

Distributor: Health Sciences Consortium

3. **Pediatrics: Administering Oral and IM Medications**
   This program describes the preparation of oral medications and the selection of sites for intramuscular injection in children of various age groups. Techniques for oral and parental medication administration are identified. Suggestions for improving the child's cooperation and compliance are offered.

Filmstrip or videotransfer:

Distributor: Concept Media

ANSWERS TO WORKSHEET

1.	a. 1650 mg	b. 1875 mg	c. 11 ml
2.	a. 1100 mg	b. No	
3.	0.11 mg		
4.	a. 48 mg	b. Yes	
5.	a. 34 mg	b. 0.68 ml	
6.	a. 81 mg	b. 4 ml	
7.	a. 0.32 mg	b. 0.32 ml	
8.	a. 80 mg	b. 2.25 ml	
9.	a. 443 mg	b. 1.8 ml	
10.	a. 8.8 mg	b. 0.44 ml	

STUDENT WORKSHEET: DRUG CALCULATIONS FOR ADMINISTERING MEDICATIONS TO CHILDREN

1. Jimmy is to receive Ampicillin 275 mg every 4 hours. He weighs 15 kg. The safe dose for Ampicillin is 125/mg/kg/day.

a. How much Ampicillin is Jimmy receiving in 24 hours?

b. What is the highest safe amount he can receive?

c. If the medication is dispensed in a preparation of 125 mg/5 ml, how many milliliters would the nurse administer to Jimmy?

2. Alice is receiving Cefazolin 500 mg every 6 hours. She weighs 22 kg. The safe dose for Cefazolin is 50 mg/kg/day. (a) What is the highest safe amount Alice should receive? (b) Is the dose Alice is currently receiving a safe dose?

3. Wanda is receiving Digoxin every 8 hours. She weighs 5.6 kg. Safe dose range for Digoxin is 0.03 to 0.06 mg/kg/day. The nurse is to administer her 8 a.m. dose. What is the highest safe amount the nurse should administer?

4. Christopher receives 12 mg of Lasix every 6 hours. He weighs 15 kg. The safe dose for Lasix is 3 mg/kg/day. (a) How much Lasix is Christopher receiving daily? (b) Is his dose within the safe dose range?

(continued)

For each of the situations listed below, calculate the following:

a. The highest safe dose (in mg) to administer based on the given weight.
b. How much of the preparation (in ml) to administer for the highest safe dose.

5. Propranolol every 4 hours — Preparation: 50 mg/ml

Child's weight: 13.6 kg — Safe amount: 15 mg/kg/day

a.

b.

6. Duiril b.i.d. — Preparation: 100 mg/5 ml

Child's weight: 6.5 kg — Safe amount: 25 mg/kg/day

a.

b.

7. Clonopin t.i.d. — Preparation: 1 mg/ml

Child's weight: 32 kg — Safe amount: 0.03 mg/kg/day

a.

b.

8. Tylenol Now — Preparation: 180 mg/5 ml

Child's weight: 8 kg — Safe amount: 10 mg/kg/dose

a.

b.

9. Penicillin G every 6 hours — Preparation: 250 mg/ml

Child's weight: 11.8 kg — Safe amount: 150 mg/kg/day

a.

b.

10. Gentamicin every 8 hours — Preparation: 20 mg/ml

Child's weight: 3.5 kg — Safe amount: 7.5 mg/kg/day

a.

b.

CHAPTER 25

NURSING MANAGEMENT OF PAIN IN CHILDREN

DISCUSSION QUESTIONS

1. How is *pain* defined by (a) the International Association for the Study of Pain and (b) from a nursing perspective? What are the limitations of each definition?
2. What do the terms *pain threshold* and *pain tolerance* mean? What factors influence an individual's tolerance for pain?
3. How is acute pain different from chronic pain? Describe the types of chronic pain individuals can experience.
4. How is pain explained by the Gate Control Theory?
5. Describe how developmental changes in (a) anatomy and physiology and (b) cognition and behavior affect pain perception and expression.
6. Summarize nursing research findings regarding pain perception in infants and children.
7. What misconceptions exist regarding pain in infants and children?
8. Describe the following pain assessment tools: (a) Eland Color Tool, (b) Poker Chip Tool, (c) Oucher, (d) Adolescent Pediatric Pain Tool, (e) Verbal 0 to 10 Scale, and (f) CHEOPS. Identify the strengths and limitations of each tool.
9. What factors influence a nurse's judgment about a child's pain?
10. What is the purpose of baseline knowledge about a child's pain-related behaviors? What information should the nurse gather to establish a baseline?
11. Identify principles for planning pharmacologic interventions for pain relief.
12. Analgesic medications are divided into two categories: (a) narcotic and (b) nonsteroidal anti-inflammatory. What are the benefits and limitations of each type? How does each act to relieve pain? What nursing considerations are important when administering drugs of each type?
13. What advantages do the following routes have for the administration of analgesics: (a) intravenous, (b) intramuscular, and (c) oral?
14. What factors influence the effectiveness of analgesic medications given on a p.r.n. schedule?
15. What questions should the nurse consider when evaluating the effectiveness of the management of a child's pain?
16. Discuss the use of patient-controlled analgesia (PCA) and epidural analgesia for pain management in children.
17. How does the developmental level of a child affect the behaviors exhibited in response to pain? What are the typical fears of each age group, and what types of comfort are effective in relieving pain and anxiety?
18. Fear and anxiety can increase a child's perception of pain. What strategies can the nurse institute that will help to reduce a child's fear and anxiety? Why is it also necessary to assist family members to be less anxious?
19. Describe non-pharmacologic interventions the nurse can use to relieve a child's pain.

CASE STUDY

Vickie, age 6 years, underwent orthopedic surgery two days ago. She is in a full spica cast. Neurovascular assessments have been normal. Vickie is restless, refuses to take oral fluid or solid food, and repeatedly asks her parents and the nurse to take the cast off.

The physician orders morphine intravenously for Vickie. Five days after surgery, despite administration of the ordered dose of morphine, Vickie continues to have frequent complaints of pain. What pain assessment tools can the nurse use to assess Vickie's pain? What information can the nurse obtain from Vickie's parents that would help with the assessment?

What principles should guide the plan for pain intervention?

What nursing actions are important in administration of morphine? If Vickie weighs 26 kg, what is the maximum safe dose she should receive?

Develop a plan for the use of non-pharmacologic interventions to assist in relieving Vickie's pain.

STUDENT LEARNING ACTIVITIES

1. Ask students to select one of the self-report pain assessment tools discussed in the textbook to assess the level of pain experienced by the children for whom they are caring. As part of the assignment, the students should write a report describing (a) why they selected the tool, (b) the child's response, and (c) the effectiveness of the tool in evaluating the child's pain.

2. As a group assignment, ask the students to construct a program using guided imagery that nurses can use with children in pain. Include in the program examples of relaxation exercises and image experiences. Ask students to explain the choice of these activities in relation to the different developmental levels. Include in the program a set of guidelines (following those stated in the textbook) that will help to achieve optimal effectiveness of the measures.

AUDIOVISUAL RESOURCES

1. **Pediatrics: Psychosocial Implications, Part 3—Alleviating Fear and Pain**
   This program identifies fears common to children at various developmental stages and discusses interventions to reduce fears or to lessen their harmful effects. Special considerations for the child experiencing pain associated with illness, diagnostic tests, and procedures are included. Also presented are techniques for recognizing both hidden and overtly expressed pain and ways for the nurse to help children deal with pain. This is a good program for students who will be caring for children in acute care settings.

Filmstrip or videotransfer: 21 minutes

Distributor: Concept Media

2. **Pediatric Pain**
   This program focuses on pain in children and describes the physiology of the pain response, techniques for pain assessment, and pain intervention options. Common misconceptions about pain and pain management in preverbal children are discussed..Ethical and legal parameters are addressed.

Videocassette: 19 minutes

Distributor: Health Sciences Consortium

3. **Patient-Controlled Analgesia**
   This program discusses the benefits of patient-controlled analgesia. A comparison between PRN pain control and patient-controlled analgesia is presented. Health risks associated with ineffectively treated pain, risks associated with patient-controlled analgesia, serum drug concentration, and patient comfort are addressed.

Videocassette: 11 minutes

Distributor: Health Sciences Consortium

4. **Why Do I Have To Cry? Assessment of Pain in Children**
   This program addresses myths and misconceptions about pain in children. Developmental differences in pain response are discussed. Research-based assessment strategies for assessing pain in children of all ages are presented. The program shows nurses and patients using three assessment tools–the Poker Chip Tool, the Oucher, and the Adolescent Pediatric Pain Tool.

Videocassette: 25 minutes

Distributor: American Journal of Nursing

CHAPTER 26

PRINCIPLES OF FLUID AND ELECTROLYTE MAINTENANCE

DISCUSSION QUESTIONS

1. Why are infants and young children at greater risk for fluid and electrolyte imbalances?
2. Describe the relationship of the following factors to fluid and electrolyte balance in infants and children: (a) body surface area, (b) metabolic rate, (c) kidney function, and (d) total body water.
3. Explain how the skin and lungs, gastrointestinal system, and cardiovascular system contribute to fluid and electrolyte regulation.
4. What is meant by intravenous fluids that are (a) *isotonic*, (b) *hypertonic*, and (c) *hypotonic?*
5. Describe the changes in pressure within the intracellular and extracellular compartments that result in edema.
6. What is the etiology of the following types of dehydration, and what effect does each have on the plasma sodium level: (a) isotonic dehydration, (b) hypertonic dehydration, and (c) hypotonic dehydration?
7. What types of conditions can result in (a) hyperkalemia, (b) hypokalemia, (c) hypercalcemia, and (d) hypocalcemia?
8. Explain how each of the following contributes to regulation of hydrogen ion concentration: (a) chemical buffers, (b) kidneys, and (c) lungs.
9. Describe the etiology of the following types of acid-base imbalances: (a) metabolic acidosis, (b) metabolic alkalosis, (c)respiratory acidosis, and (d) respiratory alkalosis. What are the typical symptoms associated with each?
10. What information would the nurse elicit from parents when fluid and electrolyte imbalance is suspected?
11. What changes in vital signs and weight could indicate a fluid and electrolyte imbalance?
12. Describe the physical assessment of a child experiencing (a) a fluid volume deficit. and (b) a fluid volume excess.
13. How is the child's neurological status affected by electrolyte imbalances?
14. Identify nursing diagnoses for the child with a fluid and electrolyte imbalance.
15. What is the formula for calculating fluid requirements for children?
16. What important observations are necessary prior to adding potassium to intravenous fluids?
17. What are the purposes of the three phases of fluid deficit therapy?
18. Discuss parent education to prevent fluid and electrolyte imbalances.
19. What are the safety and comfort considerations in intravenous line insertion and maintenance?
20. Describe the etiology of the five complications of intravenous therapy. How can the nurse minimize the occurrence of each complication?
21. What are the nursing responsibilities when caring for a child with an intravenous line?
22. Describe three venous access devices used for continuous or repeated intravenous therapy.

CASE STUDY

Randy Parker, age 2 months, is admitted to the hospital with dehydration. Robert Parker, his father, says that Randy has been having diarrhea for four days. Randy has had a 10% weight loss; his current weight is 4.8 kg. Randy's urine specific gravity is 1.038. What type of dehydration does Randy most likely have? Randy is probably experiencing what type of acid-base imbalance?

What questions should the nurse ask in obtaining the admission history from Robert? The nurse is aware that changes in Randy's weight provide important indications of his hydration status. What measures should the nurse follow to ensure obtaining accurate weights?

What typical findings would the nurse be likely to make during the exam of Randy's (a) skin, (b) anterior fontanel, and (c) eyes? How should the nurse interpret Randy's urine specific gravity of 1.038?

After Randy's hydration status is stabilized, he is started on intravenous fluid for his maintenance requirements. How much fluid should the infant receive in 24 hours? The nurse caring for Randy has what responsibilities in maintaining intravenous infusion?

STUDENT LEARNING ACTIVITIES

1. Compare nursing responsibilities for the child with (a) a heparin lock for intermittent antibiotic; (b) a continuous peripheral intravenous line; (c) a central venous catheter with an external exit such as the Broviac, Groshong, or Hickman; and (d) an implanted device such as a Protacath. Have students discuss the similarities and differences.
2. Ask students to develop a teaching plan for preparing children and families for intravenous therapy.

AUDIOVISUAL RESOURCES

1. **Fluid and Electrolyte Series**
   This five-part program discusses fluid balance, isotonic volume changes, hypotonic volume changes, hypertonic volume changes, and potassium balance. This series is not specifically directed to pediatrics but may be useful for independent student viewing.

Videocassette: 19–28 minutes each part

Distributor: Medcom/Trainex

2. **Monitoring the Patient, Documenting, Nursing Care, Managing Complications**
   This program focuses on the nurse's responsibilities in providing safe intravenous therapy. Guidelines for monitoring and documenting intravenous therapy are provided. Nursing interventions based on assessment findings are demonstrated.

Videocassette: 24 minutes

Distributor: Medcom/Trainex

3. **Pediatric IV Therapy**
   This program discusses the physiological, cognitive, and psychosocial aspects of intravenous therapy for children. Included are specific considerations of child size, metabolic rate, fluid and electrolyte balance, elimination, and acid-base balance. Teaching strategies are presented with emphasis on the child's developmental level, experience, education, and family background. Techniques for reducing fear and anxiety and for dealing with regressive behaviors in children receiving intravenous therapy are included. The film also shows the assembly of intravenous flow devices and electronic infusion pumps, nursing observation and monitoring responsibilities, and how to provide opportunities for children to participate in play activities while undergoing IV therapy. This program is comprehensive and an excellent resource for classroom or learning laboratory instruction.

Videocassette: 40 minutes

Distributor: American Journal of Nursing Company

4. **Pediatrics: Physical Care, Part 4—Fluid Balance and IV Therapy**
This program describes factors that make infants and children prone to fluid imbalances. Clinical manifestations of mild, moderate, and severe dehydration are identified. Calculations for determining intravenous fluid orders and flow rates and techniques for starting intravenous lines in children are illustrated. This program would be useful in the student learning laboratory as a demonstration of the clinical basics of pediatric intravenous therapy.

Videotransfer: 16 minutes

Distributor: Concept Media

ANSWERS TO PRETEST

1. solid dissolved in a liquid
2. liquid in which solute is dissolved
3. potential pressure resulting from two solutions with different concentrations divided by a semipermeable membrane
4. measurement of the concentration of a solution
5. movement of a solvent across a semipermeable membrane to equalize pressures on both sides of the membrane
6. hydrogen
7. plasma, water, sodium
8. potassium, protein
9. reabsorb
10. controlling blood CO_2 levels

    excretion or absorption of hydrogen ions or bicarbonate
11. pH
12. bicarbonate

    phosphate

    plasma proteins

    hemoglobin
13. absorb hydrogen ions, prevent pH changes
14. 7.35, 7.45
15. rise, alkaline

PRETEST: FLUID AND ELECTROLYTE BASICS

Define the following terms.

1. Solution: ______________________________

____

____

2. Solvent: ______________________________

____

____

3. Osmotic pressure: ______________________________

____

____

____

4. Osmolality: ______________________________

____

____

5. Osmosis: ______________________________

____

____

____

6. The ion responsible for the acidity of body fluids is ______________________________.

7. The major components of extracellular fluid are ______________________________, ______________________________, and ______________________________.

8. The major components of intracellular fluid are ______________________________ and ______________________________.

9. Secretion of antidiuretic hormone causes the kidneys to ______________________________ water.

10. Two organs participate in maintaining acid–base balance: the lungs and the kidneys. Describe what function of each organ helps maintain acid–base balance.

Lungs: ______________________________

____

Kidneys: ______________________________

____

11. Hydrogen ion concentration is measured as ______________________________.

12. The major buffers within the body are

____

____

____

____

13. The two major functions of the buffers within the body are to ______________________________ ______________________________ and ______________________________.

14. Normal pH values in body fluids range between ______________________________ and ______________________________.

15. An increase in any of the buffers causes pH levels to ______________________________ and body fluids to become ______________________________.

UNIT VI

DEVELOPMENTAL-BEHAVIORAL HEALTH CONCERNS

CHAPTER 27

UNDERSTANDING ALTERED DEVELOPMENT

DISCUSSION QUESTIONS

1. How does the 1978 and 1987 Developmental Disabilities legislation define *developmental disability?*
2. What are the provisions of the Americans with Disabilities Act of 1990?
3. What indicators gathered during the assessment should alert the nurse to a child with a developmental risk?
4. What components should be included in the yearly screening for potential developmental delay in young children?
5. What are the guidelines to follow when using a tool to assess the presence of developmental delay?
6. Describe the components of the assessment of a child with developmental disability.
7. What is the purpose and structure of early intervention programs? What population of children do such programs serve?
8. How can nurses contribute to the prevention of developmental disabilities at the primary, secondary, and tertiary levels?
9. What nursing diagnoses and interventions apply to the long-term care of an infant at risk for developmental disabilities?
10. Define *inclusion.* Why is inclusion advocated for the child with developmental disabilities in an educational setting?
11. Identify the services provided by federal and state agencies to assist individuals with developmental disabilities and their families.
12. The nurse functions in several roles when caring for the child with a developmental disability. What function does the nurse serve in each of the following roles: (a) family supporter, (b) advocate, (c) teacher, and (d) facilitating adjustment to school?
13. How is *mental retardation* defined? What behaviors are characteristic of the following types of mental retardation: (a) mild, (b) moderate, (c) severe, and (d) profound?
14. Explain the pathology of the two causes of mental retardation.
15. Develop a nursing plan for the moderately retarded adolescent admitted to the hospital for a minor surgical procedure. The care plan should focus on assisting the adolescent to maximize his self-care abilities after discharge from the hospital. What special needs for teaching do retarded adolescents have?
16. Describe the three chromosomal alterations that result in Down syndrome.
17. What are the group of physical characteristics typically found in children with Down syndrome? Describe the pattern of developmental delays exhibited by the Down syndrome child.
18. How can parents facilitate learning in their child with Down syndrome?
19. What signs are indicative of Fetal Alcohol Syndrome (FAS)?

20. Define *cerebral palsy*. Describe the characteristics of the following types of cerebral palsy: (a) athetoid, (b) spastic, (c) ataxic, (d) ridigity, and (e) mixed.
21. Identify nursing diagnoses and interventions for a child with spastic quadriplegia.
22. What is the definition of a *learning disability?* What population is at greater risk for learning disabilities?
23. What are the early warning signs seen in children with learning disabilities?
24. The family of a child with a learning disability needs to follow some general guidelines to facilitate learning and minimize emotional upset. What are these guidelines?
25. Define *dyslexia*. What are the etiologies of dyslexia? How is dyslexia diagnosed?
26. What is the best method for facilitating learning in the child with dyslexia?

CASE STUDY

Susan, age 3 years, is brought to the developmental clinic for an evaluation. She had meningitis at the age of 2 months and since then has had a seizure disorder. Susan's mother is concerned because the child is not achieving the developmental milestones for her age. After a battery of tests, Susan is found to be mentally retarded, most likely in the mild to moderate range.

Susan's parents are very upset by the diagnosis and blame themselves. They feel they should have sought treatment earlier when Susan developed the meningitis.

How can the nurse assist the parents in developing a healthy adaptation to Susan's disability? The recommendation for Susan to enroll in an early intervention program is made. How would the nurse explain the purpose of early intervention to Susan's parents?

During the physical exam, a heart murmur is noted, and Susan is admitted to the hospital for a cardiac evaluation. Construct a care plan focused on helping Susan and her parents adjust to the hospital experience.

Susan has a significant delay in language skills. Outline a teaching guide for her parents with measures to encourage Susan's language development.

Susan's mother feeds her all her meals. She explains that Susan tends to spill her food and has difficulty manipulating the utensils. What information should the nurse offer the parents regarding the benefit of Susan learning to feed herself? What measures can parents apply that will help facilitate self-feeding skills?

STUDENT LEARNING ACTIVITIES

1. Spend a day in a special class for children with developmental delays. How does the teacher structure teaching to facilitate learning?
2. Contact the agencies listed in the textbook that provide services to families and children with developmental alterations. Compile a description of the services each provides and procedures necessary for children to be seen. Construct a booklet with the information and provide copies for the nursery, clinics, physician offices, and inpatient units.

AUDIOVISUAL RESOURCES

1. **Dyslexia: Diagnosis and Prognosis**
   This program offers an overview of dyslexia that includes symptoms in preschool and school-age children, the probable cause for dyslexia, types of diagnostic testing, and types of learning assistance that allow dyslexic individuals to achieve their potential.

Videocassette: 26 minutes

Distributor: Films for the Humanities and Sciences

2. **The Handicapped Child: Infancy Through Preschool**
This eight-part program provides a detailed overview of the child with developmental alteration or delay during infancy and early childhood. The family crisis and risk factors are identified, followed by initial assessment and intervention criteria. Strategies to promote optimal growth and development are discussed with specific guidelines for sensory/motor, cognitive/language, social/emotional adaptive behavior, and interventional techniques to promote self-help skills for children who exhibit developmental alterations.

Filmstrip or videotransfer: 19–33 minutes each part

Distributor: Concept Media

3. **Child Check**
The focus of this program is early detection of developmental problems. A diary of childhood progress is used in the detection of delays. Interviews with parents of children with various emotional and physical problems illustrate how the checklist can be used to detect developmental delays.

16-mm film: 23 minutes

Distributor: Indiana University Audio-Visual Center

4. **Learning Disabilities**
This program describes the nature of learning disabilities and their warning signs. The importance of early diagnosis and treatment is emphasized. A 9-year-old child is profiled as his parents and teachers discuss the problems he faces at home and at school.

Videocassette: 19 minutes

Distributor: Films for the Humanities and Sciences

5. **Introduction to Cerebral Palsy**
This program identifies basic information about the causes, characteristics, and problems associated with cerebral palsy.

Slide–tape: 20 minutes

Distributor: Meyer Rehabilitation Institute

6. **Cerebral Palsy: A Medical Primer for the Professional**
This program details the medical aspects of cerebral palsy and the interpretation of a variety of health care professionals in a therapeutic approach to the care of the child. Strategies to facilitate communication, feeding, physical growth, and psychosocial development are discussed.

Slide–tape: 20 minutes

Distributor: Meyer Rehabilitation Institute

7. **Cerebral Palsy: What Every Parent Should Know**
This program covers the causes, symptoms, and range of possible treatments of cerebral palsy, including the relationship among physical and mental handicaps, the role of medications, and physical therapy in treatment. Selective posterior rhizotomy surgery is examined as a means of easing spasticity in certain types of patients.

Videocassette: 19 minutes

Distributor: Films for the Humanities and Sciences

8. **Feeding Infants and Young Children with Special Needs**
This program offers suggestions to make feeding children with special needs more pleasant for both the child and parent or care provider. It demonstrates positioning and feeding techniques as well as special equipment for children with motor problems.

Videocassette: 27 minutes

Distributor: Pyramid Film and Video

STUDENT WORKSHEET: DEVELOPMENTAL ALTERATIONS

Compare the developmental alterations that result from cerebral palsy, fetal alcohol syndrome, and Down syndrome.

	Cerebral Palsy	Fetal Alcohol Syndrome	Down Syndrome
Etiology			
Physical Findings			
Psychological			
Development			
Measures to Facilitate Development			
Nursing Care			

CHAPTER 28

CHILD ABUSE AND MALTREATMENT

DISCUSSION QUESTIONS

1. How is *child abuse* defined? Who is legally responsible to report suspected cases of child abuse?
2. What is the incidence of child abuse? What factors influence the ability to gather statistics on the prevalence of child abuse?
3. What are the long-term effects of physical abuse and neglect and psychological maltreatment on the child's behavior, school performance, and psychosocial development?
4. What types of behaviors are common in children who have experienced sexual abuse?
5. What is the difference between mandatory and permissive reporters in suspected child abuse?
6. What are the explanations for child abuse presented by the following models: (a) mental illness model (b) environmental stress model (c) social learning model (d) social-psychological model, (e) human-ecological model, and (f) psychological-sociological model? What are the strengths and weaknesses of each of these explanations?
7. How do the nurse's attitudes about child abuse influence his or her ability to provide optimum care to the abused child and family?
8. What information should be included in the nursing documentation of the child who has been abused?
9. What are the physical and behavioral indicators of (a) physical abuse, (b) physical neglect, (c) psychological maltreatment, and (d) sexual abuse?
10. What is Munchausen syndrome by proxy?
11. What behavioral indicators are commonly observed in the father/stepfather and mother of a sexually abused child?
12. Describe the sites of physical injuries that are highly suspected to be the result of abuse.
13. What indicators of high risk for abuse are found during the prenatal period, perinatal and postnatal periods, and neonatal period?
14. Describe the nurse's role as a child and parent advocate when dealing with abusive families.
15. What are the nursing roles in the prevention of child abuse and maltreatment?

CASE STUDY

Amanda, age 4 years, is brought to the emergency room by her mother, Rachel Boyd. Amanda has fractured her left ulnar. Her mother reports that Amanda hurt her arm after falling off of a chair. A review of the x-rays reveals several old healed fractures. Amanda has multiple bruises on her body and some small burn marks on her legs that resemble cigarette burns. Rachel states that Amanda is very active and is always hurting herself. Rachel's boyfriend was watching Amanda at the time of this most recent injury. Child abuse is suspected, and Amanda is admitted to the hospital.

What are the guidelines that the nurse performing the admission interview should follow to minimize Rachel's fear and hostility? Develop questions that provide information about (a) how the accident occurred, (b) what routine forms of discipline are used on Amanda, (c) how her mother perceives Amanda's behavior, and (d) the role of the mother's boyfriend in Amanda's care.

Write a nurse's note including all pertinent information and observations that the nurse should gather during the admission interview. What is the nurse's role in this situation? Identify goals and nursing interventions for Amanda and her family.

STUDENT LEARNING ACTIVITIES

1. Ask students to spend an afternoon or evening at a child abuse hotline and report on the types of calls received during their visit and the support and services provided by the hotline staff.
2. Interview emergency room nurses about the forms of child abuse they see. Are these cases consistent with the text's description of the child at most risk for abuse?
3. Discuss the case presented in Ethical Issues: Medicine or Child Abuse (see Chapter 28 of textbook).

AUDIOVISUAL RESOURCES

1. **Child Abuse**
This program focuses on the nurse's role in prevention, detection, and management of child abuse. Statistical information, high-risk parent profiles, and therapeutic programs are identified. The program covers recognition and assessment of various injuries, emergency room presentations, and interviewing and observational strategies for assessment of parents and children in suspected situations of child abuse. The legal responsibilities of the health care professional are also discussed.

Videocassette: 28 minutes

Distributor: American Journal of Nursing Company

2. **Child Abuse and Neglect**
This five-part program discusses the difference between abuse and neglect and explores the distinctions between discipline and abuse. Topics include common forms of abuse and maltreatment and their symptoms, traits of abusive parents, and types of help available to parents and children. This program would provide a basic introduction to classroom discussion of the nurse's role in caring for the child who has been abused.

Filmstrip or videotransfer: five parts

Distributor: The Center for Humanities

3. **Child Abuse: Physical and Behavioral Indicators**
This program shows graphic examples of child abuse. The role of the health professional in identification, initial management, and documentation of a child's injuries are discussed. Included are guidelines for family and child assessment. This program includes a comprehensive study guide that facilitates independent student viewing.

Videocassette: 28 minutes

Distributor: University of Michigan Medical Center Media Library

4. **Terrible Things My Mother Told Me**
This program depicts the suffering that verbal abuse can cause and illustrates how this kind of abuse is passed from one generation to the next. The program emphasizes that even nice people can abuse their children and reveals the importance of counseling to end the destructive cycle.

Videocassette: 31 minutes

Distributor: Coronet/MTI Film and Video

5. **Childhood Physical Abuse**
This program covers a range of problems in the area of physical abuse of children, including signs of physical abuse, effects on children, interventions to break the cycle, the distinction between discipline and abuse, and prevention of physical abuse.

Videocassette: 26 minutes

Distributor: Films for the Humanities and Sciences

6. **Systematic Assessment of Sexual Abuse in Preschoolers**
This two-part program outlines assessment guidelines and interviewing techniques. The format includes both narration and dramatization.

Videocassette: Part 1, 18 minutes; Part 2, 40 minutes

Distributor: Altschul Group Corporation

7. **Detection and Treatment of Sexually Abused Children—Part 1**
Sexual abuse is defined, and physical and behavioral signs of sexual abuse are identified. Assessment strategies and nursing interventions are discussed.

Videocassette: 28 minutes

Distributor: American Journal of Nursing Company

8. **Child Sexual Abuse: The Untold Story**
This film is narrated by female victims of sexual abuse. It shows the effects the abuse has on the girl's emotional and social development, their feelings and coping strategies, and their involvement in group therapy counseling programs.

Videocassette: 30 minutes

Distributor: American Journal of Nursing Company

9. **Sexually Misused Children: Identification, Documentation, Management**
This presentation includes physical and behavioral indicators of sexual misuse of children, guidelines for interviewing victims, physical assessment criteria, and appropriate documentation parameters. There is a comprehensive program guide that facilitates self-instruction prior to classroom discussion.

Videocassette: 26 minutes

Distributor: University of Michigan Medical Center Media Library

10. **Sexual Abuse and Harassment: Causes, Prevention...Coping**
This four-part program discusses the wide range of behaviors that can be considered sexual harassment, including unwanted touching, subtle sexual joking, and overt sexual abuse. Scenes show adolescents talking about harassment from peers, teachers, employers, and family members and their feelings of guilt, frustration, and helplessness. Also included are suggestions for addressing untoward situations and where to seek help. This program is useful for adolescent health promotion projects and for student knowledge.

Videocassette: Four parts

Distributor: The Center for Humanities

STUDENT WORKSHEET: CATEGORIES OF CHILD ABUSE

Characteristic	Physical Abuse	Physical Neglect	Psychological Maltreatment	Sexual Abuse
Etiology				
Parental Characteristics				
Clinical Manifestations				
Prevention				
Treatment				
Long-term Effects				

CHAPTER 29

ALTERATIONS IN BEHAVIOR, EMOTION, AND THOUGHT

DISCUSSION QUESTIONS

1. What variables influence a child's psychosocial functioning?
2. How is temperament pattern related to development of behavior problems? What methods can the nurse apply to assess a child's temperament?
3. Explain what is meant by *goodness of fit*. How does goodness of fit influence the development of behavior problems?
4. What are the components of a mental health assessment?
5. Identify nursing actions that focus on the prevention of behavioral disturbances.
6. What are two theories about the etiology of school phobias?
7. What behaviors are demonstrated by the child with school phobia?
8. What areas of the health history are particularly helpful when evaluating the child with school phobia?
9. What is the typical pattern of symptoms observed in children with school phobia?
10. What are the current theories on the etiology of *enuresis*?
11. What approaches can be used in the management of enuresis?
12. How is *encopresis* defined? Differentiate primary encopresis from secondary encopresis.
13. What physical manifestations are exhibited by children with encopresis?
14. What information is gathered during the history of the child with encopresis?
15. Describe the treatment regimen for encopresis.
16. Describe the behaviors of a child with *attention deficit hyperactivity disorder (ADHD)*. What are the essential features of ADHD?
17. What is the treatment of choice for children with ADHD?
18. Describe the nursing care of the child with ADHD.
19. How is a *conduct disorder* defined? What behaviors are associated with conduct disorders?
20. Identify nursing actions to help families deal with the child who lies, steals, or exhibits aggressive behavior.
21. What variables have been associated with the risk of obesity in children?
22. What physical findings are consistent with diagnosis of childhood obesity?
23. What are the current theories regarding the etiology of obesity in children?
24. What information is important to gather during the assessment of the child with obesity?
25. Describe the various methods for management of obesity in children.
26. Why is family involvement essential to the therapeutic management of a child with obesity?
27. What are the characteristics of the child with *anorexia nervosa*? What behaviors are typical in family members of the child with anorexia nervosa?

28. What are the criteria for a child to be diagnosed with anorexia nervosa?
29. Identify nursing diagnoses and interventions for the adolescent with anorexia nervosa.
30. What types of behaviors are observed in adolescents with *bulimia*?
31. Explain the relationship between substance abuse among children and adolescents and the following influences (a) developmental factors, (b) familial factors, and (c) societal factors.
32. Differentiate among the patterns of the following types of substance abuse: (a) experimental, (b) recreational, (c) circumstantial, (d) intensive, and (e) dependent.
33. What is the role of the nurse in the prevention of substance abuse?
34. What are the characteristic depressive behaviors demonstrated by children in the following age groups: (a) infancy, (b) early childhood, (c) middle childhood, (d) late childhood, and (e) adolescence.
35. What criteria are used to diagnose depression in children and adolescents?
36. Describe the nursing care of a hospitalized school-age child who is depressed.
37. What are the differences between boys and girls in the incidence of adolescent suicide and the methods of suicide chosen?
38. What factors are associated with the incidence of suicide among adolescents?
39. What warning signals are commonly observed in suicidal adolescents?
40. What are the components of a suicide assessment?
41. Describe the behavioral characteristics and medical and nursing management of the child with *autism* and the child with *childhood schizophrenia*.

CASE STUDY #1

Eight-year-old Tommy is admitted to the pediatric unit for surgical repair of a lacerated tendon. Tommy's mother tells the nurse that he has recently begun to receive treatment for excessive aggressive behavior. What questions are important to ask the mother while obtaining the nursing history?

Tommy is playing a game with two other boys on the unit. He becomes angry and throws the game across the room, then takes toys away from other children and throws them. How can the nurse best intervene to help reduce Tommy's aggressive outburst?

Tommy tells the nurse to leave him alone and yells at her, "You're ugly and fat. Leave me alone!" What are some responses that the nurse can use that will help to calm Tommy down?

CASE STUDY #2

Jennifer, age 14 years, is admitted to the hospital after a 6-week history of weight loss and poor appetite. She has lost 26 pounds and is pale and weak. A diagnosis of anorexia nervosa is made.

What signs might Jennifer exhibit that indicate a nutritional deficit? Develop a list of actual and potential nursing diagnoses for Jennifer. Construct a nursing care plan for the identified diagnosis.

STUDENT LEARNING ACTIVITIES

1. Assign students to spend an afternoon or evening in a crisis center that deals with suicidal adolescents.
2. Ask the students to construct a informational booklet for adolescents about drug and alcohol abuse and make the booklet available to the unit for helping to educate adolescents.
3. Interview adolescents about their perceptions of the dangers of drug and alcohol use. Relate these perceptions to adolescent psychosocial development.

AUDIOVISUAL RESOURCES

1. **Adolescent Anorexia**
This program explains the common psychological impairments associated with anorexia and the nurse's role in working with the anorexic adolescent. Five models of treatment used with anorexic clients are described.

Videocassette: 30 minutes

Distributor: Health Sciences Consortium

2. **Diet Unto Death: Anorexia Nervosa**
This documentary examines the causes of anorexia nervosa, explains its symptoms, and describes therapeutic management.

Videocassette or 16-mm film: 13 minutes

Distributor: Coronet/MTI Film and Video

3. **Over the Influence**
This is a two-part series focusing on substance abuse prevention programs and model treatment and recovery programs. Both parts are hosted by celebrities.

Videocassette: 47 minutes

Distributor: Pyramid Film and Video

4. **The Suicidal Adolescent—Identification, Risk Assessment, and Intervention**
This is an interactive videodisc program designed to help users recognize the signs and symptoms of teenage depression and suicidal behavior, assess the individual's suicidal risk, and decide an appropriate intervention.

Interactive optical videodisk and floppy disk with user guide

Distributor: The National Audiovisual Center

5. **Teen Suicide**
This interactive program takes viewers into high schools in California and Virginia where teens share their experiences with stress, coping with suicide of a friend, and the suicidal impulse. Preventive action is suggested.

Videocassette or 16-mm film: 22 minutes

Distributor: Coronet/MTI Film & Video

6. **Schizophrenia**
This is described as one of the most helpful programs on schizophrenia addressed to nonspecialist audiences. Adapted from a Phil Donahue program, topics include suspected causes, symptoms, prognosis for recovery, and family interventions.

Videocassette: 28 minutes

Distributor: Films for the Humanities and Sciences

7. **Bulimia**
This program is hosted by Phil Donahue includes discussions with experts and bulimic patients. Causes, consequences, and treatment of bulimia are addressed.

Videocassette: 28 minutes

Distributor: Films for the Humanities and Sciences

8. **Chemical Dependency: Risks Throughout a Lifetime**
This is a six-part series, with two parts applicable to nursing of children and adolescents. Part I, Introduction, addresses risk factors for chemical dependency and addiction. Part III, Adolescence, covers developmental factors that make the adolescent susceptible to substance abuse and early warning signs of substance abuse.

Videocassette: 105 minutes total

Distributor: Pyramid Film and Video

CHAPTER 30

THE HIGH-RISK INFANT

DISCUSSION QUESTIONS

1. Define the following terms: *preterm infant, postterm infant, small for gestational age (SGA)*, and *large for gestational age (LGA)*.
2. What age-related changes in physical development and function would the nurse expect in an assessment of a preterm infant?
3. Identify nursing diagnoses, collaborative problems, and related nursing interventions for the preterm infant.
4. What is the etiology associated with (a) SGA infants and (b) LGA infants?
5. Identify nursing diagnoses for the SGA infant.
6. Discuss the etiology and incidence of multiple gestations.
7. Why does *respiratory distress syndrome (RDS)* occur in preterm infants?
8. What is the purpose of supplemental oxygen and mechanical ventilation in the treatment of RDS? What assessments need to be made when an infant with RDS is receiving supplemental oxygen therapy?
9. What complications are associated with supplemental oxygen therapy and mechanical ventilation in the preterm infant?
10. What are the etiology and clinical manifestations of *persistent pulmonary hypertension of the newborn (PPHN)*?
11. What nursing interventions at the time of delivery minimize the risk of meconium aspiration?
12. What is the pathophysiology of *retinopathy of prematurity*?
13. What complications are associated with hypoxia/ischemia insult in the preterm infant?
14. Why are premature infants susceptible to intracerebral hemorrhage?
15. Why are preterm infants more likely to develop *hyperbilirubinemia*?
16. How is hyperbilirubinemia managed?
17. What complications are associated with phototherapy? Identify nursing interventions to prevent these complications.
18. Why are neonatal seizures difficult to diagnose in the preterm infant?
19. What is included in a septic workup? Discuss nursing care of the infant with neonatal sepsis.
20. Identify health concerns for the preterm infant after discharge from the neonatal intensive care unit.
21. Why is follow-up neurodevelopmental assessment important for the infant born prematurely?

CASE STUDY

Janie Carr is born at 28 weeks gestation and weighs 1000 g. She is the first child born to the Carrs, both of whom are 22 years of age. What is the physical appearance of the infant at 28 weeks gestation?

The infant develops respiratory distress shortly after birth and is placed on a respirator. Janie's parents ask the nurse why the infant needs the respirator. How should the nurse describe the problems with development of the premature infant's respiratory system that require the us of mechanical ventilation? How should the nurse explain that the infant is not able to receive oral feedings? Develop a care plan for Janie directed at the following: (1) infection prevention, (2) maintenance of thermoregulation, (3) nutrition, (4) respiratory function, (5) fluid and electrolyte balance, (6) promotion of parental-infant bonding, (7) appropriate stimulation, (8) skin integrity, and (9) parental support.

After three weeks, Janie is extubated and started on nasogastic feedings. The infant begins to experience three to four episodes of apnea per day. What are the common causes of apnea in the premature infant? It has been a week since her last apneic episode. In preparation for discharge, what information would the nurse give to the Carrs about caring for Janie at home?

STUDENT LEARNING ACTIVITIES

1. Arrange for a student tour of the Neonatal Intensive Care Unit (NICU). Ask students to interview a nurse working in the NICU about common health deviations of infants in the NICU, complications of treatments, and length of stay in the NICU. Have students share their findings.

AUDIOVISUAL RESOURCES

1. **The Family and the Premature Infant**
   This program identifies specific ways that nurses can counsel families with premature infants. An interview between the nurse and mother demonstrates how to help parents prepare for possible loss of their infant and anticipatory grief, how to deal with guilt and fear, and ways to plan for long-term family adjustments.

Videocassette: 30 minutes

Distributor: American Journal of Nursing Company

2. **Vulnerabilities of the Premature Infant**
   Major problems associated with premature birth are discussed. The program is designed to familiarize students with the timely medical attention that is essential to remove as much risk to the preterm infant as possible.

Videocassette: 12 minutes

Distributor: Health Sciences Consortium

3. **Apnea**
   Part of the Neonatal Problems Series, this program addresses interventions for the infant experiencing an apneic episode and the causes and treatment of apnea. It briefly discusses how to handle the infant with recurrent apneic episodes.

Slides and 14-minute Audiotape

Distributor: Health Sciences Consortium

4. **Jaundice**
   Part of the Neonatal Problems Series, this program teaches viewers how to determine if an infant has physiological jaundice or whether the condition is more serious. The program details causes of hyperbilirubinemia, diagnosis, and treatment.

Slides and 10-minute Audiotape

Distributor: Health Sciences Consortium

5. **The Low–Birth Weight Infant**
   This comprehensive program is part of the Neonatal Problems Series. It covers how to identify low–birth weight infants, recognize and stabilize respiratory distress syndrome, maintain normal temperature range, recognize two potential problems of the asphyxiated low–birth weight infant, determine whether intravenous fluid therapy is necessary, and judge and evaluate hydration.

Slides and 11-minute Audiotape

Distributor: Health Sciences Consortium

6. **Respiratory Distress**
   Part of the Neonatal Problems Series, this program addresses recognition and treatment of respiratory distress, immediate considerations in stabilizing the infant, and proper therapy for each of these considerations. It also covers treatment for the infant simultaneously experiencing respiratory acidosis, metabolic acidosis, and hypoglycemia.

Slides and 18-minute Audiotape

Distributor: Health Sciences Consortium

7. **Seizures**
   Seven signs of neonatal seizures are discussed in this program that is part of the Neonatal Problem Series. It covers diagnosis and treatment of the four main causes of neonatal seizures: metabolic, infectious, drug withdrawal, and structural disorders.

Slides and 25-minute Audiotape

Distributor: Health Sciences Consortium

STUDENT WORKSHEET: ALTERATIONS ASSOCIATED WITH DYSMATURITY

	Etiology	Clinical Manifestations	Therapeutic Management	Nursing Management
Respiratory Distress Syndrome				
Meconium Aspiration				
Hypoxic/Ischemic Insult				
Intraventricular Hemorrhage				
Hyperbilirubinemia				
Neonatal Seizures				
Sepsis				

CHAPTER 31

GENETIC PRINCIPLES AND DISORDERS

DISCUSSION QUESTIONS

1. Define the terms *mitosis* and *meiosis*.
2. Describe the two-step process of meiosis.
3. How does the concept of micropackaging relate to human genetics?
4. How can polymorphisms be helpful in human genetics?
5. Describe the three major classifications of genetic disorders.
6. What are the causes of a chromosomal disorder?
7. Why is maternal age a factor in the occurrence of chromosomal disorders?
8. Down syndrome is not always identified at birth. What factors contribute to this?
9. What characteristics may be identified during an assessment of an infant with Down syndrome?
10. What is a *single gene disorder?* Describe the characteristics of (1) autosomal dominant inheritance, (2) autosomal recessive inheritance, (3) X-linked recessive inheritance, and (4) X-linked dominant inheritance. Identify at least one disorder associated with each mode of inheritance.
11. What is meant by *disorders with multifactorial etiology?*
12. Why is the *threshold effect* an important concept in multifactorial inheritance?
13. Describe the three mechanisms that produce genetic disease associated with nontraditional inheritance.
14. How is a family history and physical assessment important in the identification of genetic disorders?
15. What information would be included in a family history and pedigree analysis for a child with a suspected genetic disorder?
16. How does the physical assessment of a child for genetic disorders vary with the age of the child?
17. What are the four categories of genetic screening?
18. Differentiate between *retrospective* and *prospective* genetic counseling.
19. What is the role of the nurse in helping families cope with the child's diagnosis of a genetic disorder?

CASE STUDY

Justin Williams is the first child born to parents who are both 28 years old. The infant is diagnosed shortly after birth with Down syndrome. The parents ask the nurse the cause of the disorder and if they are at risk for having subsequent Down syndrome children. How should the nurse answer the parents' question?

The nurse caring for the Williams family will need to provide emotional support and information on adjusting to and caring for a child with Down syndrome. What skills will the nurse need in (a) the initial diagnosis phase, (b) decision-making on further pregnancies, and (c) follow-up care for Justin?

STUDENT LEARNING ACTIVITIES

1. Assign students to children with genetic disorders. Ask each student to construct the child's family pedigree and obtain a history using the Family History Form for Genetic Assessment (at the end of this chapter).
2. Ask the students to visit the local March of Dimes Association and report on the services provided by the association on diagnosis and management of genetic disorders.

AUDIOVISUAL RESOURCES

1. From Generation to Generation: Genetic Counseling
This program explains medical genetics through the use of specific examples. Several inherited diseases are identified to illustrate the different modes of genetic inheritance. Although this program was designed for high school students, it provides a good review of genetic principles and it is useful as a teaching aid for students in health education programs on adolescents.

Slide filmstrip: 12 minutes

Distributor: March of Dimes Birth Defects Foundation

2. Healthier Babies: The Genetic Era
This documentary dramatizes the impact of birth defects arising from various genetic and/or environmental causes. The film describes the role of genetic counseling when inherited disease is present or suspected and the progress being made in the prevention, detection, and treatment of birth defects. This program illustrates the scientific advances in the study of genetics.

Videocassette or 16-mm film: 20 minutes

Distributor: March of Dimes Birth Defects Foundation

3. Between Joy and Sorrow: Parents of Children with Serious Genetic Conditions
This program focuses on five families who have children with serious genetic conditions. The parents describe how they learned of their child's condition, their reaction to the diagnosis, and how they came to accept the reality of the situation. The parents discuss the strategies they used to cope with having a child with a genetic condition. The challenge for healthcare providers is to recognize the rich, complex emotional responses that make each individual unique.

Videocassette: 27 minutes

Distributor: Health Sciences Consortium

4. Mapping the Human Genome with Genetic Markers
The use of restriction fragment polymorphisms (RFLPs) as genetic markers for assigning the location of individual genes on a chromosome is discussed by Dr. Helen Donis-Keller. This approach has been used in the analysis of such diseases as Huntington's disease, duchenne muscular dystrophy, and cystic fibrosis.

Videocassette: 54 minutes

Distributor: National Audiovisual Center

5. Parents Look at Genetic Counseling
This program presents comments from parents of children with disorders who are involved in genetic counseling at the University of Michigan Medical Center. Topics addressed include how the parents were informed of the condition, parents' reactions, positive and negative aspects of counseling, parents' opinions about genetic counseling, and plans for future children.

Videocassette: 27 minutes

Distributor: University of Michigan Medical Center Media Library

Note: The March of Dimes Birth Defects Foundation offers printed materials on genetic counseling and various genetic disorders. See the Audiovisual Resource Guide (p. 195, this manual) for the address.

STUDENT WORKSHEET: FAMILY HISTORY FORM FOR GENETIC ASSESSMENT

A. Child's Name or Initials:

B. Age of Parents

Mother:

Father:

C. Ethnic origin

Mother:

Father:

D. Potential Risks (include first- and second-degree relatives)

Stillbirths or miscarriages:

Children born with malformations:

Children who have died:

Known genetic disorders:

Conditions occurring in more than one family member:

UNIT VII

NURSING INTERVENTIONS IN PHYSIOLOGIC ALTERATIONS

Chapter 32

Altered Respiratory Function

DISCUSSION QUESTIONS

1. What are the developmental differences in the respiratory systems of infants and young children? How do these differences influence the prevalence of respiratory disorders observed in children?
2. Explain the function of surfactant in respiratory function.
3. Why is airway resistance so much higher in infants than in older children and adults?
4. What are the primary uses of pulmonary function tests?
5. What are some of the implications of oxygen therapy in infants and children?
6. What are the indications of the use of low flow oxygen therapy?
7. Describe the correct method for performing *chest physical therapy (CPT)*. What is the purpose of CPT?
8. Describe the safety precautions to follow during suctioning a child's airway.
9. What is the nursing care indicated for the child with tracheostomy in the areas of (a) skin integrity, (b) safety, and (c) suctioning?
10. Why are infants and young children so prone to respiratory infections?
11. Describe the treatment for colds in children, including (a) comfort measures, (b) reducing fever, (c) promoting rest, (d) maintenance of airway and tissue integrity, and (e) prevention of complications.
12. Why are ear infections common in children?
13. Differentiate between acute otitis media and otitis media with effusion in the following areas: (a) definition, (b) clinical signs, (c) child complaints or behavior, (d) therapeutic management, and (e) nursing care.
14. What are the indications and contraindications for tonsillectomy and/or adenoidectomy? What are important discharge instructions to provide parents of the child who has undergone a tonsillectomy?
15. Outline the nursing management for the child in the immediate postoperative period after a tonsillectomy.
16. Compare and contrast the etiology, pathophysiology, clinical manifestations, management, and nursing care of croup versus epiglottitis?
17. What are the indications of increasing respiratory distress in the child with a form of croup?
18. Provide the rationale for the use of the following therapies in the treatment of *laryngotracheo-bronchitis (LTB)*: (a) cool mist, (b) racemic epinephrine, and (c) hydration.
19. Describe the typical clinical course for bronchiolitis.
20. Describe the nursing care for the child with pneumonia.
21. Differentiate among the various bacterial pneumonias in the following areas: (a) age, (b) clinical manifestations, (c) etiology, and (d) therapeutic management.
22. What are some examples of intrinsic and extrinsic causes of asthma.

23. Describe the three changes in the airway that occur during an asthma attack.
24. What assessments are important for the nurse to make when caring for a child experiencing an acute asthma attack?
25. Describe the nursing care of a child hospitalized for an acute asthma attack.
26. Discuss the long-term management of asthma.
27. Describe the inheritance pattern for cystic fibrosis.
28. Describe the pathophysiology of cystic fibrosis. What systems are primarily involved?
29. Provide the etiology for the following common findings in the child with cystic fibrosis: (a) meconium ileus, (b) respiratory infections, (c) steatorrhea, (d) vitamin deficiency, and (e) salt depletion.
30. How is the diagnosis of cystic fibrosis made?
31. Describe the use of pancreatic enzymes in the treatment of digestive manifestations of cystic fibrosis. How is the correct amount of enzymes determined? What are examples of foods that do not require the child to take pancreatic enzymes?
32. What is the rationale for the following components of treatment for cystic fibrosis: (a) inhalation therapy, (b) chest physiotherapy, (c) breathing exercises, and (d) antibiotics?
33. Why is bronchopulmonary dysplasia (BPD) considered an *iatrogenic disorder?*
34. Describe therapeutic measures that contribute to the development of BPD?
35. What physical manifestations are observed in the infant with BPD?
36. Explain the rationale for each of the following therapies in the management of the infant with BPD: (a) high-frequency oscillatory ventilation, (b) bronchodilators, and (c) fluid restriction and diuretics
37. What is considered to be the etiology of (a) apnea of prematurity and (b) apnea of infancy? What is the therapeutic management and nursing care of these two forms of apnea?
38. What infants are at most risk for sudden infant death syndrome (SIDS)?
39. Describe the current theories of the possible causes of SIDS.
40. What forms of supportive interventions are important to provide the family who has experienced the death of an infant from SIDS?
41. Describe the clinical manifestations and medical and nursing management for (a) choanal atresia and (b) laryngomalacia.

CASE STUDY #1

Alice, who is 8 years old, is admitted to the hospital for evaluation of repeated pulmonary infections. She is scheduled for a bronchoscopy under local anesthesia in the morning. Construct a teaching plan to prepare Alice and her parents for the procedure.

When Alice returns to the floor following the bronchoscopy, her mother asks the nurse if Alice can have some juice. What factors will influence the nurse's response?

Assessment after the procedure includes observation of certain signs that indicate complications from the procedure? What are these signs?

Because Alice has experienced some airway edema, she is placed in a mist tent with 30% oxygen. Outline the important nursing interventions for Alice during the time she requires the mist tent.

CASE STUDY #2

Ken Silver brings 2-month-old Alison to the pediatrician with a history of a cold and increased labored breathing for 3 days. Ken notes that Alison was wheezing today. She refuses her bottle, and her urine output is reduced. On examination, Alison's respiratory rate is 70. No cyanosis is present, and there is an expiratory wheeze. A diagnosis of bronchiolitis is made.

Ken tells the nurse that he has a friend whose daughter has asthma and she receives epinephrine for her wheezing episodes. Ken wonders why Alison is not receiving the drug. What explanation about the action of epinephrine and its effectiveness in the treatment of bronchiolitis should the nurse give Ken?

Alison is admitted to the hospital. Outline her nursing care.

CASE STUDY #3

Tyrone, 10 years of age, is brought to the emergency room by his mother, Rosemary Kale. Tyrone has had asthma since 2 years of age. He began to experience slight wheezing one day ago, which has now progressed to a severe attack. On auscultation, Tyrone has decreased breath sounds and a prolonged expiratory wheeze. He has moderate intercostal and supraclavicular retraction. Respiratory rate is 38 and heart rate is 134.

What does the presence of retractions mean? Why is Tyrone experiencing a prolonged expiratory phase of respiration? Describe the nursing assessments and interventions provided to Tyrone upon arrival at the emergency room.

Tyrone receives an injection of subcutaneous epinephrine. After 5 minutes, his wheezing becomes louder. What does this finding indicate?

Tyrone fails to improve and is admitted to the hospital and begun on an aminophylline infusion. What signs of theophylline toxicity must the nurse watch for?

When Tyrone is discharged, he is given a prescription for cromolyn sodium. What instructions should Tyrone and his parents receive about the use of this drug? Describe the instructions the nurse should give the family on management of asthma attacks at home. What strategies can the nurse teach the family that can help to reduce the incidence of Tyrone's acute asthma attacks?

STUDENT LEARNING ACTIVITIES

1. Since asthma is a common cause of hospitalization for children, assign students to care for a child with asthma and listen to wheezing sounds. Ask students to discuss the common aspects of their patients' histories. Also ask them to discuss play activities that promote airway clearance and gas exchange.
2. Ask students to assess children without respiratory problems to assist them in identifying normal respiration. This will help them to distinguish normal breath sounds and respiratory rates in infants and small children.
3. Provide opportunities for students to care for adolescents with cystic fibrosis. How has the disease influenced the growth and development of these children? What activities common to adolescents are not possible for the individual with cystic fibrosis? How has the disease influenced their plans and goals for the future?

AUDIOVISUAL RESOURCES

1. **Acute Respiratory Care: Assessment Parameters**
   This program demonstrates and describes assessment of physical examination and history, pulmonary function tests, blood gas analysis, and x-ray procedures for respiratory assessment and evaluation. The program is not oriented toward children, but it does provide basic information and review.

Videocassette: 31 minutes

Distributor: Medcom/Trainex

2. **Suctioning Techniques for the Pediatric Patient**
This program illustrates the procedures for tracheal suctioning of the pediatric patient. Also discussed are types of tracheostomy tubes, humidification, frequency of suctioning, complications, and the emotional needs of the child. This teaching aid would be useful in the student clinical learning laboratory setting.

Videocassette: 10 minutes

Distributor: Health Sciences Consortium

3. **A Regular Kid**
This film presents interviews with children who have asthma and their families. They discuss their coping methods and concerns related to having a chronic respiratory disease. The film emphasizes a positive approach toward psychosocial adaptation to asthma. This film is geared toward children and families, but it provides information for students about coping strategies and children's feelings.

16-mm film

Distributor: American Lung Association

4. **Superstuff: Self-Help Asthma Package**
This is not a film but rather a hands-on package containing a record, poster, news magazine, book, and games designed to educate school-aged children with asthma about the disorder. The emphasis is on learning to recognize physical and environmental triggers of an asthma episode, what to do to prevent severe attacks, and how to develop healthy ways to live with asthma. This is a valuable resource for children and could be used by students involved in teaching projects for children with asthma.

Distributor: American Lung Association

5. **Assessment of Respiratory Distress in Infants and Children**
This program describes how to perform a respiratory assessment on infants and children with mild, moderate, and severe distress. Respiratory assessment has four components: level of consciousness, respiratory rate, efforts and mechanics of respiration, and evaluation of skin and mucous membranes. Several babies in respiratory distress are shown to illustrate mild, moderate, and severe distress. Differences between the pediatric and adult respiratory systems are addressed. Respiratory distress and failure are differentiated.

Videocassette: 20 minutes

Distributor: American Journal of Nursing Company

6. **Infant Cardiopulmonary Resuscitation for Parents**
This program follows American Heart Association Guidelines in demonstrating cardiopulmonary resuscitation (CPR) on an infant and what to do if choking occurs.

Videocassette: 15 minutes

Distributor: American Journal of Nursing Company

7. **Children with Croup**
This program discusses the causes, age ranges, signs, symptoms, diagnosis, and management of the various types of croup (laryngotracheobronchitis, epiglottitis, and spasmodic croup).

Slides and 9-minute Audiotape

Distributor: University of Michigan Medical Center Media Library

8. **Serous Otitis Media**
Diagnosis of otitis media through history, otoscopic and physical examinations, and hearing tests are discussed. Slides of various appearances of the tympanic membrane are included. Medical and surgical approaches to treatment are addressed. This program is geared for medical students.

Slide and 17-minute Audiotape

Distributor: University of Michigan Medical Center Media Library

9. **Issues of Cystic Fibrosis Series**
This twelve-part series offers a comprehensive picture of cystic fibrosis. Topics include the adolescent with cystic fibrosis (two parts), the newly diagnosed family, young adults, married couples, children and parents, the three-generation family, recently bereaved parents (two parts), doctors and nurses, allied professionals, and staff burnout.

Videocassette: 30 minutes each part

Distributor: Health Sciences Consortium

10. **Tonsillectomy and Adenoidectomy**
This program designed for patient education follows a young boy through his surgical experience and explains why the removal of tonsils and/or adenoids often becomes necessary. Preoperative preparation, hospitalization, and recovery are addressed. Parents are cautioned to watch for excessive bleeding, and tips on foods to offer the child during recovery are discussed.

Videocassette: 9 minutes

Distributor: Milner-Fenwick

ANSWERS TO PRETEST

1. diaphragm
2. warm, filter, humidify
3. alveoli
4. oxyhemoglobin
5. medulla, pons
6. diaphragm, intercostal muscles
7. 83–108
8. Male, 35–48, and female, 32–45
9. 7.35–7.45
10. 21–28
11. lower surface tension during expiration
12. drops below
13. two, three
14. epiglottis
15. compliance
16. pleura
17. bicarbonate ions
18. acidic
19. increases
20. bronchi, bronchiolus
21. c
22. a
23. e
24. b

PRETEST: STRUCTURE AND FUNCTION OF RESPIRATORY SYSTEM

1. The thoracic cavity is separated from the abdominal cavity by the ________________________________.

2. The upper cavity functions to ________________________, ________________________, and ________________________ inspired air.

3. Oxygen and carbon dioxide exchange occurs within the ________________________ of the lungs.

4. Oxygen is carried throughout the body in the form of ________________________.

5. The respiratory regulatory centers in the central nervous system are located in the ________________________ and ________________________.

6. The primary muscles that participate in respiration are the ________________________ and ________________________.

For questions 7–10, provide the normal range of values for each of the given components of arterial blood gas evaluation.

7. PaO_2 ________________

8. $PaCO_2$
   male: ________________
   female: ________________

9. pH ________________

10. HCO_2 ________________

11. The function of pulmonary surfactant is to ________________________________.

12. During inspiration, intrathoracic pressure ________________________ atmospheric pressure.

13. The left lung has ________________ lobes and the right lung has ________________ lobes.

14. The structure covering the opening of the larynx that prevents aspiration of liquids and foods is the ________________________.

15. The amount of force needed for lung expansion is called ________________________.

(Continued)

(Pretest continued)

16. The lungs are surrounded by the

_______________________________.

17. Carbon dioxide is transported in the body primarily in the form of ____________

_______________________________.

18. Elimination of carbon dioxide from the body prevents body fluids from becoming

_______________________________.

19. Respiratory rate ________________

____________ in response to hypercapnia.

20. The passages of the lungs are the

_____________________________ and

the _____________________________.

Match each of the following terms with the letter of the correct definition.

21. hypoxia ____________

22. apnea ____________

23. hypercapnia ____________

24. dyspnea ____________

a. cessation of breathing

b. difficult respiration

c. inadequate oxygen supply to tissues

d. normal respiration

e. increased carbon dioxide in the blood

STUDENT WORKSHEET: DIAGNOSTIC ASSESSMENT OF RESPIRATORY FUNCTION

Give the purpose of each of the diagnostic tests below, and provide an appropriate explanation of the test for the parent, preschool child, and school-age child.

Test	Purpose of Test	Explanation to Parent	Explanation to Preschool Child	Explanation to School-age Child
Posteroanterior and Lateral Chest Radiographs				
Bronchoscopy				
Computed Tomography				
Ventilatory Scan				
Pulmonary Function Tests				

STUDENT WORKSHEET: CROUP SYNDROMES AND LOWER RESPIRATORY TRACT INFECTIONS

Supply the information for the following types of croup syndromes.

	Structures Involved	Causative Agent(s)	Clinical Symptoms	Therapeutic Management	Nursing Care
Acute Laryngotracheo-bronchitis					
Spasmodic Croup					
Acute Epiglottitis					
Bronchiolitis					
Pneumonia					

STUDENT WORKSHEET: FORMS OF APNEA

	Etiology	Therapeutic Management	Nursing Care
Apnea of Prematurity			
Apnea of Infancy			

CHAPTER 33

ALTERED CARDIOVASCULAR FUNCTION

DISCUSSION QUESTIONS

1. What is the incidence and etiology of congenital heart disease? During which period of fetal development does cardiac malformation occur?
2. Plot the flow of blood in the fetus. How does fetal circulation differ from circulation after birth?
3. Explain the function of (a) ductus venosus, (b) foramen ovale, and (c) ductus arteriosus.
4. Describe the hemodynamic changes that occur after birth.
5. Define the terms *preload, afterload,* and *contractility.*
6. What typical behaviors and symptoms are assessed when obtaining the history of an infant or child with a congenital heart defect?
7. What indications of congenital heard disease are observed in the following: (a) general appearance, (b) the skin, (c) vital signs, (d) the chest, and (e) the abdomen. What procedures are applied to ensure accurate assessment in each of these areas?
8. Explain the basis for the presence of polycythemia in a child with a cyanotic heart defect.
9. What diagnostic information can be obtained from an electrocardiogram, echocardiogram, chest x-ray, and magnetic resonance imaging (MRI)?
10. What information is obtained from cardiac catheterization?
11. Describe nursing care of a child before a cardiac catheterization and postcatheterization.
12. Provide the etiology of the following clinical manifestations of congestive heart failure: (a) cardiac enlargement, (b) tachycardia, (c) tachypnea, (d) gallop rhythm, (e) decreased urine output, (f) sweating, (g) hepatomegaly, (h) failure to thrive, (i) decreased exercise tolerance, and (j) decreased peripheral pulses.
13. What are the most common signs of digoxin toxicity?
14. Besides digoxin, what medications are used in the treatment of congestive heart failure?
15. Describe the physiologic responses to hypoxemia.
16. How are congenital heart defects classified?
17. Why is there minimal shunting of blood in the infant with atrial septal defect (ASD)?
18. What factors influence closure of the ductus arteriosus? Why is the incidence of patent ductus arteriosus (PDA) higher among preterm infants?
19. What factors influence the degree of shunting that occurs with a ventricular septal defect (VSD).
20. Explain the role of pulmonary artery banding for the child with a ventricular septal defect.
21. What is the pathophysiology of atrioventricular (AV) canal defect and truncus arteriosus?
22. What is the pathophysiology of truneus arteriosus? How is this defect classified?
23. What are the treatment options for infants with hypoplastic left heart syndrome (HLHS)?

24. What are the four components of the congenital heart defect called Tetralogy of Fallot (TOF)?
25. What influences the severity of symptoms exhibited by the infant with Tetralogy of Fallot?
26. What is the function of palliative procedures for TOF?
27. What actions should be taken when a child experiences a Tet spell?
28. What is the etiology and pathophysiology of Ebstein anomaly?
29. What disturbance in blood flow occurs in infants with tricuspid atresia? How is pulmonary blood flow maintained in most infants with the defect?
30. What are the clinical manifestations of pulmonary atresia?
31. What palliative measures are used to manage the infant with pulmonary atresia?
32. How does mixing of oxygenated and unoxygenated blood usually occur in infants with transposition of the great vessels (TGA)?
33. Explain why oxygen therapy is of limited value to the infant with TGA.
34. Where is the connection of the pulmonary veins in the infant with total anomalous pulmonary venous connection? Explain how this connection affects blood flow.
35. Describe the alteration in blood flow when pulmonary stenosis is present. When aortic stenosis is present.
36. What are the signs and symptoms of pulmonary stenosis and aortic stenosis?
37. Why does the child with coarctation of the aorta have wide differences in blood pressure readings between the upper and lower extremities?
38. Describe how the nurse can prepare the child and family prior to cardiac surgery.
39. What is the nursing care in the immediate postoperative period for the child who has had cardiac surgery?
40. What information is included in the discharge instructions for the child who has undergone cardiac surgery?
41. Describe the instructions given to parents with a child receiving anticoagulant therapy.
42. How does the presence of a congenital heart defect increase susceptibility to infective endocarditis?
43. Describe the therapeutic management and nursing care of the child with infective endocarditis.
44. What information would the nurse give to parents to prevent recurrence of infective endocarditis?
45. Describe the management of hypertension in children.
46. Differentiate among the three types of cardiomyopathy.
47. What classifications of medications are used in the treatment of cardiomyopathy? What is the rationale for the use of each?
48. Identify conditions for which heart transplantation is an option for treatment.
49. How are cardiac dysrhythmias classified?
50. How is a Holter monitor useful in the diagnosis of cardiac dysrhythmias?
51. Why would a child with a cardiac dysrhythmia require a permanent pacemaker?

CASE STUDY #1

Alex, age 6 years, is admitted to the hospital for an evaluation of a heart murmur. He is scheduled for a cardiac catheterization the following day. Considering his developmental level, how can the nurse best prepare Alex for the procedure? Construct an explanation of the procedure that would be appropriate for Alex's parents.

Outline the postcatheterization care Alex will require. List the actual and potential nursing diagnoses for him after the procedure. Describe the signs that would indicate a complication related to the cardiac catheterization.

Alex's catheterization identifies a ventricular septal defect that will require surgery in the future. His parents are upset about the findings and the need for surgery. What are some of the common emotions exhibited and concerns expressed by parents of a child newly diagnosed with a congenital heart defect? How can the nurse assist Alex's parents to adjust to his disorder?

CASE STUDY #2

Megan, 6 months of age, was diagnosed at birth with atrioventricular canal defect. She is admitted now with a heart rate of 160, respiratory rate of 75, and periorbital edema. She is refusing to breastfeed and has not voided in 18 hours. Congestive heart failure is diagnosed. What explanation will the nurse give Megan's parents regarding the etiology of her symptoms?

Digoxin is ordered for Megan. What effect does the drug have on cardiac function? What signs would indicate that the Digoxin is effective?

Construct a plan of care for Megan using the Nursing Process Plan in Table 33-2, The Child with Congestive Heart Failure (see Chapter 33 of textbook) as a guide. Outline a teaching plan for the parents regarding administration of Digoxin at home.

STUDENT LEARNING ACTIVITIES

1. Provide opportunities for students to care for or assist in the care of an infant with a congenital heart defect. Ask them to describe the character of the heart sounds. How do they differ from the sounds of a normal infant's heart? What process produces the abnormal heart sound? Compare the physical and behavioral characteristics of the infant to those described in the text.

2. Does the in-patient unit have standardized teaching sheets for parents on administration of Digoxin and diuretics, home care after cardiac surgery, and warning signs of congestive heart failure? If not, ask students to develop these instruction sheets. If such teaching sheets are already available, ask the students to critique them for content, completeness, and clarity.

3. Send students to observe a child during a cardiac catheterization. Afterward, ask them to explain the rationales for the following aspects of postcatheterization care: (a) bedrest with leg straight and immobile, (b) pressure dressing checked hourly, (c) assessing the rate and character of the apical pulse, and (d) palating the pedal pulse and checking the temperature of the lower extremities.

AUDIOVISUAL RESOURCES

1. **Your Baby with a Congenital Heart Defect**
   This film shows interviews with three families in their homes as they relate their feelings and experiences associated with caring for their infants who have congenital heart defects. The families' responses to crying, cyanosis, feeding problems, developmental needs, and health care are discussed. This program is valuable for illustrating the impact and coping skills of families who have infants with significant cardiovascular alterations.

Videocassette: 29 minutes

Distributor: University of Michigan Medical Center Media Library

2. **Leonard Z. Lion Presents—Learning about Your Heart Catheterization, Learning about Your Heart Operation, and Take Care of Your Teeth to Protect Your Heart**
   These three programs are designed to explain to school-aged children the events, experiences, and participation expectations associated with cardiac catheterization and surgery and dental care for children with heart disease. The programs are informative, visually stimulating, and sensitive to the needs and fears of children who must undergo invasive cardiovascular procedures. These are helpful for patient teaching.

Videocassettes: 10–16 minutes each part

Distributor: University of Michigan Medical Center Media Library

3. **Jeannie**
This film shows an 11-year-old child during a surgical procedure for removal of a cardiac tumor. As the operation progresses, there is a voice reenactment if the child's thoughts and feelings. She expresses both fear and confusion about the operation as well as optimism about increased independence and well-being after she is well again. This program is an interesting presentation illustrating the impact of cardiac disease and surgery on a child.

Videocassette: 6 minutes

Distributor: Health Sciences Consortium

4. **Children and Heart Disease**
This program explains that as many as 30% of American children may already have high serum cholesterol levels and shows how cholesterol screening is helping children to reduce their cholesterol levels before it is too late.

Videocassette: 15 minutes

Distributor: Films for the Humanities and Sciences

5. **New Hearts for Sick Kids**
This program focuses on an 18-month-old child born with hypoplastic heart syndrome. Her parents are faced with three options: do nothing and let nature take its course, or choose between two very risky procedures—reconstructive surgery or heart transplantation. The options are analyzed in the program. The parents in this program selected transplantation, which was successful.

Videocassette: 19 minutes

Distributor: Films for the Humanities and Sciences

6. **Operation Transplant: Kids Talk About Transplants**
This program focuses on the experiences of five heart transplant recipients, ages 9 to 18 years. Topics include feelings about the transplant, medication, changes in physical appearance, reactions of friends, and social and athletic activities.

Videocassette

Distributor: University of Michigan Medical Center Media Library

ANSWERS TO PRETEST

1. left atrium
2. superior vena cava
3. right atrium
4. aorta
5. pulmonary arteries
6. left
7. mital valve
8. tricuspid valve
9. sinoatrial node, right atrium
10. myocardium
11. placenta
12. pulmonary artery, aorta
13. pericardium
14. systolic blood pressure
15. diastole
16. coronary arteries
17. e
18. g
19. c
20. d
21. h
22. f
23. b
24. a

PRETEST: STRUCTURE AND FUNCTION OF CARDIOVASCULAR SYSTEM

1. Oxygenated blood flowing from the lungs enters the ______________________________ ______________________________.

2. Blood from the upper part of the body returns to the heart by way of the __________ ______________________________ ______________________________.

3. Blood returning from the body enters the ______________________________ of the heart.

4. Oxygenated blood is pumped from the left ventricle into the ____________________ ______________________________.

5. Blood is delivered to the lungs by the ______________________________ ______________________________.

6. Pressure is highest in the ____________ ______________________ side of the heart.

7. Blood leaves the left atrium by way of the ______________________________.

8. Blood leaves the right atrium by way of the ______________________________ ______________________________.

9. The pacemaker of the heart is the ______________________________, which is located in the ____________________ ______________________________.

10. The contractile tissue of the heart is the ______________________________.

11. In fetal circulation, the major source of gas exchange occurs in the _______________ ______________________________.

12. In fetal circulation, the ductus arteriosus delivers blood from the _______________ ______________________________ to the ______________________________.

13. The heart is surrounded by a sac called the ______________________________.

14. The highest pressure generated by the left ventricle is measured by the ______________________________ ______________________________.

15. The heart fills with blood during the ______________________________ phase of the cardiac cycle.

16. The blood supply to the heart is via the ______________________________ ______________________________.

(Continued)

(Pretest continued)

List the vessels and parts of the heart in the correct order (by letter) as unoxygenated blood flows through them returning from the body.

17. ________ a. aorta

18. ________ b. left ventricle

19. ________ c. right ventricle

20. ________ d. pulmonary artery

21. ________ e. superior and inferior vena cava

22. ________ f. left atrium

23. ________ g. right atrium

24. ________ h. pulmonary vein

STUDENT WORKSHEET:
CONGENITAL HEART DEFECTS

	Hemodynamics	Clinical Manifestations	Diagnostic Findings	Therapeutic Management	Nursing Care
A. Lesions with Increased Pulmonary Blood Flow					
Atrial Septal Defect					
Patent Ductus Arteriosus					
Ventricular Septal Defect					
Atrioventricular Canal Defect					
Truncus Arteriosus					
Hypoplastic Left Heart Syndrome					

(Student Worksheet continued)

	Hemodynamics	Clinical Manifestations	Diagnostic Findings	Therapeutic Management	Nursing Care
B. Lesions with Decreased Pulmonary Blood Flow					
Tetralogy of Fallot					
Tricuspid Atresia					
Pulmonary Atresia					
C. Mixed Circulation Defects					
Transposition of the Great Vessels					
Pulmonary Stenosis					
Aortic Stenosis					
Coarctation of Aorta					

CHAPTER 34

ALTERED HEMATOLOGIC FUNCTION

DISCUSSION QUESTIONS

1. What are the age-related differences in RBC concentration and WBC count?
2. Explain the inheritance pattern for *sickle cell anemia* if both parents carry the sickle cell trait.
3. Why is the blood of the child with sickle cell anemia more viscous and have a tendency to take on a deformed shape?
4. Describe the process of *sickling* and its effect on the cells of the body.
5. What conditions can precipitate sickling?
6. Describe the pathophysiologic basis of (a) vaso-occlusive crisis, (b) sequestration crisis, and (c) aplastic crisis.
7. Explain what information is obtained from these laboratory tests: (a) Sickledex and (b) hemoglobin electrophoresis.
8. Describe the nursing care of a child experiencing a vaso-occlusive crisis.
9. Why is maintaining adequate hydration important for the child in sickle cell crisis?
10. Discuss measures to manage pain for the child experiencing a vaso-occlusive crisis.
11. What are the objectives of hypertransfusion programs for children with sickle cell anemia?
12. Describe the pathophysiological basis of *β-thalassemia.*
13. What complications are associated with the frequent blood transfusions for the child with β-thalassemia?
14. What are the clinical manifestations of *disseminated intravascular coagulation?*
15. Why is heparin administered to the child with disseminated intravascular coagulation?
16. Why does the bone marrow of the child with *idiopathic thrombocytopenia purpura (ITP)* contain normal numbers of platelets?
17. What clinical signs are exhibited by the child with ITP?
18. Why are platelet transfusions an ineffective therapy for ITP?
19. Develop a list of goals for planning the nursing care of the child with ITP.
20. Construct a list of acceptable activities for the school-age child with ITP.
21. Discuss discharge teaching for the child with ITP.
22. Describe the inheritance pattern of *hemophilia A.*
23. What are the common bleeding sites in the child with hemophilia A?
24. Describe the treatment for the child with hemophilia who has experienced a joint bleed. What is the therapeutic management for (a) controlling the bleeding, (b) pain relief, and (c) prevention of rebleeding?
25. What products are available for replacing the missing clotting factor for the hemophilic child?
26. What complications can result from replacement therapy used to treat the child with hemophilia?

27. How does *von Willebrand disease* differ from hemophilia A in respect to (a) inheritance pattern, (b) clinical manifestations, and (c) treatment?
28. What is the major consequence of anemia?
29. Why is the iron requirement greater during the first year of life?
30. Why are infants and toddlers at high risk for the development of *iron deficiency anemia?*
31. What factors relate to the incidence of iron deficiency anemia among adolescents?
32. Describe the typical physical and laboratory findings of iron deficiency anemia.
33. What interventions are important for the long-term management of iron deficiency anemia?
34. What are dietary recommendations for the prevention of iron deficiency anemia in infancy?
35. What information should parents receive about (a) administering iron supplements and (b) dietary sources of iron?

CASE STUDY #1

Eighteen-month-old Carrie is brought to the clinic for a routine visit. Her mother reports that Carrie has been well since her last visit except for a number of colds and lately she has not seemed as active as usual and appears pale. Carrie still drinks from a bottle, and her mother tells the nurse that she is a poor eater but always drinks her milk. A blood count indicates a hemoglobin of 7.8 g. Iron deficiency anemia is diagnosed.

What information should the nurse give the mother about Carrie's milk intake? Suggest some ways Carrie's mother can encourage her intake of iron-rich foods. Why is iron deficiency anemia so common during the toddler period?

Carrie is started on Fer-in-sol. If she weighs 11 kg, how much of the drug should she receive daily? What instructions should the mother receive regarding the administration of fer-in-sol?

Carrie is to return in 2 weeks for a reticulocyte count. Explain what information will be obtained from the results.

CASE STUDY #2

Robin, age 11 years, is admitted to the hospital complaining of pain in her back and knees. Robin has sickle cell anemia and is in vaso-occlusive crisis. Why does Robin have pain? Develop a list of goals for planning nursing intervention for Robin.

An intravenous line is started for hydration. Why is it important for Robin to maintain an adequate hydration level?

Provide a specific list of measures that can be taught to Robin's parents to minimize the occurrences of crisis and maximize Robin's level of health.

STUDENT LEARNING ACTIVITIES

1. Assign students to spend a day in a clinic for children with sickle cell anemia or hemophilia. Have the students list alterations in activities and family life that result from these diseases. What are the major problems caused by their diseases that the children report?
2. Have the students list activities for hemophilic children of different ages that promote healthy psychosocial development, while minimizing the chance of injury.

AUDIOVISUAL RESOURCES

1. **Blood Transfusion Today**
   This program discusses general scientific principles of the major blood groups and the RH factor; donor screening precautions; and methods used in collecting, preparing, and storing blood components. The narrator also addresses concerns associated with AIDS and blood transfusions. This film is long, but it is useful to students who require basic review.

Videocassette: 58 minutes

Distributor: National Audiovisual Center

2. **Matter of Chance**
   This film centers around a hospital-based counseling program for individuals at risk for sickle cell anemia. Genetic transmission of the disease and differentiation of sickle cell trait from sickle cell anemia are discussed. This film is useful in illustrating the risk of inheritance in sickle cell anemia and how individuals can be informed about the disorder.

Videocassette: 28 minutes

Distributor: National Audiovisual Center

3. **Sickle Cell Anemia**
   Sickle cell anemia is examined from both a human and scientific perspective. The importance of educating the black community about sickle cell anemia is stressed. Microphotography is used to show red blood cells changing into sickle cells and how they occlude blood vessels. It illustrates, through animation, how blood samples are analyzed and how normal red blood cells look compared to sickle cells.

16-mm film: 24 minutes

Distributor: Indiana University Audio-Visual Center

ANSWERS TO PRETEST

1. h
2. i
3. b
4. a
5. d
6. g
7. e
8. f
9. c

10. hematocrit
11. antibodies in immune responses
12. leukocytosis, leukopenia
13. infection, inflammation
14. B_{12}, folic acid
15. platelets, coagulation factors
16. it is the source of most coagulation factors; it contains bile salts necessary for vitamin K absorption
17. erythropoietin

PRETEST: HEMATOPOIETIC SYSTEM

In questions 1–9, match each blood component below with its primary function (a–i).

1. erythrocytes __________
2. leukocytes __________
3. plasma __________
4. prothrombin __________
5. neutrophils __________
6. eosinophils __________
7. thrombocytes __________
8. reticulocytes __________
9. basophils __________

a. precursors in blood coagulation
b. regulate blood volume via osmotic pressure
c. source of histamine and heparin
d. primary cells in fighting infection
e. hemostasis
f. mature into erythrocytes
g. respond in allergic reactions
h. supply oxygen and remove carbon dioxide from cells
i. protect against invasion of foreign matter

---

10. The ratio of packed cells to whole blood is called the ____________________.

11. Gamma globulin functions as ____________________

____________________.

12. A total leukocyte count of about 11,000/mm^3 is called ____________________, while a count less than 4,500/mm^3 is called ____________________.

13. An elevated leukocyte count generally indicates a(n) ____________________ or ____________________.

14. Erythrocytes production is dependent on vitamins ____________________ and ____________________.

15. The two components of blood that play a major role in hemostasis are the ____________________ and ____________________

____________________.

16. Two functions of the liver in blood coagulation are ____________________

____

____

and ____________________

____

____________________.

17. The hormone released by the kidneys that stimulates red blood cell production is ____________________.

STUDENT WORKSHEET:
CAUSES OF ANEMIA IN CHILDREN

	Etiology of Anemia	Clinical Manifestations	Medical Management	Nursing Management
Iron Deficiency Anemia				
Sickle Cell Anemia				
β-Thalassemia				
Aplastic Anemia				

CHAPTER 35

ALTERED DIGESTIVE FUNCTION

DISCUSSION QUESTIONS

1. Describe how the following functions differ between infants and young children: (a) intestinal absorption, (b) immune competence, (c) intestinal permeability, (d) hepatic function, and (e) digestive tract secretion.

2. What information gathered during the nursing history is specific to assessment of gastrointestinal function?

3. Explain the information regarding gastrointestinal function that is obtained from the following laboratory tests: (a) serum amylase, (b) stool trypsin, and (c) stool fat and pH.

4. How would the nurse determine the correct placement of a nasogastric tube after insertion or before initiating a gavage feeding?

5. Describe the rationale for the placement of a nasogastric tube in a child after abdominal surgery.

6. Provide the rationale for the following nursing interventions for the child with a nasogastric tube: (a) intermittent suction, (b) accurate measurement of gastric secretions, and (c) irrigate tube with normal saline.

7. Describe the procedure for gastrostomy feedings.

8. What factors are related to the incidence of cleft palate and cleft lip?

9. What factors influence the timing of corrective surgery for cleft lip and cleft palate?

10. What nutritional problems are present in infants with cleft lip and cleft palate? What techniques for feeding these infants are helpful?

11. Why are infants with cleft palate prone to ear infections?

12. Describe the postoperative nursing care for the infant who has had a (a) cleft lip repair and (b) a cleft palate repair.

13. Describe the clinical manifestations of *pyloric stenosis.*

14. Identify priority preoperative and postoperative nursing diagnoses for the child with pyloric stenosis.

15. How are oral feedings resumed after surgery for pyloric stenosis?

16. Describe the altered anatomy consistent with *esophageal atresia* with and without *tracheoesophageal fistula.*

17. Why is hydramnios during pregnancy common with infants born with esophageal atresia?

18. Describe the therapeutic management for esophageal atresia focused on (a) preventing pulmonary complications and (b) ensuring adequate nutrition.

19. What is the surgical procedure for correction of *esophageal atresia?*

20. Describe the differences in treatment and postoperative nursing care for a child with esophageal atresia with tracheoesophageal fistula versus a child with esophageal atresia without a fistula.

21. Describe the preoperative care for the infant born with *omphalocele.*

22. Describe the primary and staged surgical repair procedures for omphalocele.

23. Explain the pathophysiological basis of the following findings in an infant with a *diaphragmatic hernia:* (a) dextrocardia, (b) respiratory distress, and (c) audible bowel sounds over the chest wall.

24. Describe nursing care directed to (a) relieving respiratory distress and (b) monitoring respiratory status for the child with diaphragmatic hernia.
25. What factors influence the prognosis for the infant born with diaphragmatic hernia?
26. Describe the altered anatomy present in the male and female infant with an *inguinal hernia.*
27. What are the typical radiographic findings in the infant with intestinal atresia?
28. Describe the three abnormalities of the bowel that can occur during normal bowel rotation in the fetus.
29. Why is intestinal bleeding present in infants with *intussusception?* What is the treatment for intussusception?
30. Describe the pathophysiology and clinical manifestations of *Meckel diverticulum.*
31. Describe the basis for the intestinal obstruction experienced by the infant with *Hirschsprung's disease.*
32. What is the purpose of the colostomy for the child with Hirschsprung's disease?
33. What can be done to minimize a child's anxiety about frequent rectal examinations following surgical correction of Hirschsprung's disease?
34. Describe the four major types of *imperforate anus.* What is the therapeutic management for each?
35. Construct a nursing care plan for the infant following anoplasty.
36. Compare and contrast the pathophysiology, clinical manifestations, and medical and nursing management of *ulcerative colitis* and *Crohn's disease.*
37. Develop a list of priority nursing diagnoses for the child with inflammatory bowel disease. Provide rationale for each diagnosis.
38. Describe the three mechanisms of bacterial action associated with infectious diarrhea. Identify pathogens associated with each mechanism of action.
39. What initial and ongoing assessments would a nurse make for a child hospitalized for acute gastroenteritis?
40. How would the nurse advise parents about fluid intake and diet for a child with mild gastroenteritis?
41. Describe the processes that can lead to appendicitis.
42. List the characteristics of pain experienced by children with appendicitis.
43. Describe the pathophysiology, clinical manifestations, and medical and nursing management for the infant with *necrotizing enterocolitis.*
44. Describe the pathophysiology, clinical manifestations, and management of *irritable bowel syndrome.*
45. What dietary recommendations should be offered to parents for the prevention of constipation?
46. What are the major complications of diarrhea in infants and children, and how are these complications identified and treated?
47. What factors are thought to be associated with the presence of colic in infants?
48. Explain the various measures for preventing or reducing colic episodes.
49. Describe the medical and surgical management of *gastroesophageal reflux.*
50. What is the basis for the intestinal malabsorption seen in the child with *celiac disease?*
51. Construct a week of meals that a preschool child with celiac disease could eat.
52. What clinical manifestations are seen in the infant with lactose intolerance? How is lactose intolerance diagnosed and treated?
53. What therapeutic management is available for the infant with biliary atresia?
54. Describe the hepatic dysfunction and resulting clinical manifestations resulting from cirrhosis.

CASE STUDY #1

Jill, an infant born at 34 weeks gestation, is diagnosed at birth to have an esophageal atresia with a tracheoesophageal fistula. What symptoms did Jill most likely exhibit at birth that led to the diagnosis of esophageal atresia? What explanations will the nurse give Jill's parents as to the purpose of the Sump tube and gastrostomy tube?

Identify preoperative nursing interventions and provide the rationale for each. Develop a nursing process plan for Jill's postoperative care.

CASE STUDY #2

Calvin, an infant born full term, failed to pass meconium after birth and demonstrated signs of intestinal obstruction. After a barium enema and a rectal biopsy, Hirschsprung's disease is diagnosed.

Calvin is scheduled for surgery for a colostomy. Describe the purpose of the colostomy in terms appropriate for Calvin's parents. How can the nurse prepare Calvin's parents for the appearance of the colostomy after surgery?

Calvin remains NPO for 3 days after surgery. What comfort measures are important during this time? Construct a teaching plan for care of the colostomy at home.

Calvin returns at the age of 1 year for final corrective surgery. Describe the preoperative and postoperative nursing care. Explain the procedure in terms appropriate for Calvin's parents. What information will the nurse need to provide the parents on necessary skin care after Calvin's final discharge from the hospital?

STUDENT LEARNING ACTIVITIES

1. Provide an opportunity for all students to listen to bowel sounds in children.
2. Visit a food store and make a list of products that a child on a gluten-free diet could eat. What popular food items among children are prohibited for the child with celiac disease? What difficulties are faced by the family who plans meals for the child with celiac disease?

AUDIOVISUAL RESOURCES

1. **Life After Your Child's G-Tube Placement**
   This program offers advice and reassurance on common concerns parents have about gastrostomy tubes—keeping the tube secure, bathing and swimming, oral and skin care, sleeping, crawling, and traveling.

Videocassette: 10 minutes

Distributor: University of Nebraska Medical Center

2. **Gavage**
   Principles of gavage feeding and indications for use in patients with nasogastric or gastrostomy tubes are discussed in this program. It is not specifically designed for pediatric nursing, but it may be useful as a review for students.

Videocassette: 18 minutes

Distributor: Medcom/Trainex

3. **Ostomy Care**
   Basic ostomy care including colostomy, ileostomy, and urostomy is covered in this program. Important points the nurse needs to know before examining the patient are addressed. This program is not specific to children, but it may serve as a review of basic principles.

Videocassette: 20 minutes

Distributor: Medcom/Trainex

4. **Ulcerative Colitis**
   Designed for patient education, this program focuses on the treatment of ulcerative colitis and emphasizes that individuals with the disease can live relatively normal lives. Diagnostic testing, medications, surgery, and dietary changes are discussed. It was produced in conjunction with the National Foundation of Ileitis and Colitis.

Videocassette: 17 minutes

Distributor: Milner-Fenwick

5. **Crohn's Disease**
This program was produced in conjunction with the National Foundation of Ileitis and Colitis; it will help patients learn how Crohn's disease affects them. It covers diagnostic tests and possible treatments for this chronic condition.

Videocassette: 15 minutes

Distributor: Milner-Fenwick

6. **Preparing a Child for Appendectomy**
This program presents postoperative teaching techniques for the child who has undergone emergency appendectomy. Illustrations include the use of teaching tools to describe anatomy and physiology, procedures, wound appearance, and postoperative care procedures after abdominal surgery. This program would be useful for students prior to clinical experiences in an acute care pediatric rotation.

Filmstrip with audiocassette or videocassette: 16 minutes

Distributor: Campus Film Distributors Corp.

ANSWERS TO PRETEST

1. close off the nasopharynx
2. hydrochloric acid
3. duodenum, jejunum, ileum
4. cecum, colon, rectum, anal canal
5. digestion of fats
6. small intestine
7. mouth, starch
8. trypsin
9. lipase
10. amylase
11. pyloric sphincter
12. peritoneum

PRETEST: STRUCTURE AND FUNCTION OF DIGESTIVE SYSTEM

1. The soft palate serves to ____ during swallowing.

2. The parietal cells within the stomach secrete ______________.

3. The three segments of the small intestine are the ______________, ______________, and ______________,

4. The four segments of the large intestine are the ______________, ______________, ______________, and ______________.

5. The main function of bile is to assist ______________.

6. Most digestion and absorption of food occurs in the ______________.

7. Carbohydrate digestion begins in the ______________ with the breakdown of ______________.

8. The pancreatic enzyme responsible for protein digestion is ______________.

9. The pancreatic enzyme responsible for fat digestion is ______________.

10. The pancreatic enzyme responsible for carbohydrate digestion is ______________.

11. Food moving from the stomach into the duodenum passes through the ______________________________.

12. The lining of the abdominal cavity is called the ______________.

STUDENT WORKSHEET: THERAPEUTIC MANAGEMENT OF ACUTE INFECTIOUS DIARRHEA

Objective	Nursing Interventions	Rationale	Evaluation
Maintain or Restore Fluid and Electrolyte Balance			
Restore Bowel to Normal Functioning			
Prevent Infections of Others in Contact with Child			

CHAPTER 36

ALTERED GENITOURINARY FUNCTION

DISCUSSION QUESTIONS

1. What specific questions would the nurse ask when obtaining the history of a child with a genitourinary disorder?
2. What information is obtained from the following laboratory tests: (a) serum creatinine, (b) blood urea nitrogen, and (c) urine osmolality?
3. Explain the use of catheters, stints, and drains in the treatment of children with genitourinary disorders.
4. What anatomical alterations occur in infants with *hypospadias?*
5. What is the goal of the treatment for hypospadias? What is the rationale for the timing of the surgical repair of hypospadias?
6. What explanations by the nurse best prepare the child for a hypospadias repair, as well as minimize fears and concerns?
7. What is *cryptorchidism?*
8. Describe the medical and surgical treatment for cryptorchidism.
9. What important implications for teaching are important for the nurse to remember when caring for the child who has had treatment for cryptorchidism?
10. What are the anatomical findings and clinical manifestations observed in the child with *exstrophy of the bladder?*
11. What is the rationale for early surgical intervention for exstrophy of the bladder?
12. Describe pre- and postoperative nursing care for the infant with exstrophy of the bladder.
13. What are the causes of *hydronephrosis?* How does hydronephrosis develop?
14. How do age and gender influence the incidence and etiology of urinary tract infection in the pediatric population?
15. What typical symptoms of urinary tract infections are exhibited by (a) infants and (b) children?
16. What are the guidelines of performing radiographic studies when a child has a urinary tract infection?
17. Describe the therapeutic management of an acute, uncomplicated urinary tract infection.
18. What can the nurse teach parents and children about the prevention of urinary tract infections?
19. How is urine normally prevented from refluxing from the bladder into the ureters? How is this mechanism altered in vesicoureteral reflux?
20. Identify nursing diagnoses for the child who has undergone a ureteral reimplantation. Describe nursing actions for each nursing diagnosis.
21. Describe the etiology and pathophysiology of *renal calculi.*
22. What are appropriate nursing actions for the child with renal calculi?
23. Describe the basis for the following manifestations of *nephrotic syndrome:* (a) proteinuria, (b) hypoproteinemia, (c) oliguria, (d) generalized edema, and (e) hyperlipidemia.

24. What assessments would the nurse make when caring for a child with minimal change nephrotic syndrome? What additional assessments would be necessary if the child were receiving corticosteroids?
25. What are some conditions that can result in acute renal failure?
26. What are the principal manifestations of acute renal failure?
27. What are the three phases in the recovery of reversible acute renal failure?
28. Explain the typical metabolic imbalances seen in children with acute renal failure? How are these imbalances treated?
29. What is the etiology of the following manifestations of *glomerulonephritis:* (a) hematuria and (b) edema?
30. Compare and contrast the etiology and clinical manifestations of nephrotic syndrome with glomerulonephritis.
31. Why is the urine specific gravity elevated in glomerulonephritis? What other laboratory findings are indicative of this disorder?
32. What are the priority nursing interventions for the child during the acute phase of glomerulonephritis?
33. Describe the typical history of the child diagnosed with *hemolytic-uremic syndrome (HUS).*
34. What is the etiology of the hemolytic anemia seen in the child with HUS?
35. What laboratory findings are consistent with the diagnosis of HUS?
36. Describe the stages and symptoms associated with each stage of *chronic renal failure (CRF).*
37. What is the pathophysiology of chronic renal failure?
38. Identify nursing diagnoses for the child with chronic renal failure. Describe nursing actions for each nursing diagnosis.
39. What are the indications for instituting dialysis for the child with renal failure?
40. Describe the following modalities of treatment for end-stage renal disease: (a) hemodialysis, (b) peritoneal dialysis, and (c) continuous ambulatory peritoneal dialysis (CAPD).
41. Why is renal transplantation considered an optimal treatment choice for the child with end-stage renal disease?

CASE STUDY #1

Four-year-old Neil is admitted to the hospital with a diagnosis of minimal change nephrotic syndrome (MCNS). His mother, June, reported that over the last week she noticed Neil's clothing becoming tight around his waist, puffiness around Neil's eyes in the morning, and a decrease in his urination. Periorbital and scrotal edema are evident on physical assessment. A urinalysis shows 4+ proteinuria. What is the pathophysiological basis for these findings?

June tells the nurse, "I don't understand how Neil got this illness." How would the nurse explain the etiology of MCNS to her?

Identify nursing interventions for the nursing diagnoses (a) high risk for fluid volume excess and (b) high risk for impaired skin integrity.

Neil has been receiving Prednisone for the past 3 days. His edema is decreasing, and the most recent urinalysis revealed 1+ proteinuria. Neil is scheduled for discharge. What instructions should the nurse give to Neil's mother before the child is discharged?

CASE STUDY #2

Dean, age 10 years, is admitted to the hospital after a routine examination reveals that he has hypertension. For the past 3 weeks, Dean has had minimal urine output. Dean is a pale, quiet boy whose weight and height are at the fifth percentile for his age. His mother tells the nurse that Dean does not show an interest in active games and sports, but prefers to watch TV and read books. Past history indicates an episode of acute glomerulonephritis following strep throat 2 years ago.

The following laboratory studies are obtained: BUN, creatinine, hemoglobin and hematocrit, WBC, serum calcium and phosphorus, serum sodium, potassium, and chloride. What is the basis for Dean's hypertension? For each of the laboratory tests, describe the findings that would be consistent with end-stage renal disease? Plan a day's menu for Dean that would include typical limitations for a child with end-stage rental disease.

Dean is started on Kayexalate, Amphogel, vitamin D, calcium, and Aldomet. Provide appropriate explanations for Dean and his parents regarding the actions of the drugs he is receiving?

Dean is scheduled to start hemodialysis shortly. How would you explain the purpose of and procedures for hemodialysis to Dean and his parents?

After 8 months, Dean returns to the hospital for a renal transplant. The donor kidney is from his father. Construct a postoperative care plan for Dean.

STUDENT LEARNING ACTIVITIES

1. Assign students to spend a day in a pediatric dialysis unit. Compare the appearance and clinical manifestations of the children observed with those described in the text.
2. Ask the students to interview children and make a list of their favorite foods. How many of these foods must be eliminated from the diet of children with renal failure? What alterations or substitutes can provide children with foods they like?
3. Develop strategies for stretching the fluids for children on fluid restrictions.
4. Develop drug cards for the common drugs used to treat renal disease in children. Information should focus on child and parental learning needs.

AUDIOVISUAL RESOURCES

1. **Urethral Catheterization**
   This program demonstrates the insertion of a urethral catheter for males and females. The types of catheters and patient needs are identified. This program is self-instructional.

Videocassette: 25 minutes

Distributor: MedCom/Trainex

2. **The Indwelling Catheter: Guidelines for Nursing Care**
   This program discusses methods for preventing infection and identifying patient needs, as well as specific interventions for nursing of indwelling urinary catheters. This program is not specific to the child but provides self-instruction of basic principles.

Videocassette: 19 minutes

Distributor: MedCom/Trainex

3. **Nursing Care of the Kidney Transplant Patient**
   This program addresses important aspects of the nurse's role in caring for the physical and psychosocial needs of kidney transplant patients. Interviews with actual patients help viewers to understand and deal effectively with the range of emotions patients experience.

Videocassette: 28 minutes

Distributor: American Journal of Nursing Company

4. **Preparing a Child for Renal Transplant**
   This program dramatizes the reactions of a child during preoperative teaching prior to renal transplant, including regressive behaviors. There is a discussion of kidney anatomy and physiology, dramatic play techniques, and psychological reactions associated with hemodialysis, transplant, and postoperative body image changes. This program provides a good overview and ideas for preparing children and families experiencing a renal transplant.

Filmstrip with audiotape

Distributor: Campus Films

5. **Teaching a Child about Nephrosis**
This program describes the use of body outlines and hospital equipment to teach children about nephrosis, diagnostic tests, and management of the disease. A situation in which a child has not been prepared for hospitalization and refuses to cooperate with procedures is dramatized to emphasize the importance of preparation. This program would be useful for students involved in parent and child educational programs.

Filmstrip with audiocassette

Distributor: Campus Films

ANSWERS TO PRETEST

1. nephron
2. glomerulus
3. concentration of urine
4. 1.002 to 1.030
5. increased
6. water, nitrogenous wastes, inorganic salts
7. protein
8. calcium
9. increased
10. acid–base balance
11. increases
12. stimulated
13. decreased renal blood flow
14. raises blood pressure
15. a
16. b
17. a
18. a
19. b
20. b

PRETEST:
STRUCTURE AND FUNCTION OF GENITOURINARY SYSTEM

1. The functional unit of the kidney is the ______________________.

2. The major filtration apparatus of the kidney is the ______________________.

3. Urine specific gravity is a measure of the ______________________.

4. The normal range of specific gravity is from ______________ to ______________.

5. During dehydration, urine specific gravity is ______________________.

6. Urine is primarily composed of ______________, ______________, and ______________________.

7. Urea is the product of the final breakdown of ______________________.

8. The amount of serum phosphate influences the concentration of ______________________.

9. In renal failure, phosphate levels are ______________________.

10. By controlling the secretion of hydrogen ions and ammonia, the kidneys also help to control the ______________________.

11. The release of aldosterone ______________________ excretion of potassium by the kidneys.

12. During periods of dehydration, antidiuretic hormone secretion is ______________________.

13. Renin is produced in response to ______________________.

14. Renin catalyzes the production of angiotensin, which ______________________.

For each of the following results from a clean catch urinalysis, indicate whether the finding is (a) normal or (b) abnormal.

15. trace protein ________
16. +1 glucose ________
17. RBC 0–1 ________
18. WBC 2–4 ________
19. moderate hyaline casts ________
20. bacteria greater than 100,000 colonies/mL ________

STUDENT WORKSHEET: NEPHROTIC SYNDROME

Objective	Nursing Interventions	Rationale	Evaluation
Maintainance of Skin Integrity			
Prevention of Infection			
Reducing Edema			
Adequate Nutritional Intake			

STUDENT WORKSHEET: CHRONIC RENAL FAILURE

Clinical Manifestations	Etiology	Nursing Interventions	Rationale
Edema and Hypertension			
Hyperkalemia			
Fluid Imbalances			

(Continued)

(Student Worksheet continued)

Clinical Manifestations	Etiology	Nursing Interventions	Rationale
Anemia			
Hypocalcemia/ Hyperphosphatemia			
Growth Retardation			

CHAPTER 37

ALTERED IMMUNE FUNCTION

DISCUSSION QUESTIONS

1. Describe the following types of factors that enhance or limit immune competence: (a) genetic, (b) age-related, (c) nutritional and metabolic, (d) environmental, (e) anatomic, (f) microbial, and (g) physiological.
2. What is the basic process that results in autoimmunity?
3. What areas of the body are involved in *systemic lupus erythematosus (SLE)*? Explain the basis for the distribution of affected tissues.
4. What are the effects of SLE on body systems?
5. Describe the clinical manifestations of SLE. What findings are most commonly observed in the individual with SLE.
6. Describe the laboratory findings consistent with a diagnosis of SLE.
7. Provide the rationale for the following forms of treatment of SLE: (a) aspirin, (b) antimalarial drugs, and (c) cytotoxic drugs. What are the nursing implications of these drugs?
8. Identify nursing diagnoses for the child with SLE. Describe appropriate nursing interventions for each nursing diagnosis.
9. What are the theories on the etiology of *juvenile arthritis (JA)*?
10. What is the etiology of each of the following clinical manifestations of JA in children: (a) joint swelling, (b) joint fluid cloudiness, (c) joint stiffness and limited mobility, and (d) joint destruction?
11. What symptoms are consistent with (a) systemic onset of JA, (b) polyarticular onset of JA, and (c) pauciarticular onset of JA?
12. What drugs are currently used to treat JA? Describe their actions and side effects. What nursing interventions are important in the drug therapies used to treat JA?
13. Identify activities to maintain mobility for the child with JA.
14. Explain the theories on the etiology of *Stevens–Johnson syndrome.*
15. What is the appearance of skin lesions in children with Stevens–Johnson syndrome? What is the basis of the rash?
16. Describe nursing actions for the following nursing diagnoses identified for the child with Stevens–Johnson syndrome. Provide the rationale for the following nursing actions:

    High risk for infection

    High risk for fluid volume deficit

    Altered comfort, pain

    High risk for injury

    High risk for altered home health maintenance
17. What information is gathered during the nursing history of a child with an allergic disorder?
18. Describe the process and objectives of skin testing.
19. Construct an information sheet for parents on how to make their home allergy proof.

20. How does desensitization reduce response to allergens?
21. Identify nursing actions for the child with allergies receiving immunotherapy injections.
22. Describe the etiology, clinical manifestations, and medical and nursing management of children with (a) allergic rhinitis and (b) allergic conjunctivitis.
23. What are common food allergens in children?
24. How are foods added to an infant's diet to allow for early identification of food allergies?
25. How would an allergy to cow's milk in an infant be managed?
26. What is the etiology of the skin lesions and intense itching experienced by the child with *atopic dermatitis?*
27. Describe the characteristics and distribution of the rash in atopic dermatitis.
28. How is the pruritus and infection controlled in atopic dermatitis.
29. Compare the etiology and therapeutic management of urticaria versus angioedema.
30. What are the clinical manifestations of *allergic contact dermatitis?* What is the rationale for these manifestations?
31. Describe preventive measures for the child who experiences allergic contact dermatitis.
32. Why are adolescents a high-risk group for human immunodeficiency virus (HIV) transmission?
33. How is HIV infection classified in children?
34. Why is the individual with acquired immune deficiency (AIDS) so susceptible to infection and unable to fight infections once acquired?
35. Describe the typical clinical picture of an HIV-infected child.
36. Why is intravenous gamma globulin administered to children who are HIV positive? Describe nursing actions involved in the preparation and administration of gamma globulin.
37. For each of the nursing diagnoses listed below for the child with AIDS, give the following: (a) ways to monitor the development of the problem, (b) ways to prevent the problem, and (c) ways to treat the problem once it occurs.

    High risk for infection

    High risk for altered growth and development

    High risk for ineffective family coping

    High risk for altered home health maintenance
38. Describe the transmission of HIV and its implication for nursing actions that reduce the risk of the virus to nurses providing care for the HIV-positive child.
39. Provide the rationale for the following interventions for the child on long-term steroid therapy: (a) BP every shift, (b) no added salt diet, (c) diet high in potassium and protein, (d) administer with food, (e) test urine for glucose, (f) withhold scheduled immunizations, and (g) administer daily dose in the morning.
40. What is the etiology of *rheumatic fever?*
41. How are the Jones criteria used in the diagnosis of rheumatic fever?
42. Why is long-term penicillin prophylaxis required for the child who has had rheumatic fever?
43. What is the nurse's role in the prevention of rheumatic fever?
44. Describe the pathophysiology and clinical manifestations of *Kawasaki disease.*
45. What is the therapeutic management of Kawasaki disease?
46. Outline the nursing care for the child with Kawasaki disease.

CASE STUDY #1

Four-year-old Julie is admitted for evaluation of joint swelling and leg pain. She is diagnosed with pauciarticular onset juvenile arthritis. Julie has the following blood studies done: (a) sedimentation rate, (b) rheumatoid factor, (c) antinuclear antibodies, (d) hemoglobin and hematocrit, and (e) white blood count. Describe the typical joint and systemic manifestations of this juvenile arthritis subtype. What findings from the blood studies would be consistent with her diagnosis?

Julie will be receiving aspirin at home. She weighs 17 kg. What would be the highest safe dose of aspirin that she should receive?

Construct a discharge plan for Julie. Include interventions for teaching the parents about the administration of aspirin. What assessments should the parents be taught how to perform prior to Julie's discharge? Develop a program that the parents can use to provide both exercise and rest to Julie's affected joints.

CASE STUDY #2

Jack, 6-month-old infant, was born to an intravenous drug user who has recently died of AIDS. Jack was small for his gestational age at birth and has been hospitalized twice with failure to thrive and pneumonia. His antibody test for HIV is positive. Because of the increased severity and occurrence of infections, Jack is now considered to be exhibiting symptoms associated with AIDS.

Jack is started on intravenous gamma globulin. What is the basis for the use of gamma globulin in the treatment of AIDS? What nursing interventions are important in the preparation and administration of gamma globulin?

A foster family has been found for Jack. Develop a teaching plan for preparing the family to care for Jack at home. What information will the family need on transmission of the virus and protection of the child from infection?

STUDENT LEARNING ACTIVITIES

1. Lead a discussion of nurse's attitudes and concerns regarding caring for children with AIDS. What is the nurse's responsibility regarding these children?
2. What is the policy regarding AIDS in the hospital where your students are practicing? Are the guidelines sufficiently clear to provide protection for the infected child, staff, and other children in the unit?

AUDIOVISUAL RESOURCES

1. **Systemic Lupus Erythematosus—It Means Some Changes**
   This film shows four adult patients with SLE discussing their reactions to the diagnosis, symptoms, medications, and life style changes associated with the disease. The emotional impact on themselves and their families is also presented. This film is useful in illustrating the coping responses of people with SLE. It could also stimulate discussion of nursing strategies specific to the care of the child or adolescent with SLE.

Videocassette: 26 minutes

Distributor: University of Michigan

2. **The Terror of Anaphylaxis**
   This program describes the clinical manifestations of an anaphylactic reaction and differentiates between laryngospasm and bronchospasm. Treatment methods and precautions that decrease the risk of a serious anaphylactic reaction are identified. The program is self-instructional and includes a program guide.

Slide/tape and videotransfer: 14 minutes

Distributor: University of Michigan

3. **Allergy and Immunotherapy**
   This program shows how researchers are probing allergies and testing immunotherapy and other treatments for a variety of allergens.

Videocassette: 26 minutes

Distributor: Films for the Humanities and Sciences

4. **Allergies: The Twentieth Century Disease**
This program discusses the types, causes, and treatment of allergies through interviews with patients and physicians. Physical and psychological responses that alter lifestyle are also discussed. The film presents the controversy between allergists who practice traditional treatments and those who specialize in environmental medicine. The film suggests that our present environment, including foods and pollution, are central causative factors in allergic response. This is a good film to stimulate discussion and heighten student awareness of the various approaches to allergy treatment.

Videocassette and 16-mm film: 42 minutes

Distributor: Filmmakers Library

5. **Care of HIV-Infected Children**
This video addresses the care of HIV-infected infants and children. It presents a model of care based on patient and family needs throughout the course of the illness. A nursing care plan for HIV-infected children is illustrated. Use of universal precautions is emphasized.

Videocassette: 28 minutes

Distributor: American Journal of Nursing Company

6. **A Gift of Time (Pediatric AIDS)**
This documentary focuses on the crisis of pediatric AIDS and how if affects families. Information is conveyed through interviews with parents and the children with AIDS as well as medical experts.

Videocassette: 18 minutes

Distributor: Coronet/MTI Film and Video

7. **Kids with AIDS**
This program provides a glimpse into the lives of families who have children with AIDS. Several scenarios are presented: a typical day with a mother caring for her second child with AIDS; a professional couple raising a foster child who is HIV-positive; and two social workers who have opened a group home for children with AIDS.

Videocassette: 28 minutes

Distributor: Films for the Humanities & Sciences

8. **Ryan White Talks to Kids about AIDS**
This specially adapted Phil Donahue program shows 16-year-old Ryan White interacting with an audience of teenagers about AIDS. Ryan White had hemophilia and was infected with HIV by contaminated blood products. He tells how he dealt with the reactions of others, particularly at school. He died at the age of 18.

Videocassette: 28 minutes

Distributor: Films for the Humanities & Sciences

Note: There are many more audiovisual instructional aids designed for professional, patient, school age, and adolescent education on the topic of AIDS. See the Audiovisual Resource Guide (pp. 185–186, this manual) for additional resources.

ANSWERS TO PRETEST

1. filtering blood and lymph
2. lymphocytes, antibodies, microorganisms
3. the spread of infection
4. tears, saliva, blood plasma (lysozyme), digestive juices
5. spleen
6. tonsils, thymus
7. antigen
8. phagocytosis
9. thymus, bone marrow
10. antibodies
11. T-lymphocytes
12. histamine
13. skin, respiratory tract
14. autoimmune disease
15. increased blood flow (redness and heat), increased capillary permeability (swelling)

PRETEST: STRUCTURE AND FUNCTION OF IMMUNE SYSTEM

1. The spleen functions as part of the immune system by ____.

2. The lymph nodes are a source of ______________________ and ______________________. They filter ______________________.

3. Because of the properties given in question 2, lymph nodes prevent ______________________.

4. Two examples of body fluids that contain antimicrobial agents are ______________ and ______________________.

5. The largest lymphoid organ in the body is the ______________________.

6. Two other lymphoid organs are the ______________________ and the ______________________.

7. An agent that stimulates the immune response is called a(n) ______________________.

8. The process by which foreign substances within the body are destroyed by neutrophils and macrophages is called ______________________.

9. T-lymphocytes originate in the ______________________, while the site of development of B-lymphocytes is the ______________________.

10. B-lymphocytes respond to foreign substances by producing ______________________.

11. The lymphocytes responsible for tissue rejection are the ______________________.

12. Mast cells respond to allergic reactions by releasing ______________________.

13. Mast cells are particularly prevalent in the ______________________ and ______________________.

14. A disease involving an immune response that is directed against the body's own cells is called a(n) ______________________.

15. The chemical produced by mast cells causes ______________________ and ______________________.

CHAPTER 38

ALTERED SKIN INTEGRITY

DISCUSSION QUESTIONS

1. How is the skin's protective function affected by (a) genetic factors, (b) hormonal factors, (c) cleanliness, (d) hydration, and (e) nutrition?
2. What information would the nurse ascertain in a nursing history of a child with a skin disorder?
3. Describe the laboratory studies that can be used to assist in the diagnosis of skin disorders.
4. How should the nurse proceed with a physical assessment of the skin? What are special considerations when assessing infants and children?
5. Describe types of skin lesions that would alert the nurse to the presence of congenital problems?
6. Discuss the implications of the following developmental differences in the structure and function of the skin of infants and children: (a) thin epidermis, (b) lack of functional melanocytes, (c) more alkaline, (d) low IgA secretion from mucous membranes, (e) inactive sebaceous glands, (f) eccrine gland function immaturity, and (g) less subcutaneous fat.
7. How can the nurse help parents cope with the psychosocial aspects of having a child with a chronic skin condition?
8. Explain the rationale for the following interventions on topical treatment of skin lesions: (a) apply ointment after bath and (b) cover lesion with dressing after application of ointment.
9. What instructions should the nurse give to a parent on the prevention and treatment of diaper dermatitis?
10. What is the etiology of *seborrheic dermatitis?*
11. What areas of the body are most commonly involved in seborrheic dermatitis?
12. What are the most effective measures for the prevention and treatment of seborrheic dermatitis?
13. What is the basis for *psoriasis?*
14. Describe the characteristic lesion associated with psoriasis.
15. What are the common locations for the psoriasis lesions?
16. What is the objective of the treatment for psoriasis?
17. What is the rationale for the use of tar preparations in the treatment of psoriasis?
18. Why is the nursing diagnosis *High risk for infection* a priority when planning care for the child with psoriasis? What nursing actions apply related to this diagnosis?
19. Describe the mechanisms that result in the development of acne vulgaris.
20. What drugs are currently used to treat acne, and what is their mode of action?
21. What is the current belief about the relationship between diet and acne?

22. What information should adolescents with acne receive regarding skin care and use of topical agents?
23. What information can the nurse give to parents about sunburn prevention?
24. What is the treatment for sunburned skin?
25. What is the etiology of impetigo? Describe the progression in the appearance of the lesions associated with impetigo.
26. What are the etiology and clinical manifestations of cellulitis?
27. What are furuncles and carbuncles? What would the nurse teach parents to do when a child experiences these skin problems?
28. How do infants contract herpes simplex virus type I (HSV-1)? Which children are most susceptible to HSV-1?
29. Describe the process of the development of the lesion of HSV-1.
30. What problems are created by the gingivostomatitis caused by HSV-1? What measures are effective in treating these problems?
31. Construct a list of foods that would be most readily accepted by the child with gingivostomatitis.
32. What are the clinical manifestations of, medical care for, and nursing care for hordeolums versus molluscum contagiosum.

CASE STUDY

Shawna, age 6 years, is brought by her parents to the emergency room because of a rash. Her mother states that Shawna scratched an insect bite on her chin a few days ago. Now she has crusted draining lesions around her mouth and nose. New lesions are spreading to her chin. The diagnosis of impetigo is made. Shawna's parents ask the nurse how an insect bite could result in such a reaction. What explanations can the nurse give the parents?

Shawna complains that the lesions itch and she is seen picking at them. What interventions will reduce the pruritus, and what instructions should the parents receive on preventing the spread of lesions from scratching?

What instructions should the parents receive about watching for complications of impetigo?

Shawna is placed on erythromycin. What instructions do the parents need to ensure accurate administration of the drug? What measures will prevent the spread of the infection to other family members and Shawna's playmates?

STUDENT LEARNING ACTIVITIES

1. Construct a teaching program for adolescents on the cause and management of acne. Include diagrams and pictures of normal skin and the progressive development of acne lesions. Provide a clear rationale for the treatment of acne, as well as why such actions as the squeezing of pustules aggravates the condition. Include the interventions outlined in the textbook related to the appropriate skin care and use of topical agents.

AUDIOVISUAL RESOURCES

1. **The Integumentary System**
This program provides instructions for a methodical assessment of the integumentary system, including structure and function. Normal and abnormal findings are illustrated. It is a useful self-instructional program for the student who requires basic review.

Videocassette: 22 minutes

Distributor: MedCom/Trainex

2. **Skin, Hair, and Nails Examination**
This program covers inspection and palpation of the skin (for color, texture, temperature, hydration, turgor, and lesions) and examination of the nails and nail beds (for appearance, color, and clubbing).

Videocassette: 16 minutes

Distributor: University of Michigan Medical Center, Media Library

3. **Application of Heat and Cold**
This eight-part series introduces and details the procedures for local application of heat and cold. Included are dry heat, sterile soaks, sitz bath, compresses, and application of cold. This program is self-instructional and includes a student workbook.

35-mm filmstrips: eight parts

Distributor: J. B. Lippincott Co.

ANSWERS TO PRETEST

1. mucus
2. serous
3. dermis, epidermis
4. barrier against invasion of foreign substances; excessive water and heat loss
5. sebaceous glands produce lipid for lubrication of epidermis and hair
6. sweat glands excrete metabolic wastes and water
7. sensory receptors for touch pressure, temperature, and pain
8. redness, swelling, heat, pain
9. pus
10. necrosis
11. d
12. g
13. c
14. f
15. b
16. h
17. e
18. a

PRETEST:
STRUCTURE AND FUNCTION OF INTEGUMENTARY SYSTEM

1. The linings of body cavities and hollow organs that open to the exterior are ____________ membranes.
2. The linings of body cavities that do **not** open to the exterior are ____________ membranes.
3. The two main layers of the skin are the inner layer or ____________ and the outer layer or ____________.

For numbers 4–7, give one example of each of these functions of the skin.

4. Protection: ____________
5. Secretion: ____________
6. Excretion: ____________
7. Sensory: ____________
8. The four cardinal signs of inflammatory response are ____________, ____________, ____________, and ____________.
9. During tissue injury, the breakdown of leukocytes and necrotic tissue results in the formation of ____________.
10. Tissue destruction related to cell death is called ____________.

Match the following skin abnormalities with their descriptions (a–h) below.

11. fissure ______
12. macule ______
13. papule ______
14. vesicle ______
15. pustule ______
16. excoriation ______
17. ecchymosis ______
18. petechiae ______

a. small skin hemorrhages, pinpoint red spots
b. raised lesion containing purulent fluid
c. solid, firm, elevated lesion
d. crack or grove in skin
e. large amount of bleeding into skin
f. raised lesion containing clear fluid
g. skin discoloration without elevation
h. superficial abrasions due to trauma

CHAPTER 39

INFECTIOUS DISEASE

DISCUSSION QUESTIONS

1. Describe the immune responses elicited by (a) viruses, (b) bacteria, (c) parasites, and (d) fungi.
2. What etiologic agent is responsible for *cytomegalovirus (CMV)*?
3. What are the clinical manifestations of the following types of CMV: (a) congenital, (b) perinatal, and (c) acquired?
4. How is CMV diagnosed?
5. What are the cardinal symptoms of infectious *mononucleosis*? What other symptoms can the child with mononucleosis exhibit?
6. What guidance should the child recovering from mononucleosis be given regarding resumption of activities?
7. Compare and contrast the etiology of the clinical manifestations of the major types of *hepatitis.*
8. What symptoms of clinical hepatitis are consistent with (a) the pre-icteric stage and (b) the icteric phase?
9. What laboratory findings are consistent with the diagnosis of hepatitis?
10. What information is needed by the parents of a child with hepatitis regarding home care in the following areas: (a) activity, (b) nutrition, (c) relieving pruritus, and (d) preventing the spread of infection?
11. How is rabies transmitted to humans?
12. Describe the clinical manifestations of the three stages of rabies.
13. What is the basis for the ability of tuberculosis symptoms to recur after recovery from the initial illness?
14. What are the possible outcomes that can result from tuberculosis?
15. What is the nurse's role with the family whose child has exhibited a positive tuberculin skin test?
16. What is the limitation of the BCG vaccination for the prevention of tuberculosis?
17. What medications are used to treat active tuberculosis?
18. Identify nursing diagnoses and interventions for children experiencing *helminthic infections.*
19. What are some examples of how *pediculosis capitis* is transmitted among children?
20. Why are the following priority nursing diagnoses for the child with pediculosis capitis?

    Impaired skin integrity

    Altered comfort

    Potential for infection

    Knowledge deficit
21. What measures can the nurse teach parents that are effective in reducing the incidence of contracting pediculosis capitis?
22. What is the etiology of the pruritus and rash associated with scabies?
23. What precautions are necessary when using the lotions or shampoo prescribed for the treatment of pediculosis capitis or scabies?

24. How does congenital toxoplasmosis differ from acquired toxoplasmosis with regards to (a) clinical manifestations, (b) therapeutic management, and (c) outcome?
25. Why is the incidence of candida infections highest during the neonatal period?
26. What is the correct procedure for application of nystatin for the treatment of thrush in infants?
27. Describe the appearance of the lesion of ringworm.
28. What are preventive measures for the various forms of tinea infections?
29. Construct an instruction sheet for the child who has *tinea pedis.*
30. Describe the clinical manifestations of Rocky Mountain spotted fever.
31. Identify the clinical manifestations of Lyme disease according to stage.
32. What nursing diagnoses and interventions apply to the child with Lyme disease?
33. How does amebiasis differ from shigellosis with regard to (a) etiology, (b) clinical manifestations, (c) diagnosis, and (d) therapeutic management?
34. What measures can be taken by sexually active adolescents to prevent sexually transmitted diseases (STD)?
35. What would the nurse teach adolescents about signs and symptoms of sexually transmitted diseases?
36. What are examples of physiological alterations that can make a female prone to vaginitis?

CASE STUDY

Rhonda, age 16 years, is admitted to the hospital after a one-month-long history of purulent vaginal discharge, dysuria, fever, and abdominal pain. Rhonda has been sexually active for over a year. The diagnosis is pelvic inflammatory disease (PID).

How does PID affect fertility? What bacterial agent is most likely the cause of Rhonda's infection?

Construct a teaching plan for Rhonda focused on preventing subsequent sexually transmitted diseases and unwanted pregnancy and encouraging responsible sexual behavior.

STUDENT LEARNING ACTIVITY

1. Ask students to construct a teaching booklet to be used in teaching adolescents how to avoid sexually transmitted diseases.

AUDIOVISUAL RESOURCES

1. **Recognizing Common Communicable Diseases**
   This program provides visual illustrations of common communicable diseases of children, including measles, rubella, chickenpox, and scarlet fever. A program guide is included that contains objectives, a glossary, and learning activities with explanations. This is a very useful tool for student self-instruction in the learning laboratory.

Slides with program guide

Distributor: University of Minnesota

2. **Controlling Transmission of Infection**
   This program describes the chain of infection transmission and an overview of nosocomial infections. Category-specific and disease-specific isolation precautions are identified, along with new infection control guidelines issued by the Centers for Disease Control. This program is useful in preparing students for hospital experiences and in developing parent teaching plans for management of infection control in the home.

Videocassette: 28 minutes

Distributor: American Journal of Nursing Co.

3. **Common Neonatal Viral Infections**
This program discusses the causes, characteristics, transmission, sequelae, and management of herpes simplex, rubella, and cytomegalovirus infections in the neonate. It is useful for preparing students who will practice in the newborn nursery setting.

Videocassette: 28 minutes

Distributor: Health Sciences Consortium

4. **Infection Control and the Neonate: Hepatitis B and CMV**
This program explains isolation procedures used in nursery settings, specifically for those newborns with hepatitis B and cytomegalovirus (CMV) infections. This is useful for students in newborn nursery clinical settings.

Videocassette: 24 minutes

Distributor: Health Sciences Consortium

5. **Infectious Mononucleosis**
This program details the classic and nonclassic signs and symptoms of infectious mononucleosis. Laboratory tests used in the diagnosis of this condition are discussed. Also covered are the acute and advanced phases of the illness as well as complications.

Slide/tape: 20 minutes

Distributor: University of Michigan Medical Center, Media Library

6. **Chlamydia**
This program reviews the management and treatment of chlamydia, risk assessment, surveillance, and strategies for prevention and control of this sexually transmitted disease.

Slide set

Distributor: National Audiovisual Center

7. **Not a Game: Sexually Transmitted Diseases**
Various STDs and their symptoms, transmission, and treatment are discussed. Herpes, chlamydia, gonorrhea, human papilloma virus, venereal warts, syphilis, and AIDS are included. Safe sex practices are examined, with abstinence promoted as the best means of prevention.

Videocassette or 16-mm film: 25 minutes

Distributor: Coronet/MTI Film and Video

8. **Sexually Transmitted Diseases**
This program examines the epidemic of STDs, with a focus on chlamydia, herpes, venereal warts, and AIDS. The importance of prevention and the early detection of problems through new diagnostic tests are emphasized. Complications of STDs are addressed.

Videocassette: 19 minutes

Distributor: Films for the Humanities & Sciences

9. **Genital Herpes Simplex Infection**
Two types of herpes simplex infection are defined in this program. Characteristics of genital infection and complications are discussed.

Slide/tape: 47 minutes

Distributor: Trainex/Medcom

10. **Lyme Disease**
This program explains the symptoms of Lyme disease. The carrier tick, its life and migratory cycles, and the wildlife on which it feeds are also shown. Suggestions for avoiding tick bites and for removing the attached tick are discussed.

Videocassette: 26 minutes

Distributor: Films for the Humanities & Sciences

STUDENT WORKSHEET:
INFORMATION FOR PARENTS WHOSE CHILD HAS CHICKENPOX

Incubation period after a child has been exposed:

Determining the length of infectious period:

Common complaints the child will exhibit:

Measures to promote child comfort:

Measures to prevent complications:

Signs that should be reported to the doctor:

Chapter 40

Altered Neurologic Function

DISCUSSION QUESTIONS

1. What are the causes of primary and secondary microcephaly and macrocephaly?
2. Describe the change in skull ossification that occurs during infancy and childhood.
3. What are the age-related differences in the structure and function of the central nervous system, and what are the nursing implications related to these differences?
4. Describe the components of and the procedures for performing an acute neurological check. What is the purpose of this type of neurological assessment?
5. Why is a careful respiratory assessment an important component of assessing the status of the neurological system?
6. What questions should the nurse ask parents when gathering the nursing history of a child with a neurological disorder?
7. What are the functions of a computerized tomography (CT) scan and magnetic resonance imagery (MRI)? How do these two tests differ?
8. What information would you provide to the child scheduled to undergo a CT scan?
9. What information about neurological functioning is obtained from the following: (a) EEG, (b) EMG, (c) evoked potential, (d) doppler ultrasound, (e) myelogram, (f) cerebral angiography, and (g) digital subtraction angiography?
10. What are the two purposes of a lumbar puncture?
11. How should the nurse position the child who is undergoing a lumbar puncture?
12. Explain the process of autoregulation. What conditions affect autoregulation?
13. What is the etiology of herniation syndromes? Describe the clinical manifestations consistent with developing herniation. Why do the signs of this condition differ between infants and children?
14. What compensatory mechanism does the brain have that helps to reduce damage resulting from increased intracranial pressure (ICP)?
15. How are blood oxygen and carbon dioxide content related to ICP?
16. Explain the mechanisms that increase ICP related to (a) brain mass, (b) cerebral blood flow, and (c) cerebral spinal fluid.
17. What is the rationale for administration of the following medications in the treatment of increased ICP: (a) intravenous mannitol, (b) diuretics, and (c) pancuronium?
18. Outline the nursing care for the child with ICP, providing specific nursing interventions for the following: (a) recognition of ICP, (b) positioning, (c) temperature regulation, (d) medication administration, and (e) ensuring protection.
19. What potential complications can occur after brain surgery? How does the nurse assess for the presence of each of these potential complications?
20. What structures are present in the infratentorial portion of the brain? What problems can occur from pathology or surgery in this area?

21. What general guidelines are recommended for dealing with the following aspects of seizure activity: (a) altered sensations and (b) altered tone, mobility, or movement?
22. What information is gathered when observing seizure activity relating to (a) response to stimuli, (b) movement and tone, (c) repetitive movements, (d) altered sensation or perception, (e) postictal response, and (f) frequent and subtle seizure?
23. What should documentation of a seizure include?
24. Define *status epilepticus* and identify its causes.
25. What medications are used to manage status epilepticus?
26. Describe the nursing responsibilities for a child during a seizure.
27. Describe typical behaviors associated with the following types of seizures: (a) simple partial, (b) complex partial, (c) generalized tonic–clonic, (d) absence, (e) myoclonic, and (f) atonic.
28. Identify commonly used anticonvulsant medications and potential side effects.
29. Explain the etiology for the following risks to the child with altered responsiveness: (a) respiratory infections, (b) muscle contractures, (c) inadequate nutrition, (d) constipation, (e) urinary problems, and (f) skin breakdown.
30. What nursing interventions should be done to (a) prevent injury and (b) prevent the complications of immobility for the child with altered responsiveness?
31. What are the characteristics of *craniosynostosis* that is classified as (a) primary, (b) secondary, and (c) syndromic?
32. What findings are characteristic in infants with craniosynostosis?
33. Describe nursing care for the child who has undergone surgical treatment for craniosynostosis.
34. Describe the anatomical alterations consistent with (a) anencephaly, (b) encephalocele, (c) spina bifida cystica, and (d) spina bifida occulta.
35. How can the presence of a neural tube defect be identified in the developing fetus?
36. What priority nursing diagnoses should be identified for the infant prior to surgery for *myelomeningocele*?
37. Describe the special care required for the infant with myelomeningocele to maintain skin integrity.
38. What major problems do children with myelomeningocele experience with regards to bowel and bladder function? What are the nursing strategies related to these problems?
39. Identify nursing interventions to promote adaptive coping for the parents of an infant with myelomeningocele.
40. Trace the flow of cerebral spinal fluid from the site of production to the site of absorption.
41. What are some of the causes of (a) acquired hydrocephalus and (b) congenital hydrocephalus?
42. How do the signs of hydrocephalus differ between infants and children?
43. What types of procedures are used to drain excess cerebral spinal fluid (CSF) in the child with hydrocephalus?
44. Explain the basis for the following diagnoses for the child with hydrocephalus: (a) altered tissue perfusion, (b) potential for injury, and (c) altered nutrition?
45. Identify nursing diagnoses for the child with hydrocephalus and appropriate nursing interventions.
46. What is a Chiari II malformation? What is the currently accepted explanation for the development of Chiari II malformations?
47. Why would the child with Chiari II malformation be prone to respiratory infections or respiratory distress? What nursing interventions can be applied to reduce the incidence of these two respiratory conditions?
48. Describe the pathophysiology of neurocutaneous syndrome and neurodegenerative disorder.

49. Describe the nursing care of children with neurocutaneous syndrome and neurodegenerative disorder.
50. Describe the etiology and pathophysiology of bacterial meningitis.
51. Why does the child with meningitis complain of a stiff neck?
52. What are Kernig and Brudzinski signs? How are they evaluated?
53. What typical laboratory findings are consistent with: (a) bacterial meningitis and (b) viral meningitis?
54. Identify nursing diagnoses and appropriate interventions for the child with bacterial meningitis.
55. What clinical manifestations are associated with encephalitis?
56. Describe nursing interventions for the nursing diagnosis *Powerlessness* at it relates to the family of a child with encephalitis.
57. Identify and explain the etiology of the typical symptoms associated with Guillain–Barre syndrome.
58. Describe the different forms of head trauma.
59. How are spinal cord injuries classified?
60. Identify nursing diagnoses and related nursing interventions for the child with spinal cord injury.

CASE STUDY #1

Pedro, age 6 years, is brought to the emergency room after falling out of a second story window. On arrival at the hospital, he is unconscious, but breathing without assistance. He has lacerations on his forehead and a large hematoma on the back of his head. X-rays identify a basilar skull fracture of the occipital bone. Pedro is stabilized in the emergency room and admitted to the ICU.

What signs would Pedro exhibit that are consistent with a basilar fracture? What assessments are included in an acute neurological check? While Pedro is unconscious, what will his nursing care entail?

What priority nursing diagnoses should be identified for Pedro? Outline nursing interventions for the following goals: (a) promote optimal cerebral perfusion, (b) prevent infection, and (c) maintain adequate gas exchange.

Pedro regains consciousness 24 hours after the injury. He is maintained on IV fluids and gets nothing by mouth for another 2 days. On the third day after the injury, the physician orders a clear liquid diet for Pedro. What nursing assessments are necessary prior to beginning Pedro on oral fluids?

CASE STUDY #2

Lauren, age 3 days, was born with myelomeningocele in the lumbosacral area. She was transferred to the NICU and is scheduled for surgical repair of the myelomeningocele. What assessments would be made by the nurse assigned to Lauren? What nursing actions are taken to prevent infection preoperatively and postoperatively?

Lauren's parents visit daily and are eager to participate in her care. How can the nurse involve Lauren's parents during their infant's hospitalization?

Several days after surgery, it is noted that Lauren's head circumference has been increasing. Lauren is irritable and her fontanels are tense and bulge when she cries. ACT scan confirms hydrocephalus. Surgery is scheduled for placement of a ventriculoperitoneal shunt.

How should Lauren be positioned postoperatively? What would a neurological assessment include? What should the nurse teach Lauren's parents about shunt complications?

Lauren is discharged to the home with her parents. What long-term problems associated with myelomeningocele could Lauren's parents anticipate?

STUDENT LEARNING ACTIVITIES

1. Does the clinical agency have a seizure record form? If not, ask students to develop one that would be appropriate for recording data related to seizure activity in infants and children. If a seizure record exists, ask the students to provide rationales for the types of assessments on the record and to critique the form for content and completeness.
2. Develop teaching forms for parents who have a child with a seizure disorder.

AUDIOVISUAL RESOURCES

1. **My CAT Scan**
   This program shows a 7-year-old child undergoing computerized axial tomography (CAT) of the head during which he describes his feelings, concerns, and the physical sensations he is experiencing. The film is designed to prepare school age children for the test and includes simplified explanations. This program could be used for parent and child education.

Videocassette: 10 minutes

Distributor: American Journal of Nursing Company

2. **Nursing Management of Increased Intracranial Pressure**
   This video shows a neurological nursing assessment of an adult, explains increased intracranial pressure, and details interventions for monitoring, prevention of infection, and nursing care. This program does not address age-related differences. The discussion of the effects of nursing care procedures on a patient's intracranial pressure level and techniques for adjusting nursing activities to prevent increased pressure are appropriate for nursing students. It can be used to introduce pediatric-specific content in the identification and management of the infant or child with increased intracranial pressure.

Videocassette: 10 minutes

Distributor: American Journal of Nursing Company

3. **Assessing Levels of Consciousness: The Glasgow Coma Scale**
   In this program, a nurse is shown using the Glasgow Coma Scale to assess level of consciousness in an adolescent experiencing a drug overdose. The scoring system is explained, including description of abnormal decorticate and decerebrate posturing. Modifications of the scale for use with younger children can be provided by the instructor.

Videocassette: 7 minutes

Distributor: Health Sciences Consortium

4. **Nursing Management of Acute Head Injuries**
   This program distinguishes between minor and major head injuries using illustration and nursing diagnosis statements. Neurological assessment, Glasgow Coma Scale scoring, and ICP monitoring procedures are detailed. The nurse's role in facilitating various treatment modalities is described. This is not geared specifically to the pediatric patient, but provides a comprehensive overview of the subject.

Videocassette: 28 minutes

Distributor: American Journal of Nursing Company

5. **Complications of Spinal Cord Impairment**
   This film illustrates immobilization of the spine after an accident and distinguishes between spinal and hypovolemic shock. Respiratory, urological, gastrointestinal, cardiovascular, and autonomic system alterations associated with the level of spinal cord impairment are described with discussion of nursing management strategies. This is a useful program for student review prior to classroom content.

Videocassette: 28 minutes

Distributor: American Journal of Nursing Company

6. **Clean Intermittent Catheterization**
This video includes the anatomy and physiology of the bladder, catheter insertion for a young boy or girl, and teaching the process of self-catheterization.

Videocassette: 25 minutes

Distributor: Pyramid Film and Video

7. **Neurological Assessment of the Pediatric Patient**
This program describes the basic neurological exam for infants and children, including level of consciousness, Glasgow Coma Scale, and pupillary responses. The child's age and level of development are taken into consideration in the demonstration of the neurological examination. Signs of acute neurological deterioration, with differences between infants and children, are addressed. Techniques for adapting the exam for children with developmental delays and disabilities are included.

Videocassette: 28 minutes

Distributor: American Journal of Nursing Company

8. **Epilepsy in Children: A Primary Care Perspective**
This program describes how to differentiate between types of seizures and includes footage of actual seizures. Current treatment of seizures is addressed.

Videocassette: 22 minutes

Distributor: Medcom/Trainex

ANSWERS TO PRETEST

1. brain, spinal cord
2. cranial nerves, spinal nerves
3. synapses
4. voluntary responses
5. cardiac muscle, smooth muscle, glands
6. dura mater, pia mater, arachnoid
7. meninges
8. choroid plexuses of the ventricles
9. arachnoid villi
10. blood pressure
11. glucose
12. cervical, thoracic, lumbar, sacral, coccygeal
13. spinal cord
14. sensory, motor
15. d
16. c
17. b
18. a
19. c
20. b
21. c
22. a
23. d
24. c
25. a
26. g
27. b
28. d
29. e
30. f

PRETEST: STRUCTURE AND FUNCTION OF NEUROLOGICAL SYSTEM

1. The central nervous system consists of the ______________________ and the ______________________.

2. The peripheral nervous system consists of the ______________________ and the ______________________.

3. The transmission of an impulse from one nerve cell to another occurs at the ______________________.

4. The somatic nervous system consists of neurons for ______________________ ______________________.

5. The visceral nervous system transports impulses for functioning of the ______________________, ______________________, and ______________________.

6. The three protective coverings of the brain are the ______________________, ______________________, and ______________________.

7. The three coverings of the brain are collectively called the ______________________.

8. The primary site of cerebral spinal fluid production is the ______________________ ______________________.

9. Reabsorption of cerebral spinal fluid occurs within the ______________________ ______________________.

10. The vasomotor center within the medulla controls blood vessel diameter, which influences ______________________ ______________________.

11. The only source of energy for brain tissue is ______________________.

12. The five levels of the spinal cord are ______________________, ______________________, ______________________, ______________________, and ______________________.

13. The dorsal and ventral spinal roots connect the spinal nerves with the ______________________.

14. The dorsal root contains fibers responsible for ______________________ function, while the ventral root regulates ______________________ function.

(Continued)

(Pretest continued)

For numbers 15–23, match the part of the brain (a–d) that is responsible for each of the functions.

15. learning, thinking, memory ________
16. secretion of antidiuretic hormone ________
17. reflex centers of swallowing, vomiting, and coughing ________
18. maintenance of posture ________
19. appetite control center ________
20. respiratory center ________
21. regulation of body temperature ________
22. coordination of voluntary motor responses ________
23. speech ________

a. cerebellum
b. medulla oblongata
c. hypothalamus
d. cerebral cortex

For numbers 24–30, match the cranial nerve with the correct function.

24. oculomotor ________
25. trigeminal ________
26. facial ________
27. vestibulocochlear ________
28. glossopharyngeal ________
29. vagus ________
30. olfactory ________

a. sensation to face, teeth, forehead
b. equilibrium
c. pupil size
d. swallowing and salivation
e. parasympathetic oragn response
f. smell
g. taste anterior portion tongue, facial expression

STUDENT WORKSHEET: DRUG THERAPY FOR SEIZURE CONTROL

Drug	Common Side Effects	Nursing Implications	Implications for Parent and Child Teaching
Zarontin			
Tegretol			
Depakene			
Dilantin			
Phenobarbital			

CHAPTER 41

ALTERED MUSCULOSKELETAL FUNCTION

DISCUSSION QUESTIONS

1. Construct a list of questions the nurse should ask when gathering the history of a child with a suspected or actual musculoskeletal disorder.
2. What are the eight components of a neurovascular assessment? For each component, describe normal and abnormal findings.
3. When documenting neurovascular status, which descriptive terms should be used and which should be avoided?
4. What is the guideline for frequency of neurovascular status assessment?
5. What are the (a) physiological effects of immobilization and (b) the emotional/social effects of immobilization for the infant and child?
6. What are some of the behaviors that children exhibit in response to prolonged immobilization? How can the nurse effectively respond to these behaviors?
7. For the child who has a cast applied, what nursing actions will (a) prevent skin problems and (b) improve parental knowledge of home care?
8. What is the purpose of traction as a treatment for musculoskeletal problems? How is countertraction achieved?
9. Describe the following types of traction: (a) skin, (b) skeletal, (c) Buck extension, (d) Russell, (e) 90-90, (f) balanced suspension, (g) Bryant, (h) Dunlap, and (i) Halo.
10. What explanation is given for the greater incidence of *congenital dislocated hip (CHD)* among female infants?
11. What typical signs are observed in the infant with CHD?
12. Describe the maneuvers that are part of the assessment for the presence of CHD.
13. What therapeutic measures can be used to treat the infant with CHD? What considerations influence the choice of treatment?
14. Why is serial casting used in the treatment of clubfoot?
15. How is metatarsus adductus diagnosed?
16. What typical early behaviors are exhibited by children with *Duchenne muscular dystrophy (DMD)*?
17. What typical diagnostic findings are consistent with the diagnosis of DMD?
18. Why does the nursing diagnosis, *High risk for ineffective thermoregulation*, apply to the child with DMD? Identify appropriate nursing actions for this nursing diagnosis.
19. Identify nursing actions for the following nursing diagnosis: *Disuse syndrome related to loss of muscle strength and mobility.*
20. What is the etiology of congenital limb deformities?
21. How is leg length measured? How can leg length discrepancy be treated?
22. What are torsional deformities? How are they evaluated, and what is their therapeutic management?
23. What is the normal development progress of genu varum and genu valgum?

24. Describe the anatomical alteration consistent with *slipped capital femoral epiphysis (SCFE)?*
25. What is the rationale for the following aspects of treatment for SCFE: (a) non–weight bearing, (b) Buck traction, and (c) surgical stabilization?
26. What are the three major types of *scoliosis?*
27. Why is scoliosis most commonly diagnosed during adolescence?
28. What characteristics differentiate structural from nonstructural scoliosis?
29. What is the etiology of the lateral deviation of the spinal column seen in scoliosis?
30. Describe the screening procedure for identification of scoliosis.
31. Describe the two methods of treatment of scoliosis: (a) bracing and (b) surgery.
32. What difficulties related to promotion of self-image can be associated with the bracing treatment of scoliosis?
33. Identify nursing diagnoses and interventions for the adolescent who has undergone a posterior spinal fusion for scoliosis.
34. What are *kyphosis* and *spondylolisthesis?* How are these spinal deviations different from scoliosis?
35. What are the clinical signs of *Legg-Calve-Perthes disease?*
36. What is the rationale for the following aspects of the treatment for Legg-Calve-Perthes disease: (a) non–weight bearing and (b) long leg cast and abduction?
37. What is the pathophysiology of *osteomyelitis?*
38. What is the treatment for osteomyelitis?
39. Identify nursing diagnoses and nursing actions for the child experiencing either osteomyelitis or septic joint.
40. Describe the management of knee injuries.
41. What types of complications can result from fractures in children?
42. How do the typical forms of management of fractures relate to the characteristics of bone structure in children?

CASE STUDY

Nellie, age 9 years, is brought to the emergency room after being struck by a car on her way home from school. She is complaining of pain in her left leg. On examination, a large degree of swelling is noted in the left thigh. X-ray reveals a fractured femur.

On arrival at the pediatric unit, Nellie is placed in Russell's traction. How would the nurse explain the function of this form of traction to Nellie and her parents? What position should Nellie maintain during the time she is in traction? What measures by the nurse will help to ensure the maximum desired effect of the traction?

Construct a form to assess Nellie's neurovascular status. What findings would indicate neurovascular compromise?

After 7 days Nellie is placed in a spica cast. On return to the floor, what important aspects of nursing care should be instituted? Nellie is discharged two days after application of her cast. Develop a teaching sheet for Nellie's parents on the care of Nellie at home.

STUDENT LEARNING ACTIVITIES

1. Ask students to construct an information sheet for parents on activities and means of stimulation of the infant or child in a cast or who requires prolonged immobilization.
2. Arrange for students to care for a child in traction or in a spica cast. Identify nursing diagnoses and appropriate nursing actions for the child.
3. Arrange for students to observe cast application or cast removal. How are children prepared for the experience? How was the child's cognitive development a factor in the preparation?

AUDIOVISUAL RESOURCES

1. **Orthopedic Assessment**
This program demonstrates physical assessment of the musculoskeletal system in a healthy adult. Special aspects of assessing children, emergency room patients, and individuals with orthopedic alterations are included. This film is comprehensive, includes a study guide, and can be used for students in the learning laboratory for independent instruction.

Videocassette: 28 minutes

Distributor: American Journal of Nursing Company

2. **Nursing Care of Patients with Casts**
The first part of this two-part program details the purposes, types, application, and removal of casts, emphasizing nursing care responsibilities. Part II covers priorities of care including preventing complications, reducing pain, increasing mobility, and providing information. The nursing process format is stressed throughout. It is a comprehensive program for self-instruction or supplementation of lecture material.

Videocassette: 28 minutes each part

Distributor: American Journal of Nursing Company

3. **Caring for the Child in a Hip Spica Cast**
This parent education program describes the application of a hip spica cast and related care measures. Included are techniques for keeping the cast clean and dry, checking circulation, protecting the skin, planning play activities, and ensuring safety. This program can be used to instruct both parents and students.

Slide/tape: 19 minutes

Distributor: University of Michigan Medical Center Media Library

4. **Children in Traction**
This program explains the physical care needs of the child in traction. There is also a thorough discussion of the psychological problems imposed by immobilization and nursing care strategies to meet the psychological needs of children in traction. This is a comprehensive program designed specially for nursing education.

Videocassette: 27 minutes

Distributor: Health Sciences Consortium

5. **Traction: Checks and Balances**
This program depicts various types of traction, including manual, skin, and skeletal traction. Topics addressed include the purpose of traction, key nursing observations, assessment techniques, and interventions. The content is not specific to children but could offer students useful information.

Videocassette: 28 minutes

Distributor: American Journal of Nursing Company

6. **Taking Care of Your Plaster Cast**
This program includes how casts are made and how to care for a wet cast. Important aspects of home cast care are addressed, including circulation checks, skin care, keeping the cast clean, diversional activities, and safety. This program could be useful for patient and parent education.

Slide/tape: 13 minutes

Distributor: University of Michigan Medical Center Media Library

7. **Spinal Fusion: What You Need To Know**
This patient education program shows an adolescent recalling her experiences preoperatively, immediately postoperatively, and during the period of immobilization while in a body case following spinal fusion surgery. The content of this film is informative for students who will be caring for adolescents hospitalized for spinal fusion. The discussion of body casting should be reviewed since the use of a body brace allowing increased mobility is now more common.

Videocassette: 18 minutes

Distributor: University of Michigan Medical Center Media Library

ANSWERS TO PRETEST

1. periosteum
2. epiphyses
3. diaphysis, epiphysis
4. ossification
5. epiphyseal plate
6. calcium, phosphate
7. hard, rigid
8. fontanels
9. body, processes
10. spinous processes
11. manubrium, body, xiphoid process
12. ulnar, radius
13. olecranon process of the ulnar
14. ilium, ischium, pubis
15. ATP, creatine phosphate, carbohydrate metabolism

PRETEST: STRUCTURE AND FUNCTION OF MUSCULOSKELETAL SYSTEM

1. The tough connective tissue that covers the outer surface of most bones is called the ______________________.
2. Prior to puberty, lengthwise growth of bones occurs at the ______________________.
3. The shaft of long bones is called the ______________________, while the term for the ends is the ______________________.
4. Replacement of membranous tissue or cartilage by bone is called ______________________.
5. Lengthwise growth ceases when the ______________________ ______________________ closes.
6. A large portion of bone is made up of the inorganic salts ______________________ and ______________________.
7. The inorganic salts serve to make bones ______________________ and ______________________.
8. In the fetus and young infant, the cranial bones are separated by membranes called ______________________.
9. A vertebra is made up of a large rounded portion called the ______________________ and seven projections called ______________________.
10. The projections that can be felt when palpating the middle of the back are the ______________________.
11. The three portions of the sternum are the ______________________, ______________________, and ______________________.
12. The bones of the forearms are the ______________________ on the medial side and the ______________________ on the lateral side.
13. The elbow is formed by the ______________________.
14. The pelvic girdle is composed of three bones: the ______________________, ______________________, and ______________________.
15. The three sources of energy for muscle contraction are ______________________, ______________________, and ______________________.

CHAPTER 42

NEOPLASMS/CANCER

DISCUSSION QUESTIONS

1. How do malignant cells differ from normal cells with respect to structure and function?
2. How is the function of the immune system thought to influence growth of malignant tissue?
3. What is the process by which cancer cells spread through tissues of the body?
4. Provide explanations appropriate for a young child about the procedure for and the purpose of the following diagnostic studies: (a) bone marrow aspiration, (b) bone, liver–spleen scan, (c) ultrasound, (d) intravenous pyelogram, and (e) lymphangiogram.
5. How does radiotherapy reduce or destroy malignant tissues?
6. What are the properties of (a) cycling cells, (b) nondividing cells, (c) resting cells, and (d) stem cells?
7. How does each of the following forms of chemotherapeutic agents function and on what types of malignant cells are they most effective: (a) cell cycle specific and (b) cell cycle nonspecific?
8. Describe the action of the following classifications of chemotherapeutic agents: (a) alkylating agents, (b) alkaloids, (c) antimetabolites, (d) synthetic hormones, and (e) enzymes.
9. Why is combined chemotherapy treatment most effective in treating cancers?
10. What is the advantage of using a central venous access device for chemotherapy administration?
11. What is the purpose of a bone marrow transplant? What are the different types?
12. Explain the basis of *graft versus host disease (GVHD)*. What symptoms does the child with GVHD exhibit?
13. How can the nurse support the child and family during the diagnosis of cancer?
14. Identify children's reactions to treatments of cancer.
15. What are the five most commonly found late effects of therapeutic treatment for childhood cancers?
16. How is the *absolute neutrophil count (ANC)* determined? What information is obtained from the ANC value?
17. Explain the process of normal white blood cell production and maturation. How is this process defective in the child with leukemia?
18. What conditions place a child at greater risk for leukemia?
19. What is *pancytopenia?* Why is this condition often present in the child with leukemia?
20. Why is treatment for *acute lymphoblastic leukemia (ALL)* directed toward preventing a relapse?
21. Describe the following components of the treatment regimen for ALL: (a) induction, (b) CNS prophylaxis and consolidation, and (c) maintenance.
22. Identify nursing diagnoses and the related nursing interventions for the child with ALL.

23. What is the incidence of testicular leukemia? What symptoms does the child with testicular leukemia exhibit? How is this form of malignancy treated?
24. Why is early diagnosis of brain tumors in children often difficult?
25. What modalities are used in the treatment of brain tumors in children?
26. What factors influence the effectiveness of chemotherapy as a component in the treatment of brain tumors?
27. Why is it important to monitor for increased intracranial pressure postoperatively for a child who has undergone an excision of a posterior fossa brain tumor? Identify nursing interventions to prevent increased intracranial pressure.
28. Explain why the child with an infratentorial brain tumor is often positioned lying flat after surgery, while the child who has had surgery for supratentorial tumor is positioned with the head elevated.
29. Describe the site where found and the treatment for the following types of brain tumors: (a) medulloblastoma, (b) cerebellar astrocytoma, (c) brain stem tumor, (d) cerebral astrocytoma, (e) optic pathway tumor, and (f) optic nerve glioma.
30. Rhabdomyosarcoma is a malignancy of which type of tissues? Where are the common sites for this form of malignancy?
31. What forms of treatment are available for the child with *osteogenic sarcoma?* What factors influence treatment choice?
32. What role does citrovorum play in the treatment of osteogenic sarcoma?
33. What are the common sites for *Ewing's sarcoma?*
34. What are some of the adverse effects of radiotherapy for the treatment of Ewing's sarcoma?
35. What is the typical history of the child diagnosed with *Wilms' tumor?*
36. Describe the characteristic findings in each of the four stages of Wilms' tumor.
37. What priority nursing care strategies are there for the child with Wilms' tumor (a) preoperatively and (b) postoperatively? What is the rationale for each strategy?
38. Which structures are involved in the malignancy of *Hodgkin's disease?*
39. What typical clinical manifestations are exhibited by the individual with Hodgkin's disease?
40. How is staging used in the diagnosis of Hodgkin's disease?
41. What is the rationale of the following measures for the child undergoing treatment for non-Hodgkin's lymphoma: (a) assess kidney function and (b) ensure adequate hydration?
42. *Neuroblastoma* is a malignancy of the cells of the neural crest and adrenal gland. Where are these structures located, and how does their location relate to the symptoms exhibited?
43. How is neuroblastoma diagnosed? What is its treatment?
44. Explain the etiology of the development of *retinoblastoma.*
45. Explain the mechanisms involved in the extension tumor cells in retinoblastoma.
46. What is the etiology of the cat's eye reflex observed in the child with retinoblastoma?

CASE STUDY

Nine-year-old Cheryl is brought to the pediatrician with a 3 week history of pallor, fever, and malaise. Today her mother noted bruises on Cheryl's arms and legs. Also, Cheryl has noted that when she brushes her teeth, her gums bleed. On examination, the physician notes that Cheryl's liver and spleen are enlarged and that she complains of generalized body aches. A complete blood count indicates hemoglobin at 6.8, a hematocrit of 28%, and a white blood count of 100,000 with 95% blasts. Cheryl is admitted to the hospital with the tentative diagnosis of acute lymphoblastic leukemia (ALL).

What factors will influence Cheryl's prognosis for long-term remission? What is the basis for Cheryl's fever, bruising and bleeding, body aches, and enlarged liver and spleen?

Cheryl is scheduled for a bone marrow aspiration. How best can the nurse prepare Cheryl and her family for this procedure?

After the diagnosis of ALL is confirmed, Cheryl is started on the induction phase of treatment. Which drugs are typically a component of this stage of therapy and what are their major side effects? What nursing strategies are important for the child undergoing induction therapy?

STUDENT LEARNING ACTIVITIES

1. Construct teaching sheets that can be given to families with children on the different chemotherapeutic agents. Include the signs of toxicity to watch for and report, management of side effects, and dosage schedules.
2. Construct drug cards for the commonly used chemotherapeutic agents. Include drug action, side effects, pertinent nursing strategies, and teaching needs of parents and child.
3. Ask students to attend a support group for families of children with cancer. What are common fears, concerns, and problems expressed by families? How does the group assist families in coping with the stress of having a child with a malignancy?

AUDIOVISUAL RESOURCES

1. **Camp Star Trails: Just Like Other Kids**
   This program offers an explanation of the summer camp for children with cancer at the University of Texas M. D. Anderson Cancer Center.

Videocassette: 24 minutes

Distributor: M. D. Anderson Cancer Center

2. **Caring for the Myelosuppressed Child**
   This program details the cellular alterations and manifestations of myelosuppresion in children receiving chemotherapy. Transfusion therapies and nursing strategies for different types of treatment, management, support, and evaluation of an affected child and family are discussed. This is a comprehensive program that includes a study guide.

Videocassette: 28 minutes

Distributor: American Journal of Nursing Company

3. **Coping with Cancer**
   This four-part series details the developmental coping responses of children with cancer and their siblings. Strategies for nurses to use to promote understanding, reduce fear and anxiety, and facilitate coping with cancer experiences and sequelae are included. In the early school-age program, children are shown acting out their feelings in play therapy. Middle school-age children are filmed in a therapeutic group setting where they discuss their feelings about cancer, pain, fear, hair loss, returning to school, dealing with friends, overprotective parents and teachers, and maintaining independence. Siblings are shown discussing the changes in their lifestyles and their feelings experienced during their sibling's treatment for cancer.

Videocassette: 20–37 minutes each part

Distributor: American Journal of Nursing Company

4. **Julie and John**
   In this program, two terminally ill teenagers with cancer reveal their thoughts and feelings from different perspectives. Julie is shown in a music video she developed in which she chronicles the events of her illness. The portion of the program concerning John is a series of edited tapes that he recorded as a permanent and private legacy for his family. Viewer discretion is advised due to the poignant nature of the subject and the tone and concept of the presentation.

Videocassette: 35 minutes

Distributor: Health Sciences Consortium

5. **I'm Still the Same Person: Teenagers with Cancer**
   This program presents interviews with two adolescents, Jenny, diagnosed with osteogenic sarcoma resulting in a leg amputation, and Bob, diagnosed with Hodgkin's disease. The adolescents discuss their views about family and friends' responses to their illnesses, hospitalization experiences, effects of chemotherapy, adjustments to the diagnosis and treatment of cancer, and their plans for the future.

Videocassette: 29 minutes

Distributor: University of Michigan Medical Center, Media Library

6. **Only One Road: Three Families Coping with Childhood Cancer**
   Interviews are presented with three children and their families who are past the initial stages of diagnosis and treatment of cancer. A special focus of this program is discussion of the problems that occur outside the hospital or treatment setting. A program guide is available that contains a summary, objectives, discussion questions for parents and health professionals, and recommended readings.

Videocassette: 53 minutes

Distributor: University of Michigan Medical Center, Media Library

STUDENT WORKSHEET: PEDIATRIC CANCERS

Cancer	Clinical Manifestations	Rationale	Therapeutic Management
Acute lymphoblastic leukemia			
Brain tumors			
Neuroblastoma			
Retinoblastoma			
Rhabdomyosarcoma			

(Continued)

(Student Worksheet continued)

Cancer	Clinical Manifestations	Rationale	Therapeutic Management
Osteogenic sarcoma			
Ewing's sarcoma			
Wilms' tumor			
Hodgkin's disease			
Non-Hodgkin's lymphoma			

CHAPTER 43

ALTERED ENDOCRINE FUNCTION

DISCUSSION QUESTIONS

1. How does *growth hormone deficiency* influence the pattern of growth?
2. Why does the child with growth hormone deficiency experience difficulties in blood glucose maintenance?
3. What are the components of screening and definitive testing for growth hormone deficiencies?
4. What are the nursing responsibilities for the child with growth hormone deficiency during the time of (a) assessment and (b) treatment?
5. What psychosocial problems can the child with growth hormone deficiency experience? What approaches are best for dealing with these problems?
6. What characteristic findings are consistent with *diabetes insipidus* with respect to (a) urine specific gravity, (b) serum sodium, and (c) serum osmolality? What is the basis for these findings?
7. What is the objective of water deprivation tests? What result would be consistent with the diagnosis of diabetes insipidus?
8. What is the role of DDAVP in the treatment of diabetes insipidus? Outline the instructions that would be provided to the family who will be administering DDAVP at home?
9. Describe the process of normal pubertal development. How is this process altered in *precocious puberty?*
10. What are the common causes of precocious puberty?
11. Describe the pharmacological management of precocious puberty.
12. What is the normal function of the hormones affected by *adrenal hypoplasia (CAH)?* What are the clinical manifestations exhibited by the child with CAH, and what is the basis for these manifestations?
13. What is the rationale for the use of corticosteroids in treating CAH?
14. What are the signs and symptoms of acute adrenal insufficiency?
15. What factors can precipitate an adrenal crisis? What is the therapeutic management of these crises?
16. What is the etiology of Cushing disease? What clinical findings are associated with this disease?
17. Adrenal tumors typically produce what types of clinical manifestations? Why?
18. Why does the child with pheochromocytoma experience tachycardia and hypertension?
19. What findings in the neonatal period are typical of infants with *congenital hypothyroidism?*
20. What signs indicate excessive levothyroxine dosage in infants who are receiving the drug for congenital hypothyroidism?
21. What are the causes of acquired hypothyroidism?
22. Why does the child with *Graves disease* exhibit increased appetite along with weight loss, heat intolerance, and nervousness?
23. What are options for the treatment of Graves disease?

24. What are the indications of hypocalcemia after surgery for Graves disease? Why does thyroid surgery place a child at risk for hypocalcemia?
25. What are the manifestations of parathyroid hormone deficiency, and what is the rationale for these manifestations?
26. What are the nursing responsibilities for the child experiencing an episode of acute hypocalcemia?
27. What findings are consistent with the diagnosis of ambiguous genitalia?
28. What are the etiology of and clinical manifestations and treatment for (a) premature thelarche and (b) gynecomastia?
29. What are the typical causes of hypoglycemia in the (a) newborn, (b) infant, and (c) young child?
30. What are the current research findings regarding the etiology of type I diabetes mellitus?
31. Explain the role of glucose in the body. How does insulin relate to glucose function?
32. What are the classic symptoms associated with *diabetes mellitus*? What is the basis for these symptoms?
33. Explain the etiology of the acidosis and accumulation of ketone bodies in the process of ketoacidosis.
34. Describe the clinical manifestations consistent with the following stages of diabetes mellitus: (a) ketoacidosis, (b) ketosis, and (c) hyperglycemia. What nursing strategies are appropriate for each stage?
35. The therapeutic approach for the child with diabetes mellitus is focused toward meeting what three goals?
36. For the child with insulin-dependent diabetes mellitus, identify nursing diagnoses relating to (a) metabolic control, (b) psychosocial impact of the disease, and (c) self-care management.
37. How does exercise influence glucose metabolism?
38. What are the limitations in the use of urine testing to monitor glucose levels?
39. Why is blood glucose testing a more effective method for evaluating glucose levels?
40. Which sites are preferred for insulin administration? What areas should be avoided?
41. Describe the procedure for preparing and administering insulin.
42. What type of diet should the child with diabetes mellitus follow?
43. What is the rationale for encouraging children with diabetes mellitus to consume a high fiber diet?
44. What are the symptoms and treatment of (a) hypoglycemia and (b) hyperglycemia?
45. Why does the diabetic child experience hyperglycemia with episodes of infection?
46. Describe the nursing care of an adolescent in *diabetic ketoacidosis (DKA)*.
47. Describe the etiology and management of the following long-term complications of diabetes mellitus: (a) atherosclerosis, (b) retinopathy, (c) kidney infections and nephropathy, and (d) neuropathy.
48. What factors influence the level of compliance to therapy by the diabetic child and his family?

CASE STUDY

Linda, age 9 years, is admitted to the hospital for evaluation of an 8-week history of weight loss, excessive thirst, and frequent urination with bed wetting. Linda is found to be in the diabetic ketosis stage. She will receive a combination of regular and NPH insulin. Outline the medical and nursing management appropriate for this stage. How would you explain the cause of Linda's weight loss, thirst, and frequent urination to Linda and her parents?

Explain the rationale for the combination of regular and NPH insulin, and the time of onset and duration of action of each type of insulin.

Construct a teaching plan for Linda and her family. Include information about the disease, insulin administration and action, diet, and identification and management of hypoglycemia and hyperglycemia. What other information is important to include in the teaching plan?

What specific concerns about the diagnosis of diabetes would be consistent with Linda's developmental level? What actions by the nurse could help Linda adjust to her disease?

STUDENT LEARNING ACTIVITIES

1. Have students role play the nurse's role in caring for the infant with ambiguous genitalia. How should the nurse respond to the following questions: (a) siblings, relatives, and friends who ask if the child is a boy or girl; and (b) the parent who asks, "What's wrong with my baby?"
2. Assign students to care for children with diabetes mellitus. Have students assess the child's knowledge about diabetes management and compliance to the therapeutic regimen. Students should develop and implement a teaching plan for any identified learning needs.
3. Ask students to interview nurses about teaching the child with a new diagnosis of diabetes mellitus and her family. What information is included? How is information presented? How is learning evaluated?

AUDIOVISUAL RESOURCES

1. **Evaluation of the Child with Small Stature**
   This film describes the use of growth charts, history, and physical examination and diagnostic tests for evaluation of small stature in children. Common syndromes of growth disorders are also reviewed. This is a medically oriented program and may only be useful for illustration of diagnostic procedures and criteria.

Videocassette: 27 minutes

Distributor: University of Michigan Medical Center Media Library

2. **Detecting Diabetes**
   This program profiles and 11-year-old child with insulin-dependent diabetes mellitus. The program discusses the etiology, pathophysiology, clinical manifestations, and management of this form of diabetes.

Videocassette: 19 minutes

Distributor: Film for the Humanities & Sciences

3. **Diabetic Emergencies**
   This program compares and contrasts two kinds of diabetic emergencies: diabetic coma and insulin shock. Signs of symptoms and emergency care for both are discussed.

Videocassette: 15 minutes

Distributor: Films for the Humanities & Sciences

4. **Listen to the Kids—Adolescents Talk about Diabetes**
   This program is designed to help health professionals and parents understand the special problems facing the adolescent with a chronic illness such as diabetes. Interviews with adolescents about how diabetes affects their lives are included.

Videocassette: 15 minutes

Distributor: University of Michigan Medical Center Media Library

5. **Diabetes Ketoacidosis: Management in Children**
   The incidence, pathophysiology, clinical manifestations, and treatment of diabetic ketoacidosis in children are described in this program. Precipitating factors are outlined and suggestions for prevention are stressed. A case study is used to illustrate management principles. This program is oriented toward the physician but is valuable for nursing students as well.

Slide/tape or videotransfer: 27 minutes

Distributor: University of Michigan Medical Center Media Library

6. **Amy—An Adolescent with Diabetes**
This program identifies problems frequently seen in the adolescent who has diabetes, including noncompliance, lack of knowledge, rebellion, family conflicts, and lack of independence. An interdisciplinary approach is demonstrated as valuable in assessment and intervention for promoting self-care, responsibility, and a positive lifestyle. This is a good film for illustrating the team approach and nursing care strategies for the adolescent with diabetes.

Slide/tape: 15 minutes

Distributor: University of Michigan Medical Center Media Library

7. **Diabetic Care Series**
This is an twelve-part series covering issues and concerns related to diabetes. Several programs may be useful in pediatric nursing: (1) Listen to Your Body: Hypoglycemia and Hyperglycemia; (2) Your Child and Diabetes; (3) The Insulin Pump: A New Option in Diabetes Management; (4) Type 1 Diabetes: One Man's Story as Student, Husband, Father; (5) You're in Control; and (6) Insulin Use and Management.

Videocassette or 16 mm film: 18–40 minutes each part

Distributor: Medcom/Trainex

8. **Survival Skills for Diabetic Children**
This program prepares nurses in helping children with diabetes to develop the necessary survival skills of proper nutrition, blood glucose monitoring, maintaining normal blood sugar levels, insulin administration, and understanding diabetic emergencies.

Videocassette: 28 minutes

Distributor: American Journal of Nursing Company

ANSWERS TO PRETEST

1. e, increases available glucose for energy
2. g, growth and function male reproductive system, stimulates synthesis of bone and muscle
3. f, growth and function of female sex characteristics
4. a, stimulate water reabsorption by the kidneys
5. e, promotes transport glucose, amino acids, fatty acids from blood into cells; enhances synthesis glycogen from glucose
6. d, electrolyte and water balance, blood pressure regulation
7. b, regulates metabolism
8. b, calcium and phosphorus metabolism
9. a, stimulates production of glucocorticoids, utilization of amino acids and glucose by muscle cells
10. a, stimulates bone and soft tissue growth
11. d, inhibits inflammatory responses, conserves glucose supplies
12. target cells
13. adrenal glands, sodium, potassium
14. insulin, glucagon

PRETEST: STRUCTURE AND FUNCTION OF ENDOCRINE SYSTEM

For each of the hormones in questions 1–11, give (A) the letter of the site of production from the list at the bottom (a–g) and (B) the function(s) of the hormone.

1. Glucagon

   A. _______

   B. ______________________________

   ____

2. Androgens

   A. _______

   B. ______________________________

   ____

3. Estrogen

   A. _______

   B. ______________________________

   ____

4. Antidiuretic hormone

   A. _______

   B. ______________________________

   ____

5. Insulin

   A. _______

   B. ______________________________

   ____

6. Mineralocorticoids

   A. _______

   B. ______________________________

   ____

7. Thyroxine

   A. _______

   B. ______________________________

   ____

8. Calcitonin

   A. _______

   B. ______________________________

   ____

9. Adrenocorticotropic hormone

   A. _______

   B. ______________________________

   ____

10. Growth hormone

    A. _______

    B. ______________________________

    ____

11. Glucocorticoids

    A. _______

    B. ______________________________

    ____

---

a. pituitary gland
b. thyroid gland
c. parathyroid gland
d. adrenal gland
e. pancreas
f. ovary
g. testes

(Continued)

(Pretest continued)

12. Although hormones reach all tissues of the body, they produce an effect on only specific structures called ____________________.

13. Aldosterone, a hormone secreted by the ____________________ assists with fluid and electrolyte balance by stimulating reabsorption of ____________________ and excretion of ____________________.

14. A rise in blood glucose levels stimulates the release of the pancreatic hormone ____________________, while a drop in blood glucose stimulates the release of ____________________.

CHAPTER 44

ALTERED METABOLIC FUNCTION

DISCUSSION QUESTIONS

1. What is the biochemistry associated with inborn errors of metabolism?
2. How is genetics related to inherited metabolic disorders?
3. What are the principles of treatment for metabolic disease?
4. Describe the genetic inheritance pattern of *phenylketonuria (PKU).*
5. Describe the normal process of phenylalanine metabolism. How is this process altered in the child with PKU?
6. What is the most damaging result of untreated screening for PKU?
7. What is the rationale for the timing of the screening for PKU?
8. How do the following forms of PKU differ: (a) atypical, (b) benign persistent, (c) biopterin cofactor defect, and (d) maternal?
9. Discuss dietary management of PKU for (a) infants and (b) young children. What foods must be avoided in the diet?
10. What is the basis for the maple sugar smell of the urine and the mental retardation exhibited by the child with *maple sugar urine disease (MSUD)?*
11. Why is the child with MSUD at risk for serious problems even during times of minor illness? What types of measures help to reduce serious responses to illness?
12. What is the etiology of pathophysiology for the group of disorders known as of *organic acidemias?*
13. What are the symptoms of *ornithine transcarbamylase (OTC) deficiency?*
14. What is the basic defect present in *galactosemia?*
15. What types of formulas are fed to the infant with galactosemia?
16. What is the etiology and pathophysiology of *medium-chain acyl-CoA dehydrogenase deficiency (MCADD)?*
17. What is the clinical presentation of MCADD?
18. What is the dietary management of MCADD?
19. Describe the typical physical appearance of the child with Hurler syndrome.
20. What actions by the nurse can facilitate family adaptation to the child with a metabolic disorder? What nursing interventions assist family understanding of the child's disease process?
21. What strategies can parents apply to get the cooperation and active participation of their child in adhering to dietary restrictions?

STUDENT LEARNING ACTIVITIES

1. Ask students to report on the various special formulas available for the infant with a metabolic disorder discussed in the text. How readily available are these formulas? What is their cost compared to regular infant formulas?

AUDIOVISUAL RESOURCES

1. **Hidden From View: PKU in the Teenager**
   The aim of this program is to answer adolescent's questions about phenylketonuria (PKU), including how this metabolic disease is acquired and how it affects the body. Emphasis is placed on decisions and lifestyle choices facing the adolescent with PKU, such as explaining PKU to friends, deciding whether to have children, and choosing a career.

Videocassette: 13 minutes

Distributor: University of Michigan Medical Center Media Library

ANSWERS TO PRETEST

1. chemical reactions within and outside of cells
2. catabolism, anabolism
3. metabolic
4. transformation, exchange
5. ATP
6. enzymes, coenzyme
7. glucose
8. amino acids
9. glycogen, fat
10. monosaccharides: glucose, fructose, galactose
11. disaccharides: maltose, sucrose, lactose
12. polysaccharides: cellulose, starch, glycogen

PRETEST: METABOLIC FUNCTION

1. Metabolism can be described as a process of ______________________________ ______________________________ ______________________________.

2. Metabolism consists of two phases: ______________________________, in which complex chemicals are broken down into simpler ones, and ______________________________, in which complex chemicals are built from simpler building blocks.

3. The end-product of each of the phases of metabolism is called a ______________________________.

4. The result of all metabolic reactions is either ______________________________ or ______________________________ of energy.

5. Energy resulting from the oxidation of food is not directly available to cells but is converted to ______________________ for energy supply.

6. Metabolic reactions necessary for body functions are catalyzed by substances called ______________________ or ______________________________.

7. The primary product of carbohydrate metabolism is ______________________.

8. The building blocks of proteins are the ______________________________.

9. Carbohydrates not used as energy are stored as ______________________ or ______________________________.

Carbohydrates can be grouped into three categories. Give these categories and an example of a substance in each.

10. Category: ______________________
Example: ______________________

11. Category: ______________________
Example: ______________________

12. Category: ______________________
Example: ______________________

Chapter 45

Sensory and Communication Alterations

DISCUSSION QUESTIONS

1. What is the current thought regarding the newborn's visual acuity? What developmental factors are related to infant visual acuity?
2. What are the characteristics of vision development from birth to 3 years of age?
3. What is the rationale for the current use of erythromycin rather than silver nitrate drops in the eyes of the newborn?
4. What behaviors may alert the nurse that a young child is experiencing reduced visual acuity?
5. Explain the processes of refraction, accommodation, and convergence.
6. What is the basis for the following types of refractive errors and what alteration in visual acuity does each produce: (a) hyperopia, (b) myopia, and (c) astigmatism?
7. What is *strabismus?* What terms are used to describe strabismus?
8. How do the clinical manifestations of nonparalytic and paralytic strabismus differ?
9. Identify nursing diagnoses and interventions for the child with strabismus.
10. How do miotic preparations function in the treatment of strabismus?
11. What are the negative aspects of the use of miotic preparations for treating strabismus?
12. What is the rationale for patching an eye prior to corrective surgery for strabismus?
13. What diagnostic sign is indicative of *amblyopia?*
14. Describe the conditions that can cause amblyopia.
15. What assessment procedures are used to identify cataracts in infants?
16. Why is the surgical procedure used for adults with cataracts not used for children?
17. Explain the basis for the (a) increased intraocular pressure and (b) optic nerve atrophy produced by glaucoma.
18. What is the effect produced by goniotomy in treating glaucoma?
19. Why are mydriatic agents used after surgery for glaucoma?
20. What are the criteria for the following visual conditions: (a) blindness, (b) partial sight, (c) visual handicap, and (d) residual vision?
21. Why does the partially sighted child often exhibit (a) delayed mobility and (b) inattention and irritability?
22. Why are there potential problems related to parental attachment when an infant is blind?
23. What alterations in motor development are typical of blind infants? What activities can parents use to facilitate their blind infant's motor development?
24. How can socialization and play skills be promoted in blind children?
25. How does a hearing impairment affect (a) orientation responses, (b) vocalization, (c) visual attention, and (d) emotional and social behavior?

26. What is the basis for (a) central hearing losses and (b) peripheral hearing losses?
27. What high-risk factors are associated with hearing loss in infants?
28. How can hearing function be assessed in the following: (a) newborns and young infants, (b) toddlers and preschoolers, and (c) school age children?
29. What are the benefits of promoting the *total communication method* for deaf children?
30. How is speech–language impairment defined according to the Education of All Handicapped Children Act?
31. Why do children exhibit stuttering during the toddler to preschool years?
32. Describe receptive and expressive language development at 12 months, 18 months, and 24 months of age.
33. Identify signs of language and speech problems in young children.
34. How does normal nonfluency differ from stuttering?
35. What can the nurse teach parents about facilitating the child's language development?

CASE STUDY

Danny, age 4 years, has been profoundly deaf since birth. He is admitted to the hospital for a cervical abscess that is to be surgically drained. What difficulties might Danny experience adapting to the hospital setting and the other children? How can the nurse facilitate his adjustment? What information gathered during the nursing history can help plan Danny's adjustment to the hospital experience?

What aspects of the operating room experience will most likely induce anxiety for Danny?

Construct a plan for preparing Danny for medical procedures such as drawing blood, insertion of the IV, blood pressure monitoring, and the operating room experience.

STUDENT LEARNING ACTIVITIES

1. Visit a school for the visually or hearing impaired child. What difficulties did the teacher experience maintaining student attention? What is an explanation for the student behaviors observed? How did the teacher structure her teaching to compensate for the student's sensory deficits?
2. Ask students to prepare a program for preparing a blind child and a deaf child for the hospital experience. On which senses did the students focus their teaching to compensate for the hearing or visual deficit?

AUDIOVISUAL RESOURCES

1. Can Your Patient Hear?
This program teaches screening techniques for potential hearing impairments in children up to the age of 6 years. Simple questions, anatomical and physical indicators, and conversational techniques for use with children during a routine history and physical examination are described as they relate to assessment of speech, language, and hearing. This film is valuable for illustration of assessment criteria for detection of hearing impairment.

Videotape: 32 minutes

Distributor: Health Sciences Consortium

2. Children and Deafness
This three-part series focuses on the needs of families with children who have profound hearing loss. Family reactions at the time of diagnosis through acceptance are explored. Options for testing, treatment, education, and systems of communications are described, including the use of hearing aids. This comprehensive program is valuable for enhancing student sensitivity and knowledge about the impact and assessment of children with hearing alterations and their families.

Videotape: 30 minutes each

Distributor: Pyramid Film and Video

3. **Language and Hearing Impaired Children**
This film explains the difference between normal language development and language development in the child who is hearing impaired. Vignettes of children in learning situations are used to describe a total communication approach to promote language, social, and motor development in children with alterations in hearing ability. This program is clearly illustrated and contains both simple and complex strategies useful for the student working with such children and their families.

Videocassette: 15 minutes

Distributor: Health Sciences Consortium

4. **Crossing the Silence Barrier**
This program examines technological advances the help the hearing disabled, including a system that enables a deaf person to see another's sign language over the telephone and speech recognition and synthesis, which will permit total communication between the deaf and the hearing.

Videocassette: 26 minutes

Distributor: Films for the Humanities & Sciences

5. **Strabismus and Amblyopia**
This program describes the physiological processes of how the retina perceives an image and how both eyes work to produce a binocular image. Deviations in the optical system that inhibit fusion (strabismus) are discussed. Diagnostic tests and management are identified. This program is directed toward a physician or medical student audience.

Slide/tape: 15 minutes

Distributor: University of Michigan Medical Center, Media Library

ANSWERS TO PRETEST

1. sclera, cornea
2. focus light rays
3. choroid, ciliary body, iris
4. iris
5. cones, rods
6. cones
7. fovea centralis
8. vitreous humor, aqueous humor
9. near and far vision
10. transparency, elasticity
11. malleus, incus, stapes
12. conduct sound into inner ear
13. eustachian tubes
14. tympanic membrane
15. hearing, equilibrium

PRETEST: STRUCTURE AND FUNCTION OF THE EYE AND EAR

1. The outer layer of the eye consists of the ______________________ and ______________________.
2. The major function of the cornea is to ______________________.
3. The middle or vascular layer of the eye contains the ______________________, ______________________, and ______________________.
4. The structure regulating the amount of light that enters the eye is called the ______________________.
5. The retina contains two types of photoreceptor cells: the ______________________, which function in night vision, and the ______________________, which function in bright light and color vision.
6. The photoreceptor cells responsible for visual acuity are the ______________________.
7. The ______________________ is the portion of the retina where the sharpest visual images are transmitted.
8. The posterior cavity of the eye contains a jelly-like substance called ______________________, while the anterior cavity contains a watery fluid called ______________________.
9. The lens of the eye functions to focus light rays for ______________________.
10. The properties of the lens that are necessary for optimal function are ______________________ and ______________________.
11. The three bones of the middle ear that form the auditory ossicles are the ______________________, ______________________, and ______________________.
12. The function of the ossicles is to ______________________.
13. The middle ear is connected to the nasopharynx by the ______________________.
14. The ______________________ separates the outer and middle ear.
15. The inner ear contains structures for the functions of ______________________ and ______________________.

CHAPTER 46

THE INJURED CHILD

DISCUSSION QUESTIONS

1. What developmental differences are related to the child's respiratory responses to injury, his circulatory responses to injury, and his thermal regulatory responses to injury?
2. What anatomical characteristics of children are related to the location of injuries?
3. Describe the processes of performing (a) a primary survey and (b) a secondary survey on an injured child.
4. What is the objective of *triage?* What is included in a triage assessment?
5. What event usually precedes most cardiac arrests in children? How does this factor influence preventive actions?
6. What are the current guidelines for managing airway obstruction in children?
7. What information would the nurse give to parents about caring for cuts, scrapes, and puncture wounds?
8. What is the immediate care for a child who has sustained a snake bite?
9. What are the guidelines regarding closure of dog bite wounds?
10. What is the major risk after a human bite?
11. How does cold cause tissue damage? What are the degrees of frostbite?
12. What information can children and parents receive that can help prevent frostbite?
13. Describe the process of rewarming after frostbite. What is the rationale of this form of treatment?
14. Explain the measures that should be instituted after a child has knocked out a permanent tooth.
15. Explain the rationale of the following nursing strategies for the child experiencing epistaxis: (a) keep firm pressure over nostrils, (b) position sitting with head tilted forward, (c) encourage to spit out rather than swallow blood, and (d) use humidified air during sleep.
16. What are the symptoms exhibited by the child who has a foreign body in the (a) larynx, (b) trachea, and (c) bronchi?
17. After removal of a foreign body, what signs would indicate to the nurse that the child is experiencing a secondary obstruction? What is the cause of secondary obstruction?
18. What is the procedure for removing live insects from a child's ear?
19. Why are miniature batteries a special hazard when placed by a child in her ear?
20. Describe the immediate management of the following types of poisonings (a) ocular, (b) topical, and (c) inhalation.
21. What measures are used in the treatment of ingested poisons to achieve the following goals: (a) decreasing absorption and (b) hastening elimination?
22. Describe the pathophysiology of *salicylate poisoning.*

23. What clinical manifestations would the nurse expect to observe in a child who has ingested a toxic dose of salicylates?
24. Why are the following measures important when caring for the child experiencing salicylate poisoning: (a) reduce fever gradually and (b) test urine pH?
25. What organ is primarily affected in acetaminophen poisoning?
26. How does mucomyst function in acetaminophen ingestion?
27. What is the recommended therapeutic management of (a) corrosive substances and (b) hydrocarbon substances?
28. How does diet relate to lead absorption?
29. What are the primary sources of the lead responsible for lead poisoning in children?
30. In what organs does lead produce the most toxic effects?
31. Explain the process by which the drugs BAL and CaEDTA remove lead from the blood and tissues.
32. Identify nursing actions for the child receiving chelation therapy which help to (a) relieve discomfort from frequent injections and (b) maintain fluid balance and renal flow.
33. What common residual effects can result from lead poisoning?
34. How do the following factors relate to the prognosis of a near-drowning victim: (a) age of the child and (b) temperature of the water?
35. Describe nursing care for the child who has had a submersion injury.

CASE STUDY

Brittany, age 3 years, is brought to the Emergency Room by her father who reported that his daughter swallowed a great deal of baby aspirin. What information about the ingestion would the nurse gather from Brittany's father? What initial assessments would the nurse make about her condition?

What is the basis for respiratory alkalosis and metabolic acidosis by salicylate poisoning? What diagnostic procedures can identify the presence of salicylate ingestion? What is the emergency management of salicylate ingestion?

Identify nursing diagnoses for Brittany. Describe nursing care to (a) minimize physiologic injury and (b) maintain fluid balance. Develop a teaching plan for Brittany's family to prevent future ingestion of poisonous substances.

STUDENT LEARNING ACTIVITIES

1. Make assignments for students to spend a day in an emergency room. What were the most common injuries experienced by children seen in the emergency room? What was the nurse's primary role in this setting? Did students identify other roles that the nursing staff could have performed to meet the child's and family's needs? Does the emergency room have a triage system? Are nurses provided with clear criteria for assigning degree of urgency to illness and injury?
2. Are instructions available in your hospital for home care after treatment of the common forms of childhood injuries? Are the instructions complete, accurate, and clear? If such instructions are not available, ask students to prepare them.

AUDIOVISUAL RESOURCES

1. **Pediatrics Physical Care: Evaluating Children**
   The focus of this program is an interview with Mary Fran Hazinski about the nurse's role in obtaining baseline data and recognizing early and late signs of physiological distress. Also discussed are the three important complications of illness and injury-poor systemic perfusion, respiratory distress, and alterations in consciousness.

Videotransfer: 20 minutes

Distributor: Concept Media

2. **The ABC's of Pediatric Trauma Nursing**
   This program offers a systematic approach to assessment and stabilization of the child with multiple injuries and includes an actual case vignette. The needs of pediatric trauma victims are differentiated from the adult, with emphasis on pharmacological and psychosocial considerations.

Videocassette: 28 minutes

Distributor: American Journal of Nursing Company

3. **Pediatric Mock Code**
   This videotape demonstrates two simulated pediatric codes. The first shows everything that can go wrong when personnel are not prepared or do not follow procedures properly. The second simulation gives a clear picture of how to respond to a pediatric code, showing how smoothly an arrest can be handled when the proper steps are taken.

Videocassette: 28 minutes

Distributor: Health Sciences Consortium

Chapter 47

The Child with Burns

DISCUSSION QUESTIONS

1. What factors are associated with a high incidence of burns?
2. What physiological changes occur in the following body systems as a result of a burn injury: skin, respiratory, metabolic, gastrointestinal, and tissue and fluid balance?
3. What are the clinical manifestations of (a) inhalation injuries and (b) skin injuries in the burned child?
4. Describe the four categories of diagnostic assessment for the burned child.
5. In assessing the severity of a burn, how does one determine (a) the extent of the burn and (b) the depth of burn.
6. What are the criteria needed for a burn to be assessed as (a) a minor burn and (b) a major burn?
7. What are the three stages of therapeutic management of the child with burns? What are the goals for each phase?
8. How is *hypovolemia* treated? What is the guideline for fluid resuscitation in the infant and child?
9. What are the nursing responsibilities for the burned child undergoing fluid resuscitation?
10. Identify nursing actions to promote effective breathing patterns and gas exchange for the child with burns.
11. Describe interventions for the initial management of burn wounds.
12. Describe the management of major burn wounds.
13. Why is nutrition an important component in the care of a burned child? Identify nursing actions to promote nutrition for a child with major burns.
14. How is the burned child's pain managed?
15. How can the nurse help the child with burns cope with changes in body image as a result of a burn injury?
16. What two major considerations are the focus of the rehabilitative period after the burn injury?
17. When would the child's burn injuries be evaluated for indications of child abuse?

CASE STUDY

Casey, age 4 years, is brought into the emergency room after his clothes caught fire while he was playing with matches. He has second- and third-degree burns covering the entire anterior portion of his chest and abdomen, shoulders, upper arms, and both hands. Assessment reveals no burns about the face or any respiratory distress. Casey is stabilized in the emergency room and then transferred to the burn unit.

How would Casey's burns be classified? What assessments would the nurse make about: (a) burn wounds, (b) respiratory status, (c) fluid and electrolyte balance, (d) gastrointestinal function, (e) metabolic requirements, and (f) nutritional needs? How are Casey's fluid needs determined in the emergent phase?

A foley catheter is inserted. The urine obtained is black in appearance. What does the black urine indicate? What measures would the nurse expect to initiate after notifying the physician?

Considering the extent and distribution of Casey's burns, construct a list of actual and potential nursing diagnoses that would be appropriate for Casey. What nursing actions are pertinent for each identified diagnosis?

After 5 days, Casey's condition is improved and daily burn care is instituted. What measures can the nurse apply to help minimize Casey's discomfort during his wound care? In what position should Casey be placed to prevent skeletal deformities?

STUDENT LEARNING ACTIVITIES

1. Arrange for students to observe the care of children with burn injuries at a burn center. Ask students to describe (a) the treatments they observed, (b) nursing care of the child with burn injuries, (c) children's reactions to treatments, and (d) their personal reactions to this observational experience.

AUDIOVISUAL RESOURCES

1. **Emergency Management of Acute Burns**
   This program explains what the nurse must consider in the management of burn patients. Burn categories and classifications are discussed. Also addressed are fluid replacement as well as therapeutic measures.

Videocassette: 57 minutes

Distributor: Health Sciences Consortium

Audiovisual Resource Guide

Altschul Group Corporation
Health and Safety Division
1560 Sherman Avenue, Suite 100
Evanston, Illinois 60201
(708) 328-6700 or (800) 421-2363
Fax: (708) 328-6706

American Journal of Nursing Company
555 West 57th Street
New York, New York 10019-2961
(212) 582-8820
Fax: (212) 586-5462

American Lung Association
1740 Broadway
New York, New York 10019

Campus Film Distributors Corp.
24 Depot Square
Tuckahoe, New York 10707
(914) 961-1900

The Center for Humanities
Box 3000
Mount Kisco, New York 10549
(800) 431-2266

Concept Media
2493 Du Bridge Avenue
Irvine, California 92714
(714) 660-0727 or (800) 233-7078

Coronet/MTI Film & Video
108 Wilmot Road
Deerfield, Illinois 60015
(800) 621-2131
Fax: (708) 940-3640

Family Communications
Marketing Department
4802 Fifth Avenue
Pittsburg, Pennsylvania 15213
(412) 687-2990
Fax: (412) 687-1226

Filmakers Library
124 East 40th Street
New York, New York 10016
(212) 808-4980
Fax: (212) 808-4983

FilmFair Communications
A Division of the Altschul Group Corp.
Health and Safety Division
1560 Sherman Avenue, Suite 100
Evanston, Illinois 60201
(708) 328-6700 or (800) 421-2363
Fax: (708) 328-6706

Films for the Humanities & Sciences
P.O. Box 2053
Princeton, New Jersey 08543-2053
(800) 257-5126
Fax: (609) 452-1602

Health Sciences Consortium
Jack Adcox
201 Silver Cedar Court
Chapel Hill, North Carolina 27514-1517
(919) 942-8731
Fax: (919) 942-3689

Indiana University Audio-Visual Center
Bloomington, Illinois 47405-5901
(800) 552-8620 (outside Indiana)
(800) 942-0481 (in Indiana)

J. B. Lippincott Company
Department of Audiovisual Media
227 East Washington Square
Philadelphia, Pennsylvania 19106-3780
In Pennsylvania and Canada, call collect
(215) 238-4443
(800) 523-2945

MDA-TV
M. D. Anderson Cancer Center
1515 Holcombe Boulevard
Houston, Texas 77030
(713) 792-7287
Fax: (713) 794-1724

March of Dimes Birth Defects Foundation
1275 Mamaroneck Avenue
White Plains, New York 10605
(914) 428-7100

Medcom/Trainex
P.O. Box 3225
12601 Industry Street
Garden Grove, California 92641
(714) 891-1443 or (800) 877-1443

Meyer Rehabilitation Institute
University of Nebraska Medical Center
600 South 42nd Street
Omaha, Nebraska 68198-5450
(402) 559-7467
Fax: (402) 559-5737

Milner-Fenwick, Inc.
2125 Greenspring Drive
Timonium, Maryland 21903
(800) 432-8433
Fax: (410) 252-6316

National Audiovisual Center
8700 Edgeworth Drive
Capital Heights, Maryland 20743-3781
(301) 763-1891

Pyramid Film and Video
Box 1048
Santa Monica, California 90406
(213) 828-7577 or (800) 421-2304

University of Michigan Medical Center
Media Library
1327 Jones Drive
Ann Arbor, Michigan 48105-1899
(313) 998-6140

University of Minnesota
Media Distribution
Box 734 UMHC
420 Delaware Street SE
Minneapolis, Minnesota 55455
(612) 624-7906

Strategies for Clinical Instruction

INFORMATION TO GET FROM THE STUDENTS

1. Find out their past experiences with children, such as caring for younger siblings or babysitting. Students who have only minimal experiences will require more assistance and supervision in routine care activities such as holding and feeding infants.
2. Get their correct phone numbers. Often the number recorded in the school is the parent's home number. Ask students to be sure to give the number where you can reach them if the clinical experience is canceled.
3. Ask students prior to starting their rotation what their goals are related to the experience and how the instructor can assist them in meeting these goals.
4. The clinical agency may request specific health information from each student (such as dates of MMR and hepatitis B immunization).

INFORMATION TO PROVIDE TO THE STUDENTS

1. How can they reach you if they are ill or will be late arriving? Before what time must they call you in the morning? What is the telephone number that they can call at the hospital if they miss you at home? Must students make up clinical absences? What is the procedure for making up missed time? If weather is bad or you are going to cancel clinical for other reasons, set up a system where you call one student, who then calls the next, and on down the line. Then you won't need to personally call all students.
2. What are the dates and times for the clinical rotation? If the experience contains a mixture of days and evenings or weekends, make sure the students understand the schedule.
3. What are the guidelines of student attire? Jewelry such as dangling earrings should be discouraged. What attire is required when they visit the hospital to read their patient's chart prior to the clinical day? Name tags should be worn whenever students are on the hospital unit.
4. How are breaks and meals arranged? Can students bring lunch?
5. What time will the instructor have assignments made out? Does the unit have specific times when they ask students not to come to review charts, such as at report time?
6. When are written assignments related to clinical due? Be specific and consistent.
7. What constitutes a satisfactory clinical performance? Review clinical evaluation tools with students.

CLINICAL ORIENTATION TO THE UNIT: WHAT TO INCLUDE

1. Stress the need for safety. Include the following guidelines:
   a. Children wear slippers when they are out of bed.
   b. Crib side rails always completely up.
   c. Infants and toddlers restrained when in high chairs or strollers.
   d. Small children supervised at all times.
   e. Leave no small items within reach that an infant or small child could swallow or aspirate. Do not leave solutions such as alcohol or iodine at the bedside.
   f. Make sure infants are securely positioned in infant seats.
   g. Check temperature of warmed formula prior to feeding.
   h. Place infant on side or back after feedings; do not prop bottles.
2. Review the need for confidentiality. Students should not discuss their patients in public places, such as elevators. Provide guidelines regarding what is appropriate to discuss with the child's family.
3. Give students a tour of the unit or send students on a scavenger hunt of the unit. For the scavenger hunt, have pairs of students locate several different items and share their findings with the rest of the group. Suggestions for items to find on a scavenger hunt include
   a. restrooms for staff use
   b. location of student assignments
   c. linens
   d. crash cart
   e. nursing kardex(es) (where located and how divided)
   f. urine specimen container
   g. phone number(s) for the unit
4. Review patient charts and kardexes with students. If they are required to come to the unit on the day before clinical to gather information about their assigned patient(s), they will need to know where to find important information.
5. Provide students with the phone numbers for a code or fire. What is their role in each of these emergencies?
6. Tell students which occurrences they need to report immediately to the instructor or staff nurse. Students may not realize that they need to report that an infant refuses his bottle or that a child is febrile.
7. Review the general routine for patient care. Although patient needs will differ, all students should begin their shift with a patient assessment. Vital signs are done first. What are mealtimes on this unit? Also remind students to weigh patients before meals. To help students develop organizational skills, have them prepare a schedule for carrying out care. Review the schedules in conference. What measures need to be performed close to a specific schedule, and which can be performed whenever there is time?
8. What is the policy on administering medication? Can students give all types of drugs, including those administered intravenously? Are all drugs administered only with the instructor present?
9. Have students prepare drug cards on all the drugs ordered for their assigned patient. The student should include the specific reason that their patient is receiving the drug, rather than list all the uses of the drug. Is the drug dose appropriate for the child? Have students calculate safe dosages for all the drugs that they administer.
10. Go over the charting that is used on that unit. If the unit has sheets for charting IV infusions hourly, it helps the students to practice with these prior to using the sheets on the floor.
11. What should students include in their report to the nurse when they are leaving the floor for the day? Review the procedure for nurse's notes. Provide the students with a sample nurse's note. Do the students write the note on a piece of scrap paper to review with the instructor prior to placing it on the chart?

STUDENT PREPARATION FOR CLINICAL EXPERIENCES

Give clear instructions on how the students should prepare for the clinical experience. Providing students with the Clinical Preparation Worksheet (p. 192 in this manual) will help them to understand the type of information they need to gather and prepare for each clinical assignment. Practice in identifying information needed can be provided during the orientation. Examples of questions to give students include

a. Why is the child in the hospital? What events lead up to the hospitalization?

b. If you are assigned this patient tomorrow on the day shift, what medications and procedures will you be responsible for?

c. Find the procedure book and look up the procedure for nasogastric feeding and chest percussion.

d. What diet is the child on? What is the infant's feeding schedule?

Many more questions can be developed by reviewing the patient charts the day the students are present for orientation.

PROVIDING FOR STUDENT EXPERIENCES

Decide what types of experiences you want all the students to have. It usually is not possible to ensure that each student has identical types of patients or the opportunity to practice identical skills, but careful planning can provide all students with varied experiences. It may be possible to assign all students to patients

a. requiring complex care

b. for whom the focus is on family or patient teaching

c. experiencing an acute illness

d. experiencing a chronic illness

e. with whom developmental assessment skills are practiced,

f. requiring postoperative care

g. who have a running IV

h. receiving several drugs

i. on isolation.

APPLICATION OF CLASSROOM MATERIAL TO CLINICAL PRACTICE

Students can be required to perform an extensive assessment and develop a care plan on one specific child for whom they are assigned to provide nursing care. Other weeks, the students can be required to complete the Weekly Care Plan (p. 191 in this manual). The students are instructed that the Weekly Care Plan be done on the major focus of their care for that experience.

ONGOING EVALUATION

Offer students frequent feedback about the strengths and weaknesses of their clinical performance, including knowledge of pathophysiology or growth and development, skills in assessment, documentation, organization or communication, and nursing care plans.

Students can complete the Clinical Student Self-Evaluation (p. 194 in this manual) each week, which provides the instructor with information on the student's perception of their performance and learning.

CLINICAL PREPARATION WORKSHEET

Patient Name:

Age:

Date of Admission:

Surgical Procedures:

Chief Complaint:

Diagnostic Procedures:

Medical Diagnosis:

Diet:

Pertinent Laboratory Data:

Activity:

IV Therapy:

Medical Regimen: List treatments and current medications

Pathophysiology of Medical Diagnosis:

Clinical Manifestations: Underline signs and symptoms manifested by this patient

WEEKLY CARE PLAN

Name: ______________________________

Date: ______________________________

Nursing Diagnosis:

Assessment Data

Subjective:

Objective:

Outcomes	Nursing Strategies	Rationale	Evaluation

CLINICAL STUDENT SELF-EVALUATION

Name: ______________________________

Week Number: ______________________

Dates: ______________________________

For items 1–5, be sure to include those areas with which you are particularly pleased and those that you feel need improvement.

1. Interpersonal skills (with patients and their families, instructor, peers, and nurses on the unit):

2. Ability to identify priorities of care and organizational ability:

3. Performance of physical care and procedures:

(Continued)

(Clinical Student Self-Evaluation continued)

4. Ability to perform accurate physical, developmental, and family assessments

5. Demonstration of accountability (clinical preparation, reporting to pertinent people, participation in conference, and handing in assignments on time):

6. Identify methods through which your instructor can facilitate your learning (be specific):

7. Learning objectives for next week:

Test Items

INTRODUCTION

Evaluating nursing knowledge is a serious responsibility for nursing faculty. Evaluation means assessing the student's mastery of curriculum content, which ultimately ensures the safety of recipients of nursing care. This evaluation process includes assigning grades that accurately reflect the students' level of mastery of skills and knowledge. Testing is a vital part of the evaluation process. As most faculty agree, test construction is a time-consuming and arduous task for faculty and support staff. We hope this collection of approximately 700 test questions covering all 47 chapters of the Betz, Hunsberger, and Wright textbook will make the task of test construction more efficient and effective for all nursing faculty who use the book.

Rationales are given for the correct answer to each question. Also, the cognitive learning level is given for each question as knowledge, interpretation, or application, which are defined as follows:

- **Knowledge:** These questions test the student's recollection of facts, principles, theories, terms, or procedures; fact questions.
- **Interpretation:** These require the student to demonstrate some understanding or interpretation of the subject matter (to interpret, explain, distinguish, and/or predict). Within the context of this manual, these questions often require students to apply knowledge to a specific clinical situation.
- **Application:** These questions require students to synthesize pertinent information on a subject area and to demonstrate their understanding by making appropriate interpretations, judgments, or evaluation. Within this manual, application questions often present clinical situations in which students are required to make progressive decisions about nursing care

EXAMASTER

ExaMaster software is available to qualified adopters of *Family-Centered Nursing Care of Children*, second edition, for convenience in adapting the questions in this manual to your own curriculum needs. Contact your local W. B. Saunders representative or write on your school letterhead to

Textbook Department
W. B. Saunders Company
The Curtis Center
Independence Square West
Philadelphia, PA 19106-3399

CHAPTER 1

ITEM 1 Cognitive Type: Application

Knowledge of infant and child mortality and morbidity statistics assists the nurse in

a. recognizing changes in adaptation.

b. identifying age groups at risk for disease or injury.

c. developing a commitment to family advocacy.

d. alleviating parental anxiety about childhood illness.

ANSWER

b. The nurse can apply childhood disease statistics to the practice of health promotion and protection.

ITEM 2 Cognitive Type: Knowledge

Which of the following is the leading cause of death for children under 19 years of age?

a. Congenital anomalies

b. Diseases of the heart

c. Injuries

d. Malignant neoplasms

ANSWER

c. The nurse recognizes which problem causes the highest risk of mortality for children.

ITEM 3 Cognitive Type: Knowledge

Which of the following is the leading cause of hospitalization in the United States of children 1 to 9 years of age?

a. infectious diseases

b. diseases of the respiratory system

c. injuries

d. diseases of the heart

ANSWER

b. Respiratory system diseases lead the causes of hospitalization for ages 1 to 9 years, while injury is the leading cause for ages 10 to 14 years.

ITEM 4 Cognitive Type: Knowledge

Which of the following statements is true about the incidence of poverty in the United States?

a. People on welfare make up the majority of American poor.

b. Children living in poverty-level environments are provided with government support for adequate food and shelter.

c. The "working poor" are concentrated in central city areas.

d. The poorest age group in the American population is children.

ANSWER

d. The nurse can identify factual information regarding poverty statistics in the United States.

ITEM 5 Cognitive Type: Interpretation

Which of the following is a function of advocacy in pediatric nursing?

a. Assuming total responsibility for a hospitalized child's care.

b. Working with the family to obtain optimum services for a sick child.

c. Acting as a legal consultant for ethical decision making.

d. Expecting the well child to participate in self-care activities.

ANSWER

b. The nurse can distinguish which activity reflects responsibilities for advocacy in the care of children.

ITEM 6 Cognitive Type: Interpretation

Health teaching in pediatric nursing is primarily directed toward

a. facilitating the use of well child services.

b. meeting a criterion of professional nursing.

c. decreasing the cost of pediatric health care services.

d. assisting the child and family in applying health-promoting activities.

ANSWER

d. The nurse can distinguish the most important aspect of health teaching.

ITEM 7 Cognitive Type: Knowledge

Which of the following has had the most significant influence on infant and child health care?

a. Regulation of child labor laws

b. Scientific advances in the study of growth and development

c. Pasteurization of milk

d. Establishment of health maintenance organizations

ANSWER

b. Increasing knowledge about the physiology and psychology of childhood emphasizes the historical and societal changes contributing to the health care of children.

ITEM 8 Cognitive Type: Interpretation

Information about an infant's altered patterns of elimination communicated to the nurse by the mother would be included in the nursing process plan as

a. a potential problem statement.

b. objective assessment.

c. a defining characteristic of the problem.

d. subjective assessment.

ANSWER

d. The nurse recognizes subjective assessment as data supplied by another person and not directly observed by the nurse examiner.

ITEM 9 Cognitive Type: Interpretation

Which of the following should receive priority when implementing the care plan of an infant who requires gavage feedings at home?

a. Initiate a teaching schedule with the parents for instructions in gavage feeding procedures.

b. Demonstrate alternative oral stimulation techniques for the infant.

c. Meet with the family to ascertain their acceptance of the proposed plan.

d. Assess the family's cognitive and emotional ability to cope with the problem and carry out the plan.

ANSWER

c. The nurse recognizes that the first phase of implementation is to discuss with the family their perceptions and acceptance of the plan. This ensures cooperation and prevents value conflicts.

ITEM 10 Cognitive Type: Interpretation

Which of the following is the most effective means of evaluating the success of nursing strategies in pediatric practice?

a. Elicit feedback from the child and family.

b. Validate goal achievement through objective assessment.

c. Determine potential problem areas.

d. Explain the care plan to the family in simple terms.

ANSWER

a. The nurse recognizes that goal achievement is determined by child and family responses and outcomes that are best evaluated when input is given by the client.

ITEM 11 Cognitive Type: Interpretation

Consider the following nursing diagnosis: Activity intolerance related to discomfort associated with illness. The next step in the nursing process would be to

a. identify defining characteristics.

b. instruct in fatigue sparing activities.

c. assess the child's discomfort.

d. state expected outcomes.

ANSWER

a. The parts of a nursing diagnosis can be remembered with the acronym RRED: *r*esponse, *r*elated to risk, *e*tiologic factors, and *d*efining characteristics. Defining characteristics of each response are included in published lists of nursing diagnoses.

CHAPTER 2

ITEM 1 Cognitive Type: Knowledge

A limitation of examining the family from the developmental model is

a. the impact of society on the family is not included in this framework.

b. the model is based on the assumption of the nuclear family.

c. problems such as child abuse and neglect cannot be explained in this model.

d. changes in family patterns are linked to critical role transitions.

ANSWER

b. The nuclear family represents a small portion of American families. Societal trends are such that the emphasis on individual life span issues may not fit with the model of the family's lifestyle.

ITEM 2 Cognitive Type: Interpretation

Which of the following statements offers the best description of contemporary American families?

a. The nuclear family represents a minority of American families.

b. The majority of U.S. families consist of a breadwinner father and a homemaker wife and their children.

c. There is a move toward extended families.

d. A breakdown of the institution of the family is evidenced by an increase in single parent households.

ANSWER

a. The majority of American households no longer fit the nuclear family model.

ITEM 3 Cognitive Type: Knowledge

Which of the following statements is a basic assumption for nurses working with families?

a. The family must be actively involved in the plan of care.

b. Once a family understands their problems, change will occur.

c. The family may need help perceiving the reality of a situation.

d. The presence of psychosocial problems suggests that the family will require intervention.

ANSWER

a. A basic assumption about families is that they should be full participants in their care. Psychosocial problems may actually serve a positive family function.

ITEM 4 Cognitive Type: Interpretation

In the multidisciplinary approach to working with families at risk for health problems, the first person who has contact with the family should

a. arrange for the other team members to meet the family.

b. assist the family in identifying their needs.

c. contact community resources for the family.

d. conduct an in-depth assessment of family functioning.

ANSWER

b. The initial intervener should first identify the needs of the family with them. Then resources currently used by the family are identified.

ITEM 5 Cognitive Type: Application

A facilitative nursing intervention for an impoverished family whose 2-year-old child is noted to have small rodent bites is to

a. have the child admitted to the hospital to prevent additional neglect.

b. assist the family in contacting the housing authorities for home inspection and extermination.

c. make arrangements for the child to be placed in foster care until a home investigation is completed.

d. teach the family how to enclose the crib in mesh sheeting while projecting an air of sympathy toward their situation.

ANSWER

b. The nurse recognizes that intervening with families at risk includes a developmental role of educating about available resources and a facilitative role in assisting them to gain access to the services.

ITEM 6 Cognitive Type: Interpretation

The nurse elects to use the Family APGAR for collecting information from a family. This information will assist the nurse in determining

a. the specific types of communication problems the family is having.

b. the difficulties the family is having in allocating time for family functions.

c. the individuals in the family who may be dissatisfied with the way the family is functioning.

d. the specific ways that family members respond to the expression of emotion in the family.

ANSWER

c. The Family APGAR is a tool that can quickly measure a family's satisfaction with their general state of functioning.

ITEM 7 Cognitive Type: Knowledge

Which of the following types of information should be included in the construction of a genogram?

a. Children's health histories

b. Family relationships with community agencies

c. Indications of the quality of the parents' relationships with their family members

d. Indications of the quality of the family members' relationships with one another

ANSWER

a. The genogram provides an orderly way of organizing the family and their history so that the family and nurse can identify key association, such as the transfer of a specific disease or characteristic within the family.

CHAPTER 3

ITEM 1 Cognitive Type: Application

The nurse evaluates the developmental norms of a child based on

a. the chronological age of the child.

b. the family's perception of the child.

c. the individual behaviors of the child.

d. the physical appearance of the child.

ANSWER

c. The nurse knows that care should be based on the child's individual behavior rather than on his or her chronological age.

ITEM 2 Cognitive Type: Interpretation

Mary Jo, age 1 year, has learned how to hold and drink from her plastic cup. The nurse gives her a paper cup full of juice. Mary Jo holds on tightly and crushes it, spilling the juice. According to Piaget, this is an example of

a. assimilation.

b. accommodation.

c. equilibrium.

d. organization.

ANSWER

a. The nurse understands the meaning of assimilation, which is the process of allowing the individual to adapt to her environment through the use of already existing behaviors, in this case, holding a paper cup with as firm a grip as a plastic cup.

ITEM 3 Cognitive Type: Knowledge

The individual who has contributed most toward an understanding of cognitive development is

a. Alfred Bandura.

b. Sigmund Freud.

c. Erik Erikson.

d. Jean Piaget.

ANSWER

d. The nurse knows that Piaget developed a theory of cognitive development.

ITEM 4 Cognitive Type: Interpretation

The nurse notes that 3-month-old Andrew has been sucking his thumb periodically. This is an example of which of the following sensorimotor period behaviors?

a. Object permanence

b. Primary circular reactions

c. Secondary circular reactions

d. Tertiary circular reactions

ANSWER

b. The nurse understands the characteristics of Piaget's sensorimotor period. Primary circular reactions are activities repeated for the pleasure they bring.

ITEM 5 Cognitive Type: Application

The statement "I was a bad boy so I got sick" reflects which of the following preoperational thought patterns?

a. Transductive reasoning

b. Deductive reasoning

c. Centration

d. Decentration

ANSWER

a. The nurse understands the meaning of transductive reasoning—particular to particular—and realizes that it can cause illogical thinking in the preschool child.

ITEM 6 Cognitive Type: Interpretation

While 8-year-old Jonathan is hospitalized, he spends a lot of time working on his dinosaur sticker collection. The nurse would expect Jonathan's collection to be

a. arranged in a rather disorganized fashion.

b. arranged very orderly.

c. arranged only according to size.

d. arranged only according to type.

ANSWER

b. The nurse understands the characteristics of Piaget's concrete operational period. Classification skills are enhanced and decentration is possible. Children in this stage invest much energy in efforts to order and classify experiences in their lives, as evidenced by collections and scrapbooks.

ITEM 7 Cognitive Type: Interpretation

A mother is concerned because her 3-year-old son has started using unacceptable words she often hears her husband say. The nurse can base explanations of this behavior on which theory of language development?

a. Innate theory

b. Reinforcement theory

c. Social learning theory

d. Operant conditioning theory

ANSWER

c. The nurse understands that social learning theory describes the development of language as a modeling process, resulting in a child's imitation of adult remarks.

ITEM 8 Cognitive Type: Application

A mother reports to the nurse that her 4-year-old son continually asks "why" about everything. Recalling Erikson's psychosocial theory of development, the nurse could respond,

a. "Children of this age feel the need to use language skills to learn about everything."

b. "He's an unusually curious child."

c. "Try not to answer all of his questions because he will just ask more."

d. "Preschool children like to irritate their parents with lots of questions to assert their independence."

ANSWER

a. The nurse understands that questioning is one of the behaviors indicative of Erikson's sense of initiative, the psychosocial task of preschool age children.

ITEM 9 Cognitive Type: Application

In caring for an 8-year-old hospitalized child, the nurse can best reflect Erikson's theory of school age developmental tasks by

a. providing the child with opportunities to keep up with his school work.

b. making sure that the mother has liberal visiting opportunities.

c. providing him with an opportunity to take part in the care of a younger patient.

d. making sure that the child has a chance to talk with the doctor everyday so he can ask any questions he might have.

ANSWER

a. The nurse knows that the psychosocial task of the school age child is the development of industry or productivity and this is best accomplished with the completion of school assignments.

ITEM 10 Cognitive Type: Interpretation

Amy, who is 5-years-old, was overheard telling 4-year-old Jay, "You have to take your medicine because the doctor said so and he will give you a shot if you don't." Amy's statement reflects which of Kohlberg's phases of moral development?

a. Conventional morality

b. Principled morality

c. Preconventional morality

d. Postconventional morality

ANSWER

c. The nurse identifies a preschool child's perception of rules as absolute and having a punishment and obedience orientation. This reflects the preconventional stage of morality defined by Kohlberg.

ITEM 11 Cognitive Type: Knowledge

Temperament is best defined as

a. one's behavioral style.

b. one's response to frustration.

c. one's innate capabilities.

d. one's genetic make up.

ANSWER

a. The nurse knows that temperament is described as a behavioral style that makes one's approach to people and situations unique.

ITEM 12 Cognitive Type: Knowledge

Jason has always been difficult for his parents to manage. His mother described him as screaming during his first few baths, spitting out new foods, and seemingly generally irritable most of the time. The nurse might conclude that

a. Jason's parents' anxiety has caused him to become anxious.

b. Jason's mother didn't want to have a baby.

c. Jason probably possesses a difficult temperament.

d. Jason is probably a hyperkinetic child.

ANSWER

c. The nurse recognizes the characteristics of a child with a difficult temperament: slow to adapt to new situations, predominance of negative moods, and intense reactions.

ITEM 13 Cognitive Type: Knowledge

Being able to hold up one's head before being able to use the pincer grasp to pick up small items represents an example of

a. simple development.

b. complex development.

c. cephalocaudal development.

d. proximodistal development.

ANSWER

c. The nurse recognizes an example of cephalocaudal development—an infant gains head control before being able to control the movement of the limbs.

ITEM 14 Cognitive Type: Knowledge

In counseling parents about patterns of television viewing, the nurse could suggest that

a. children should be rewarded for good behavior with an opportunity to watch their favorite television program.

b. television can be used as a babysitter if the parents are busy, but only for a few hours a day.

c. parents should have input into their children's viewing habits.

d. parents should not impose their own values about television viewing on their children because it would confuse the child's decision-making process.

ANSWER

c. The nurse is familiar with recommendations based on research findings of the effects of television viewing, namely, that television should not be used as a reward or punishment, television should not be used as a babysitter, and parents should have input into their children's viewing habits.

ITEM 15 Cognitive Type: Knowledge

One behavior associated with the increased amount of children's television viewing might be

a. greater responsibility for sexual behavior.

b. more realistic attitudes about women and minorities.

c. healthy nutritional practices.

d. interest in violent acts and weapons.

ANSWER

d. Research suggests aggressive and antisocial tendencies are stimulated by viewing television violence.

CHAPTER 4

ITEM 1 Cognitive Type: Application

Which of the following nursing actions helps to facilitate the paternal identification and attachment process immediately after the birth of a new baby?

a. Instruct the father in careful handwashing, change of clothes, and the need to keep the baby carefully wrapped.

b. Send the father off quickly to inform the extended family of the good news.

c. Hand the baby to the father and encourage him to unwrap and inspect the infant.

d. Allow the father to stay with the mother while the baby is taken to the nursery for routine care.

ANSWER

c. The nurse understands that father–infant bonding is facilitated when the father is present in the delivery room.

ITEM 2 Cognitive Type: Knowledge

Which behavior alerts the nurse to a possible problem in the development of maternicity?

a. Absence of passive reaching

b. En face positioning

c. Touch regression

d. Cooing behaviors

ANSWER

a. Identification of behaviors of maternicity are necessary to evaluate mother–infant attachment.

ITEM 3 Cognitive Type: Application

An infant's initial assessment at birth showed a heart rate of 142, regular respirations, a facial grimace, arms and legs pulled into the body but not actively moving, and pink body color with pale extremities. Her Apgar score would be

a. 6. b. 7. c. 8. d. 9.

ANSWER

b. The nurse shows that she can properly apply the correct criteria for Apgar scoring.

ITEM 4 Cognitive Type: Application

Straightening the back with slight hyperextension of the head while in ventral suspension would be an indication of neuromuscular maturity according to

a. the Denver Developmental Screening Test.

b. Apgar scoring.

c. the Neonatal Behavioral Assessment Scale.

d. the Dubowitz Assessment of Gestational Age.

ANSWER

d. Understanding the Dubowitz Assessment tool for determining gestational age is needed to assess the newborn properly.

ITEM 5 Cognitive Type: Knowledge

Which of the following findings noted on physical assessment of a newborn girl alerts the nurse to a possible problem?

a. Hair tufts at the base of the spine

b. Small, white nodules on the nose

c. Blood-tinged mucoid discharge from the vagina

d. Fine, downy hairs covering the shoulders and back

ANSWER

a. The nurse is able to differentiate between normal and abnormal findings in the neonatal physical assessment.

ITEM 6 Cognitive Type: Application

You are assigned to care for a newborn boy in the newborn nursery. Which of the following nursing actions is necessary to assist him in maintaining stable body temperature?

a. Limit his exposure to visitors.

b. Stimulate the baby frequently to increase his activity.

c. Keep him covered at all times.

d. Put the baby under a warmer for 72 hours.

ANSWER

c. The nurse recognizes actions that prevent heat loss and maintain thermal balance in the newborn.

ITEM 7 Cognitive Type: Application

A newborn's care plan includes nursing interventions to maintain optimal hydration. The nurse recognizes which of the following as a contributing factor to the neonate's potential for dehydration?

a. Inability to utilize iron stores

b. Immature immune system

c. Limited ability to concentrate urine

d. Incomplete myelinization

ANSWER

c. The nurse understands that large amounts of water are lost with the excretion of solutes in the urine of the newborn. This is the result of immature kidney function and limited production of concentrated urine.

ITEM 8 Cognitive Type: Knowledge

On physical assessment of a newborn girl, the nurse notes the presence of diffuse edema of the soft tissues of her scalp that cross suture lines. These findings are indicative of

a. molding.

b. hemangioma.

c. caput succedaneum.

d. cephalhematoma.

ANSWER

c. Recognition of common deviations from normal is necessary when assessing the neonate.

ITEM 9 Cognitive Type: Knowledge

When teaching how to take a rectal temperature, the nurse instructs the parent to leave the thermometer in place for

a. less than 2 minutes.

b. 3 minutes.

c. 5 minutes.

d. as long as the baby will tolerate it.

ANSWER

b. Accurate thermometer readings result from holding the thermometer in place for the correct amount of time.

ITEM 10 Cognitive Type: Interpretation

A small amount of yellow-green drainage at the base of the umbilical cord stump is an indication of

a. infection.

b. imminent separation.

c. proper healing.

d. the need to apply a belly band.

ANSWER

a. The nurse must readily recognize signs of infection in the neonate.

ITEM 11 Cognitive Type: Interpretation

An important reflex elicited by touching the baby's lips with the breast or nipple is the

a. Moro reflex.

b. swallowing reflex.

c. suck reflex.

d. gag reflex.

ANSWER

c. Neurological assessment is important in newborns, and assessment of reflexes necessary for survival is vital.

ITEM 12 Cognitive Type: Knowledge

Which of the following is a guideline for bathing and skin care for neonates?

a. Do not immerse the infant in water until the umbilical cord has fallen off.

b. Schedule bathing immediately before or after a feeding.

c. Baby powders can be used to minimize perspiration.

d. Vigorous scrubbing with soap and water will remove vernix.

ANSWER

a. Sponge bathing is recommended until the umbilical cord has dropped off and the stump has healed.

CHAPTER 5

ITEM 1 Cognitive Type: Knowledge

Which is the correct sequence for the introduction of solid foods for a 4– to 6-month-old child?

a. Rice cereal, fruits, vegetables, meats

b. Fruits or vegetables, rice cereal, meats

c. Vegetables, meats, fruit, rice cereal

d. Egg yolks, rice cereal, fruits, vegetables

ANSWER

a. Rice cereal is introduced first because it is the least allergenic of all cereal grains, followed by fruits and vegetables, with meats introduced last.

ITEM 2 Cognitive Type: Application

Adam's birth weight was 7 lb 8 oz. Based on your knowledge of physical growth during the first year, which weight at 1 year of age would indicate that Adam is growing satisfactorily?

a. 14–16 lb

b. 18–20 lb

c. 22–24 lb

d. 27–30 lb

ANSWER

c. Birth weight is generally tripled by 1 year of age.

ITEM 3 Cognitive Type: Knowledge

Assessment of fine motor development in an 11-month-old would most likely reveal that he can

a. pick up a rattle with a raking motion of the hand.

b. use the index and middle finger to pick up Cheerios.

c. grasp objects with the right hand most of the time.

d. stack four to six blocks.

ANSWER

b. The pincer grasp develops at approximately 8–9 months.

ITEM 4 Cognitive Type: Knowledge

According to Piaget, a 5-month-old infant is in which stage of the sensorimotor period?

a. Primary circular reactions

b. Secondary circular reactions

c. Use of reflexes

d. Coordination of secondary schema

ANSWER

b. Secondary circular reactions are the third substage of the sensorimotor period (4–8 months of age).

ITEM 5 Cognitive Type: Knowledge

The central task of psychosocial development during infancy is

a. trust.

b. adjustment.

c. bonding.

d. adaptation.

ANSWER

a. Infants must learn to trust others to achieve a sense of trust in themselves.

ITEM 6 Cognitive Type: Knowledge

When teaching a group of new parents about nutrition, the nurse includes information on introducing solid foods at about

a. 2 months.

b. 6 months.

c. 10 months.

d. 14 months.

ANSWER

b. An important issue with parents is solid food introduction. Anticipatory guidance will promote healthy development.

ITEM 7 Cognitive Type: Application

Which of the following actions taken by the mother of a 6-month-old infant, who is experiencing discomfort associated with teething, indicates that the nurse's teaching plan has been successful?

a. She provides the infant with a hard rubber toy to bite on.

b. She reports that the baby was less irritable after placing an aspirin against the erupting tooth.

c. She gives the baby an ice cube to suck on.

d. She promises to put the whiskey and sugar lotion suggested by her grandmother on the baby's gums only at bedtime.

ANSWER

a. The nurse recognizes safe interventions for teething pain and can apply this knowledge to the evaluation of successful teaching strategies.

ITEM 8 Cognitive Type: Knowledge

During a well baby visit to the clinic, the nurse would expect the mother of a normal 7-month-old boy to report that he is

a. walking nearly unassisted.

b. creeping up and down four steps.

c. sitting alone for brief periods.

d. beginning to hold his head erect.

ANSWER

c. Gross motor developmental milestones should be easily recognized by the nurse.

ITEM 9 Cognitive Type: Interpretation

The mother of a 3-month-old infant calls the office nurse with a concern about the baby's stools. She is sure the child is constipated because she strains and turns red in the face with every stool. Her stools are mushy yellow and occur three to four times a day. Which of the following is the nurse's best response?

a. "Yes, she does sound constipated. Try giving her a little prune juice each day."

b. "Babies do strain during bowel movements because their muscle coordination is still immature. Your baby's stooling pattern is normal."

c. "No, she is not constipated. All babies get red in the face. Try not to worry so much."

d. "Why don't you bring her in so the doctor can look at her."

ANSWER

b. Nursing knowledge of normal elimination patterns can help relieve parental anxiety.

ITEM 10 Cognitive Type: Application

A new mother wonders when she should start weaning her 7-month-old infant. Which information should be included in the nurse's teaching plan?

a. Weaning should not be initiated until after the first birthday.

b. The infant can begin to have finger foods such as carrot and celery sticks.

c. Drinking from a cup is possible at this age and can be gradually substituted for the breast or bottle.

d. The optimal time for weaning is when solid foods are preferred by the child.

ANSWER

c. The nurse recognizes expected developmental skills of a 7-month-old child that accommodate weaning. These include the ability to grasp, hand-to-mouth movements, and ability to sit. Solid foods are not the sole preference of infants, and the finger foods mentioned are dangerous because raw vegetables require strong chewing ability.

ITEM 11 Cognitive Type: Application

The father of a 5-month-old infant asks the nurse for information about activities that will foster his child's development. Which of the following suggestions is appropriate?

a. Provide the infant with toys or household items that she can stack.

b. Give the infant large stuffed animals to play with in her crib.

c. Play simple hide-and-seek games with the infant.

d. Put the infant in a program that teaches movement and swimming skills.

ANSWER

c. The nurse recognizes the developmental capabilities of the 5-month-old and is able to choose appropriate activities for infants at this stage of development.

ITEM 12 Cognitive Type: Knowledge

Health promotion for a 4-month-old infant during a well child visit would include

a. DPT, OPV, and HbCV immunizations.

b. lead screening.

c. screening for iron deficiency anemia.

d. MMR vaccine and DPT booster.

ANSWER

a. The 4-month-old infant should receive DPT, OPV, and HbCV immunizations according to the currently recommended immunization schedule.

ITEM 13 Cognitive Type: Application

Joshua is 10 months old and weighs 23 pounds. He is crawling and pulling himself to a stand. Which of the following statements suggests that his parents are knowledgeable about infant safety?

a. "When I'm driving, I put Joshua in a rear-facing carseat right next to me."

b. "We have a gate at the top and bottom of the stairs in our house."

c. "Joshua loves to play with the clowns and string on the mobile we put on his crib."

d. "Joshua's favorite foods are hot dogs and carrot sticks."

ANSWER

b. The nurse recognizes that this infant is at risk for falling and that the parents have taken the proper precautions.

ITEM 14 Cognitive Type: Application

The mother of an 11-month-old reports that her infant is waking at night. How should the nurse advise this mother?

a. Place a bottle of juice in the crib at bedtime.

b. When the infant awakens, offer formula or breastmilk.

c. Do not let the infant nap during the day.

d. Let the infant cry for 5 minutes, then go to the infant.

ANSWER

d. Nightwaking is usually a transient development phase. When parents respond to the awake infant by holding them at night, the infant learns to expect conforting. Crying is reinforced by the secondary gain of being held. To break this pattern, parents need to decrease this reinforcer.

ITEM 15 Cognitive Type: Application

How would the nurse promote parent–infant attachment for a hospitalized 3-month-old whose parents and siblings live 2 hours away from the hospital?

a. Have the parents hold the infant for the entire length of their visit.

b. Allow the parents to sit with their infant after visiting hours.

c. Take a photograph of the infant for parents to take home.

d. Play an audiotape of the parents' voices to the infant in their absence.

ANSWER

d. The nurse can facilitate parent–infant attachment during hospitalization with a variety of nursing strategies, one of which is asking parents to record their voices on tape and then playing the tape to the infant when the parents cannot be with their child.

CHAPTER 6

ITEM 1 Cognitive Type: Knowledge

Which of the following is characteristic of the physical development of a 15-month-old child?

a. Has a bowed leg appearance.

b. Primary dentition is complete.

c. Can use a spoon to feed self.

d. Dresses self without assistance.

ANSWER

a. Understanding the physiological changes in the toddler is especially helpful when providing anticipatory guidance to parents.

ITEM 2 Cognitive Type: Knowledge

The nurse should expect to observe healthy toddlers playing

a. alone with a solitary game.

b. beside one another but not together.

c. with an imaginary friend.

d. cooperatively with one another.

ANSWER

b. Toddlers are still developmentally egocentric and prefer to play alongside other children rather than to share.

ITEM 3 Cognitive Type: Knowledge

During the toddler stage of psychosocial development, a child is struggling to achieve a sense of

a. trust.

b. object permanence.

c. initiative.

d. autonomy.

ANSWER

d. According to Erikson, the toddler is struggling to relieve the crisis of autonomy versus doubt and shame.

ITEM 4 Cognitive Type: Knowledge

Energy requirements during the toddler years are affected by which of the following?

a. Decreased growth rate and decreased protein needs.

b. Decreased metabolic rate.

c. Increased growth rate and increased activity levels.

d. Increased activity rate and decreased growth rate.

ANSWER

d. The nurse must understand nutritional needs in relation to growth parameters.

ITEM 5 Cognitive Type: Interpretation

Fifteen-month-old Susie continually drops food from her high chair onto the floor. Her mother is convinced that she does this on purpose and asks for advice on what to do. The nurse's answer is based on an understanding that during this stage of cognitive development, toddlers

a. often misbehave to gain attention.

b. learn about spatial relationships and causality by manipulating objects in their environment.

c. repeat negative actions that are not immediately punished.

d. are able to use thought processes to experience events and actions.

ANSWER

b. Understanding levels of development will help in understanding behavior.

ITEM 6 Cognitive Type: Knowledge

Negativism and dawdling are common behaviors for toddlers. To assist parents in avoiding undue stress from these behaviors, the nurse should suggest that they

a. avoid requesting completion of tasks when the toddler is tired or hungry.

b. finish tasks for the child.

c. take time to reason with the child about negative behavior.

d. avoid social contact so others are not subjected to the toddler's behavior.

ANSWER

a. Parents often need anticipatory guidance on how to deal with negativism.

ITEM 7 Cognitive Type: Knowledge

Michael is 2 years, 3 months old. He has been walking and running well for quite some time. He enjoys imitating and can understand and express himself with words. The nurse recognizes that Michael's development indicates readiness for

a. self-care responsibility.

b. toilet training.

c. relinquishing bedtime rituals.

d. associative play.

ANSWER

b. Anticipatory guidance and recognition of development will assist parents in making toilet training a positive experience.

ITEM 8 Cognitive Type: Knowledge

Sex role identification during the toddler years is learned through

a. imitation and responses to behavior received from parents.

b. anatomical differences between males and females.

c. developing a close relationship with both parents.

d. behaviors that show appropriate male and female orientation.

ANSWER

a. During the toddler years, gender identity and sex-role identification are primarily influenced by experiences within the family.

ITEM 9 Cognitive Type: Interpretation

Energy depletion in families with toddlers can be avoided by

a. providing autonomous play activities for the child.

b. childproofing the family residence.

c. equalizing the division of labor among family members.

d. enrolling an especially inquisitive or energetic child in a day care program.

ANSWER

c. The nurse recognizes that keeping up with a busy toddler requires distribution of labor resources in the family to avoid energy depletion in one or more of its members.

ITEM 10 Cognitive Type: Application

To promote socialized eating behaviors in the toddler, parents should be counseled to

a. provide nutritious between-meal snacks for the child who is not hungry at mealtimes.

b. encourage family members to remain at the table throughout a meal.

c. create a mealtime environment that includes stimulating activities such as music or manipulative toys.

d. avoid correcting the table manners of siblings during a meal.

ANSWER

b. A toddler needs total concentration to accomplish the skills of self-feeding. Persons leaving and returning to the table distract a toddler from the task at hand.

ITEM 11 Cognitive Type: Application

The parents of a 2-year-old boy report that he holds his breath whenever he has a temper tantrum. When counseling them, the nurse should

a. teach the parents how to perform mouth-to-mouth resuscitation.

b. advise the parents to give in to the child's demands since breath-holding can result in anoxia.

c. recommend that parents ignore the behavior since the child will resume breathing as a reflex.

d. provide the parents with ways to reason with the child by appealing to his feelings of attachment toward them.

ANSWER

c. If temper tantrums are accompanied by breath holding, parents need to know that this behavior will not result in harm to the child.

ITEM 12 Cognitive Type: Knowledge

Alison, 22 months of age, sits quietly and says "car, car" while pointing at an automobile in her picture book. Later in the day, when Alison sees a moving automobile on television, she runs to the door, bangs on it, and says "car, car." Alison's behavior illustrates which of the following characteristics of language development in the toddler?

a. Expressive jargon

b. Telegraphic expression

c. Holophrastic speech

d. Egocentric speech

ANSWER

c. Holophrastic speech refers to using one-word utterances to convey whole ideas.

ITEM 13 Cognitive Type: Knowledge

During a well child visit, Teresa Lee reports she is frustrated by her 2-year-old son's negative behavior. What suggestions could the nurse offer Teresa to help her cope with her son's negativism?

a. Negativism should be resolved by the age of 2 years. Hang in there.

b. Do not phrase a request as a choice if there is no choice available.

c. Don't tell the child what you are going to do. Just perform the task.

d. Discipline the child when the negative behavior occurs.

ANSWER

b. Negativism is a typical toddler behavior present from 18 months to 3 years. The parent–toddler relationship is facilitated when parents know to expect negativism and how to handle it.

ITEM 14 Cognitive Type: Knowledge

According to the immunization schedule, the measles-mumps-rubella (MMR) vaccine and the hemophilus B conjugate (HbCV) vaccine should be administered at what age?

a. 15 months

b. 18 months

c. 24 months

d. 36 months

ANSWER

a. MMR and HbCV are administered at 15 months, although MMR may be administered at 12 months to toddlers living in a high-risk area. The measles vaccine may be administered to infants as young as 6 months during a measles outbreak in a high-risk area. If the child is immunized before 12 months, reimmunization is done at 15 months.

CHAPTER 7

ITEM 1 Cognitive Type: Knowledge

In Erikson's third stage of emotional development, preschool age children are striving to develop a sense of initiative. This task refers to

a. the determination to master tasks and feel good about one's self.

b. the channeling of energy to plan and undertake activities or enterprises.

c. a sense of selfhood.

d. becoming someone who is able to trust others.

ANSWER

b. Recognition of developmental tasks to be accomplished by the preschooler provides the nurse with guidelines for developing strategies to foster optimal growth and development.

ITEM 2 Cognitive Type: Knowledge

The nurse should expect to observe a preschool age child playing

a. cooperatively with other children.

b. quietly alongside other children.

c. with manipulative objects such as nesting blocks.

d. alone with a hand-held computer toy.

ANSWER

a. Cooperative play is a characteristic of preschoolers.

ITEM 3 Cognitive Type: Knowledge

Cognitive thinking of the preschool age child in the preoperational period includes

a. conservation.

b. classification.

c. centration.

d. assimilation.

ANSWER

c. Centration is the ability to focus on only one aspect of a situation at a time.

ITEM 4 Cognitive Type: Interpretation

When assessing a 4-year-old's gross motor development, the nurse would ask the child to demonstrate

a. hopping on one foot for 10 seconds.

b. climbing steps by holding onto the rail.

c. walking backward heel to toe.

d. jumping rope five times.

ANSWER

a. By age 4 years, the child can run easily, hop on one foot, climb steps without holding onto railing, and sometimes skip.

ITEM 5 Cognitive Type: Knowledge

Nursing interventions to help prevent injury to a preschooler should include advising the parents to

a. check the child's play environment periodically for hazards such as dangerous hiding places and unsafe toys.

b. structure all play time carefully.

c. allow the child to remain home alone only with other siblings.

d. provide opportunities for imaginary play when the child must wait alone in a car.

ANSWER

a. Safety is increasingly important as the child becomes more independent.

ITEM 6 Cognitive Type: Interpretation

Four-year-old Maria's mother is concerned because Maria has recently had trouble going to bed at night because she thinks that the big oak tree near her bedroom window is mean and wants to hurt her. When counseling her mother, the nurse should

a. suggest that Maria be seen by a psychiatrist for evaluation and treatment.

b. advise the mother to close the curtains and leave a night light on in her room.

c. recommend that Maria stop watching TV and avoid spicy foods at dinner time.

d. encourage the family to cut down the oak tree.

ANSWER

b. Children's vivid imagination at this age can cause nighttime fears.

ITEM 7 Cognitive Type: Interpretation

Which of the following statements by parents suggests that they understand dental care for their preschool child?

a. "We stopped our child's thumbsucking so it would not affect his baby teeth."

b. "Our 4-year-old girl just can't seem to floss her teeth without our help."

c. "We plan to take our child for his first dental examination when he starts first grade."

d. "Our daughter brushes her teeth at least once a day."

ANSWER

d. Anticipatory guidance should include information about dental care. Parents should monitor and assist their preschooler with brushing teeth at least once a day.

ITEM 8 Cognitive Type: Interpretation

Which of the following characteristics noted in a 5-year-old child indicates readiness for school?

a. A vocabulary of at least 1000 words

b. Highly imaginative play behaviors

c. Ability to wait for and take turns

d. Skilled in dressing and undressing without assistance

ANSWER

c. The ability to tolerate frustration if not given immediate attention and to wait for attention in the form of taking turns is necessary prior to attending school.

ITEM 9 Cognitive Type: Application

Which behavior by the mother of a 5-year-old boy should alert the nurse to the need for teaching about safety?

a. She allows the child to play with cooking utensils and to assist with meal preparation.

b. She encourages him to climb on the monkey bars in the park while she stands just below him.

c. She allows the child to walk home from school with a 12-year-old sibling.

d. She asks him to find them seats inside the movie theater while she purchases popcorn in the lobby.

ANSWER

d. The preschooler should not be left alone because at this age the child is not yet able to assume responsibilities that require judgment skills.

ITEM 10 Cognitive Type: Knowledge

Which of the following most accurately describes the preschooler's moral reasoning? An action is judged

a. in relation to its intent.

b. according to subjective values.

c. in terms of its consequence.

d. in light of the needs of others.

ANSWER

c. Conscience begins developing in the preschool years as children learn what behaviors are acceptable to parents. They judge their actions based on consequences.

ITEM 11 Cognitive Type: Application

When talking with the mother of a 4-year-old boy, the nurse notices her embarrassment when the child begins to touch his genitalia. The nurse should

a. tell the mother that masturbation is normal in a 4-year-old.

b. ask the mother if anyone has been touching him inappropriately.

c. advise the mother to remind the child that he will lose television privileges if he continues to touch himself.

d. gather information about the mother's values and beliefs concerning sexuality.

ANSWER

d. The nurse recognizes a sensitive approach to counseling the family about sexual inquisitiveness in the preschooler.

ITEM 12 Cognitive Type: Knowledge

The mother of a 3-year-old boy tells the nurse that her son recently seems to be jealous of his father. According to Freudian theory, this behavior is known as

a. Electra complex.

b. Oedipal complex.

c. penis envy.

d. castration anxiety.

ANSWER

b. The Oedipal complex resolves with the child's identification with the same sex parent.

CHAPTER 8

ITEM 1 Cognitive Type: Knowledge

Which finding should the nurse expect when assessing physical growth in school age children?

a. Decreasing amounts of body fat and muscle mass

b. Yearly weight gain averaging 2.5 kg (5.5 lb)

c. Little change in bodily appearance from year to year

d. Progressive linear growth averaging 4 inches per year

ANSWER

b. The nurse recognizes normal patterns of physical growth during the school age years.

ITEM 2 Cognitive Type: Interpretation

Which is the best way for the nurse to assess lateral preference in a school age child?

a. Ask the child to throw a ball.

b. Check the child's spelling skills.

c. Perform a visual screening examination.

d. Observe the child's ability to imitate the movements of another.

ANSWER

a. The nurse knows that lateral preference is usually established by early school age and can identify an assessment technique used to observe a child's preference for the right or left hand.

ITEM 3 Cognitive Type: Application

Which of the following is a characteristic of peer group relationships in the 8- to 9-year-old child?

a. Activities are organized around competitive games and sports.

b. Informal socialization occurs between both sexes.

c. Loyalty and strong affiliations to a particular group of the same sex are apparent.

d. Activities are focused around shared interests with a best friend.

ANSWER

c. The nurse recognizes the progressive stages of socialization in the school age years and identifies middle childhood peer interactions.

ITEM 4 Cognitive Type: Interpretation

In response to a father's inquiry about whether he should allow his 9-year-old daughter to join the soccer team at school, the nurse would

a. explain that this activity is appropriate since it will allow the child to practice motor skills and feel proud of her strength.

b. recommend that he encourage her to join the Girl Scout troop instead.

c. suggest that he develop an intensive training program for her to practice running and ball kicking skills.

d. advise the father to give his permission only if he can attend her practice sessions to monitor the child's safety.

ANSWER

a. School age children explore the world with their bodies and take pride in their increasing skills.

ITEM 5 Cognitive Type: Knowledge

To promote responsibility in an 8-year-old, the nurse could recommend to the parents that they have the child

a. take full charge of pet care duties.

b. make his own bed.

c. get a summer job.

d. prepare dinner for younger siblings.

ANSWER

a. Providing safe age-appropriate tasks that can be easily accomplished helps promote responsibility and independence.

ITEM 6 Cognitive Type: Interpretation

When planning a developmental health promotion program for a group of parents with school age children, the nurse should include strategies to assist parents in

a. learning to "let go" of their child.

b. giving comprehensive instruction and assistance with homework.

c. correcting a child's mistakes so that they are not repeated.

d. relaxing rules and limits to accommodate their child's request to be allowed to do what other children are allowed to do.

ANSWER

a. Parental advancement through developmental tasks that encourage communication and foster increased independence are necessary in the school age period.

ITEM 7 Cognitive Type: Interpretation

Which of the following statements best describes the gross motor development of a 7-year-old child?

a. Boundless energy and refining skills in running and jumping.

b. Energetic but clumsy with skipping and bicycling.

c. Well-developed muscular control and skill in all gross motor activities.

d. Cautious yet intent on acquiring foot movement sequencing, throwing, and catching skills.

ANSWER

d. Refinement of six gross motor skills—running, jumping, sequencing foot movements, balancing, throwing, and catching—occurs during the school age period. The 7-year-old child is more cautious, quiet, and intent as she refines these skills.

ITEM 8 Cognitive Type: Knowledge

The nurse assessing language development in 6-year-old children would expect

a. speech to be 75% fluent.

b. correct articulation of all speech sounds.

c. inconsistent use of correct grammar.

d. formation of five- to six-word sentences.

ANSWER

d. The 6-year-old child speaks clearly and uses grammar correctly; he can form five- to six-word sentences with a vocabulary of 2500–3000 words.

ITEM 9 Cognitive Type: Knowledge

One characteristic of the concrete operational stage of cognitive development is

a. scientific reasoning.

b. egocentrism.

c. competency.

d. conservation.

ANSWER

d. Principles of conservation begin now and have increased application as the child moves through the school age period.

ITEM 10 Cognitive Type: Knowledge

Nine-year-old Courtney's height is at the 25th percentile and her weight is at the 95th percentile. Strategies to reduce the risk of obesity include

a. maintenance of a 2100-calorie diet with daily exercise.

b. instituting an immediate weight reduction program.

c. skipping breakfast and eating a good lunch at school.

d. changing eating habits to small frequent meals and snacks.

ANSWER

a. The nurse understands that daily exercise coupled with calorie maintenance are the best ways to avoid abesity into adulthood.

ITEM 11 Cognitive Type: Knowledge

Ten-year-old Gary's mother asks the nurse what she can do about her son's habit of fingernail biting. The nurse should advise her to

a. offer alternatives to Gary such as pounding a punching bag.

b. tell Gary there is nothing for him to worry about.

c. point out that fingernail biting is disgusting and childish.

d. buy something Gary wants if he stops biting his nails.

ANSWER

a. The nurse understands nail biting is an anxious behavior and that the individual must find other outlets for the anxiety.

ITEM 12 Cognitive Type: Knowledge

Which of the following temperament categories describes a child's awareness of visual and auditory stimuli in the environment?

a. Intensity of reaction

b. Distractibility

c. Threshold for stimuli

d. Approachability

ANSWER

c. An understanding of the factors involved in temperament will help the nurse to provide anticipatory guidance for decreasing stress areas.

ITEM 13 Cognitive Type: Knowledge

According to Erikson, if a school age child is not given the opportunity to engage in tasks and activities that they can carry through to completion, they are likely to develop a feeling of

a. guilt.

b. shame.

c. isolation.

d. inferiority.

ANSWER

d. Erikson's fourth stage, industry versus inferiority, is the major concept of psychosocial development in the school age period.

ITEM 14 Cognitive Type: Interpretation

When responding to a teacher's inquiry about techniques to use with a child whose temperament is slow to warm, the nurse should recommend that the teacher

a. ensure that the child be the leader often.

b. avoid eye contact with the child to prevent a withdrawal response.

c. allow the child to be included in activities without assigning responsibility until the child initiates active participation.

d. be critical of exaggerated reactions.

ANSWER

c. Recognizing temperament style and allowing the child to move at his or her own pace will be richly rewarded.

CHAPTER 9

ITEM 1 Cognitive Type: Interpretation

The central psychosocial task of adolescence involves developing a stable identity to avoid

a. feelings of guilt.

b. doubt and shame associated with sexuality.

c. role confusion.

d. mistrust in society.

ANSWER

c. According to Erikson, the central task of the adolescent period is identity versus role confusion. The adolescent either develops a stable identity or remains confused about her identity during adulthood.

ITEM 2 Cognitive Type: Application

Physical assessment findings for an 11-year-old girl include the presence of sparse, dark, slightly curled pubic hair and breast development without contour separation. The nurse concludes that this child is in which stage of sexual maturation as described in the Tanner rating scales?

a. First

b. Second

c. Third

d. Fourth

ANSWER

c. The nurse must recognize physical characteristics of sexual development.

ITEM 3 Cognitive Type: Knowledge

Female adolescents usually experience a growth spurt

a. at the same time as males.

b. 2 years earlier than males.

c. just prior to the onset of puberty.

d. that increases height by 4 inches per year.

ANSWER

b. The nurse recognizes that normal physical development in female adolescents involves a growth spurt earlier than that in males.

ITEM 4 Cognitive Type: Interpretation

As 14-year-old Marcie is getting ready for school, she calls frantically for her mother because she can't find her contact lenses. "I can't wear those horrible glasses on my first day of high school!" Marcie's behavior is an example of which characteristic of adolescent cognitive development?

a. Reality versus possibility

b. Combinational thinking

c. Use of implication

d. Adolescent egocentrism

ANSWER

d. Adolescent egocentrism refers to the self-consciousness adolescents feel over situations adults and younger children find insignificant.

ITEM 5 Cognitive Type: Interpretation

Nursing interventions to assist parents in promoting positive attitudes about sex in their adolescent children include

a. encouraging parents to assist their teens in securing birth control measures since many sexual urges cannot be controlled during adolescence.

b. identifying ways for parents to promote self-esteem and problem-solving skills in their teenager.

c. assisting parents in allowing their teenager to experience the natural consequences of sexual experimentation.

d. emphasizing the need for parental discipline and limit setting regarding sexual activity.

ANSWER

b. Parents can help adolescents to think through difficult situations in advance and consider the potential consequences of their actions.

ITEM 6 Cognitive Type: Knowledge

Kelly, a 16-year-old girl, has come to the clinic for birth control information. She has reviewed literature about different methods and has decided to use the diaphragm. What information should be included in the nurse's teaching plan?

a. This method of contraception requires a complete physical examination with Pap smear, hct, B/P, and blood tests for syphilis and GC.

b. This method of contraception is also helpful in preventing the spread of venereal disease and AIDS.

c. This method of contraception requires that it remain in place for at least 6 hours after intercourse and no douching should be done.

d. An appointment will be necessary to fit this device, and it should be done during menstruation to facilitate insertion.

ANSWER

c. The nurse understands the correct information about the safe and effective use of a diaphragm for contraception.

ITEM 7 Cognitive Type: Knowledge

When conducting an information program about adolescent sexuality and contraception use, the nurse should consider which of the following?

a. Teenage pregnancy is usually the result of rebellion against parental authority.

b. Most adolescents who seek birth control have already been sexually active for 6 to 12 months.

c. Teenagers in today's society value sexual freedom and are knowledgeable about the physiological processes associated with reproduction.

d. Sexual experimentation is necessary for the adolescent to develop a sense of personal identity and self-worth.

ANSWER

b. The nurse should provide information that is accurate and relevant to the sexuality of the adolescent.

ITEM 8 Cognitive Type: Interpretation

Your next door neighbor, who has a 14-year-old son, complains that lately he finds fault with everything she does and says. She's worried that their once close relationship is in danger but doesn't understand what she is doing wrong. Your response is based on your understanding that during this stage of cognitive development

a. an adolescent creates psychological distances from parents so as to begin the separation process.

b. parents must change their value system to meet the needs of the adolescent if they expect to remain close to their child.

c. the adolescent's most significant relationship continues to be with the parent even if their conflicts are unresolved.

d. parents should relinquish responsibility for the adolescent's social development to teachers or friends of the same sex whom they admire.

ANSWER

a. The nurse can correctly identify and interpret the stresses of psychosocial changes in adolescents when dealing with their families.

ITEM 9 Cognitive Type: Knowledge

Matt, age 17 years, tells the school nurse that his friend got a disease after he had sexual intercourse. How would the nurse advise Matt about safe sex?

a. The female partner should apply a spermicide before intercourse.

b. A latex condom should be worn during intercourse.

c. Both partners should cleanse the genital area immediately before intercourse.

d. Matt should refrain from sexual activity until he is more mature.

ANSWER

b. Condoms are very effective in preventing sexually transmitted disease, but abstaining from sex is the only way to prevent disease.

ITEM 10 Cognitive Type: Knowledge

Research studies have shown that, in comparison to children of older mothers, the offspring of adolescent mothers experience

a. poorer self-esteem.

b. more academic difficulties.

c. less physical problems during childhood.

d. greater opportunities for mother–child interaction.

ANSWER

b. The nurse knows that according to research by Davis (1988), some of the problems experienced by offspring of adolescent mothers include academic difficulties, low intellectual functioning, and more behavior problems in school.

CHAPTER 10

ITEM 1 Cognitive Type: Application

The community health nurse can best promote adaptation and stability in the family who has a baby with Down syndrome by

a. discussing the genetic cause of the child's disorder.

b. performing a Denver Developmental Screening frequently to evaluate the child.

c. referring the child to an infant stimulation program that includes family guidance.

d. referring the parents to a genetic counseling agency.

ANSWER

c. From a framework of adaptation, nursing intervention is aimed at restoring adaptive behavior or reducing the impact of environmental stressors. The correct action here helps the child and family to progress beyond a crisis toward achieving optimal potential for functioning.

ITEM 2 Cognitive Type: Interpretation

Immunization against the polio virus is an example of which type of health promotion activity?

a. Primary prevention

b. Secondary prevention

c. Tertiary prevention

d. Wellness promotion

ANSWER

a. Primary prevention activities aim to decrease the probability of encountering illness or to ward off specific illness that may threaten the quality of life or longevity.

ITEM 3 Cognitive Type: Application

The school nurse identifies that more than half of the seventh and eighth grade boys in the elementary school are using snuff. Drawing from expectancy theory, the nurse should attempt to promote behavior changes in these boys by

a. beginning a health class that deals with the effects of tobacco on the respiratory tract and tissues of the mouth.

b. discussing the effect of stained teeth and bad breath on social life.

c. reporting the children's behavior to the principal.

d. sending notes home to the children's parents related to their child's behavior.

ANSWER

a. The nurse is able to apply interventions based on an understanding of expectancy theory as it relates to children's health behaviors.

ITEM 4 Cognitive Type: Application

When counseling the mother of an 11-year-old boy who is overweight, the nurse would

a. suggest that she provide his favorite foods on weekends as a reward for calorie counting during the week.

b. advise her to allow the child to engage in occasional food binges with his friends.

c. recommend that she encourage the child to join a weight reduction support group of children of the same age.

d. explain the importance of enrolling the child in an aerobics exercise class.

ANSWER

c. Although a child may go off on a binge with peers occasionally, this should not be used as a motivation technique. A group of supportive peers is the best answer.

ITEM 5 Cognitive Type: Interpretation

Fifteen-year-old Jane is a cheerleader and a member of the National Honor Society. She has recently been diagnosed with diabetes mellitus and tells the school nurse that she is having a difficult time adjusting her lifestyle to meet the physiological requirements of diabetes control. The nurse would

a. assess her understanding of the relationship among activity level, diet, and insulin requirements.

b. urge her to give up cheerleading because this strenuous activity increases caloric energy requirements.

c. provide her with a list of foods she should not eat, such as concentrated sweets.

d. counsel Jane's close friends about the importance of helping her cope with this disorder.

ANSWER

a. Assessment of understanding is the first step in problem solving to arrive at action alternatives. The nurse is then able to understand and support decisions made by the child.

ITEM 6 Cognitive Type: Interpretation

A camp nurse can best help young campers make appropriate use of the health clinic by

a. providing an orientation program on the health services available for campers.

b. completing physical assessments on all campers to determine possible health problems.

c. discussing health information needed by campers with parents prior to the children's camp experience.

d. enforcing rules related to hygiene.

ANSWER

a. The nurse can best support the children's ability to be responsible for their own health maintenance by informing them of the available services.

ITEM 7 Cognitive Type: Application

During a well child examination, the nurse notes that Annie, age 14 months, looks toward her mother for reassurance and smiles whenever her mother praises her for cooperating with the examination. Physical findings reveal the presence of a severe diaper rash and malodorous hair and scalp. How should the nurse initiate health promotion in this situation?

a. Ask the mother how often she washes Annie's hair.

b. Explain to the mother why she should change Annie's diaper more frequently.

c. Praise the mother's supportive interaction with Annie.

d. Tell the mother that Annie's development is normal except that she should be more independent for her age.

ANSWER

c. Effective health promotion activities are supported by promoting confidence and self-esteem in the parent and by giving positive reinforcement for a parent's credibility as capable caretaker.

ITEM 8 Cognitive Type: Knowledge

The Sabin oral polio vaccine (OPV) is the recommended drug for routine immunization against polio in the United States. Which of the following agents is used in the preparation of this vaccine?

a. Killed bacteria

b. Killed virus

c. Live, attenuated virus

d. Bacterial toxoid

ANSWER

c. The nurse can identify which type of agent is used to prepare the Sabin oral polio vaccine.

ITEM 9 Cognitive Type: Knowledge

Toxoids are given to induce which type of immunity?

a. Artificial active immunity

b. Natural passive immunity

c. General immunity

d. Artificial passive immunity

ANSWER

a. A toxoid is a bacterial toxin that has been treated to destroy its toxic properties while retaining its ability to stimulate antibody production. This way of acquiring protection against specific illness is called artificial active immunity.

ITEM 10 Cognitive Type: Interpretation

A healthy 4-month-old infant arrives at the well child clinic for immunizations. The nurse would expect to administer which of the following?

a. Td, HBV, MMR

b. DPT, HIB, MMR

c. DT, HBV, TOPV

d. DPT, TOPV, HIB

ANSWER

d. The nurse knows the recommended schedule for active immunization for normal infants and prepares accordingly.

ITEM 11 Cognitive Type: Application

Which of the following represents the correct administration of the DPT vaccine to a 2-month-old infant?

a. Intradermally in the upper arm

b. Intramuscularly in the anterolateral thigh

c. Orally followed by a formula feeding

d. Subcutaneously in the vastus lateralis muscle

ANSWER

b. The nurse applies knowledge of administration of immunizing agents to safe site selection for infants receiving intramuscular injections.

ITEM 12 Cognitive Type: Application

Nursing strategies to assist the parent of an infant in managing possible reactions to a DPT immunization should include

a. instructions on how to reduce fever and inflammation at the injection site.

b. explanation about dietary restrictions to prevent vomiting and diarrhea.

c. reassurance that infants will probably not experience any reaction to DPT immunization.

d. teaching how to prepare and administer saline nose drops to alleviate nasal congestion.

ANSWER

a. The nurse recognizes fever and localized inflammation as typical reactions to DPT immunization and teaches parents accordingly.

ITEM 13 Cognitive Type: Knowledge

It is important to obtain information about allergies from the parents of a 15-month-old who is scheduled to receive the MMR immunization because

a. reactions are common in children with hay fever.

b. the vaccine is live, attenuated virus prepared in an egg medium.

c. many children develop hypersensitivity to toxoids administered subcutaneously.

d. the intended effect of the immunization is diminished in the presence of milk intolerance.

ANSWER

b. MMR immunization may be contraindicated if a child is allergic to eggs. The nurse recognizes why obtaining information about true allergies is important prior to the administration of the MMR vaccine in its usual form.

ITEM 14 Cognitive Type: Application

Brian was brought to the well child clinic for his 18-month check-up and immunizations. He has a fever of 102°F but no other physical symptoms. The nurse's best action is to

a. give the immunization since Brian has no physical symptoms.

b. tell Brian's mother he can skip this immunization as it is not an important one.

c. administer the immunization and reschedule Brian for a follow-up examination the next day.

d. withhold the immunization and tell his mother to bring Brian back when his fever has subsided.

ANSWER

d. Children with febrile illness should not be immunized because the fever may be symptomatic of a more serious condition.

ITEM 15 Cognitive Type: Application

In which of the following situations should the caregiver seek health care for their child?

a. A 2-year-old has a rectal temperature of 100.8°F but is playful and taking oral fluids.

b. A 9-month-old has a cold, is cranky, and is not eating or sleeping as usual.

c. A 12-month-old vomited once after breakfast, but took 8-ounce bottle 1 hour later without problems.

d. For the past week, a 2-year-old eats well one day and then barely eats at all the next day.

ANSWER

b. Parents should seek health care if they notice a combination of changes in their child.

CHAPTER 11

ITEM 1 Cognitive Type: Interpretation

Which of the following is most important for the nurse to consider when attempting to communicate effectively with children?

a. Physical health or illness state

b. Level of language and cognitive development

c. Nonverbal expressions of need

d. Family patterns of interaction

ANSWER

b. Effective communication with children involves all of these, but an understanding of a child's level of language development and cognition is fundamental to effective observation and listening when a child and an adult are communicating.

ITEM 2 Cognitive Type: Application

After her mother has denied 13-year-old Amy's request for money to purchase a trendy new item of clothing, Amy responds, "You're awful—you never let me do anything. I hate you!" How should her mother respond?

a. "Now Amy, we all wish we could have everything we want, but we just can't."

b. "Amy, in light of what you just said, I'm not very fond of you at this moment either."

c. "I know you're really upset with me, but I feel I must budget money for clothing."

d. "How could you speak to me that way? I just bought you new shoes yesterday."

ANSWER

c. In relating to any age child, an adult should respect the child's emotions, be honest in a caring way, and be able to set limits.

ITEM 3 Cognitive Type: Application

The nurse should include which of the following statements in her teaching about communicating with their 2-week-old infant?

a. A high-pitched cry indicates that the infant is tired.

b. Do not speak to the infant in "baby talk."

c. Speak softly and rock the infant during feedings.

d. Crying usually means the infant is hungry.

ANSWER

c. The infant learns to experience pleasure in response to a soft-spoken voice. Holding and rocking communicate feelings of attachment.

ITEM 4 Cognitive Type: Application

Which of the following statements made by the nurse would most likely encourage 9-year-old Timothy to talk about his past experiences with hospitalization?

a. "How old were you when you were in the hospital?"

b. "I know you were in the hospital. Tell me what happened when you were there."

c. "Do you remember if you liked the hospital?"

d. "Why did you have to be in the hospital?"

ANSWER

b. To encourage dialogue about a past experience, the nurse should refer to the incident and reflect on the meaning of the experience that includes the child's feelings about the event.

ITEM 5 Cognitive Type: Application

During the preoperational stage of development, children engage in pretending as a form of communication. This practice

a. allows a child to act out feelings and past experiences.

b. has no relationship to the real world or events.

c. demonstrates the child's need for an interpretive response from an adult.

d. is the child's attempt to interact with others prior to the development of conversational language.

ANSWER

a. Children's natural tendency to act out their feelings and experiences helps them to cope with the real world.

ITEM 6 Cognitive Type: Application

Which nursing action should be included in the plan of care for an 8-year-old child who requires surgery and speaks only Spanish?

a. Use storytelling and books to prepare the child for surgical experiences.

b. Arrange for the child and the family to attend classes to learn to speak English prior to the surgical experience.

c. Use an interpreter and a bilingual dictionary to communicate with the child and family.

d. Use touch and gestures to explain the preoperational procedure.

ANSWER

c. To promote understanding and acceptance in the child with cultural or language differences, the nurse may need to enlist the aid of an interpreter and bilingual dictionary to foster effective communication.

ITEM 7 Cognitive Type: Knowledge

Which of the following principles would the nurse use to facilitate effective communication with children?

a. Touch the child's hand as soon as you meet her.

b. Minimize or play down painful procedures.

c. Use an open-ended question to start the conversation.

d. Stand close to a sitting child while speaking.

ANSWER

c. The nurse knows that open-ended questions give the child options for answering and stimulate him to think and express his ideas.

ITEM 8 Cognitive Type: Application

While discussing future diagnostic testing with a 14-year-old, the nurse makes the following statement: "You said you had some questions about the bone marrow aspiration you are going to have tomorrow." The nurse's statement is an example of which strategy to encourage conversation?

a. Focusing

b. Informing

c. Sustaining

d. Enabling

ANSWER

d. Enabling refers to statements that enable and help the child to move toward an extended meaning of a particular situation.

CHAPTER 12

ITEM 1 Cognitive Type: Interpretation

Consistency in parenting practices assists the child in developing

a. greater freedom and mastery of the environment.

b. a moral conscience.

c. attitudes and emotional expressions of admired others.

d. a sense of security and respect for rules and authority.

ANSWER

d. Consistency, an essential element of parenting, fosters respect for rules and authority and provides a sense of security since the child knows what is expected.

ITEM 2 Cognitive Type: Interpretation

Which of the following is the most effective method of teaching rules to infants and toddlers?

a. Limit setting

b. Direct verbal communication

c. Nonverbal communication

d. Environmental control

ANSWER

d. The best method of conveying rules to infants and toddlers to ensure their safety is environmental control.

ITEM 3 Cognitive Type: Interpretation

Which of the following negative reinforcement methods can be used to help children recognize self-regulation as a personal responsibility?

a. Allow them to experience the natural consequences of their actions.

b. Have them apologize for an inappropriate behavior.

c. Remind them of their wrongdoings.

d. Remove them from situations that prompt unacceptable behavior.

ANSWER

a. Allowing children to experience the natural consequences of their actions fosters their ability to take responsibility for self-control.

ITEM 4 Cognitive Type: Interpretation

Which of the following actions would concern the nurse about a parent's use of negative reinforcement?

a. The parent punishes the child in a calm, matter-of-fact manner.

b. The parent explains why he disapproves of the child's behavior.

c. Physical punishment is not used as a method of negative reinforcement.

d. The 3-year-old child is sent to her room for 3 hours.

ANSWER

d. As a general rule, isolation periods of longer than 1 hour breed contempt for the parent rather than redirecting the child's behavior. Isolation is not a preferred method before preschool age.

ITEM 5 Cognitive Type: Interpretation

When counseling parents about the use of rewards as a means of enforcing rules or setting limits, the nurse should

a. recommend that token rewards be given when the child promises to not misbehave.

b. explain that recognizing and acknowledging the child in a spontaneous act of being good is a reward that can eliminate many parent–child conflicts.

c. suggest that social rewards be given only if the child is able to repeat a desired behavior on several occasions.

d. explain that personal rewards given by another can be effective in helping the child who has a poor self-concept.

ANSWER

b. Positive reinforcement (reward) increases the likelihood that a child will repeat a desired behavior. Accentuating the positive aspects of behavior fosters the child's perception of the parent as a supporter of the growing self.

ITEM 6 Cognitive Type: Application

To promote positive functioning in the child whose temperament has been defined as easy, the nurse should counsel parents to

a. introduce new rules gradually and repeatedly to enhance learning.

b. use a democratic approach when setting limits to encourage cooperation.

c. clearly define and consistently endorse expectations to avoid confusion for the child.

d. provide for repeated exposure to new situations to avoid conflict between the child and the environment.

ANSWER

c. The easy child adapts to almost any parenting approach and is easy to manage as long as expectations are clearly defined and consistently enforced.

ITEM 7 Cognitive Type: Knowledge

How can the nurse advise parents about safety for the home-alone child?

a. Whenever possible, limit the time alone to less than 2 hours.

b. The parent should review the after-school routine with the child.

c. A child under 12 years of age should not be left home alone.

d. Arrange for several friends to come over after school.

ANSWER

b. Children should not be left alone without first establishing that they are ready for it. Safety is a primary concern for the home-alone child. The parent should walk through the after-school routine with the child.

ITEM 8 Cognitive Type: Interpretation

Which of the following is important for achieving success in stepparenting?

a. Assume parenting responsibility for the stepchild early on.

b. Establish trust with the stepchild before making or enforcing rules.

c. Allow stepchildren to manipulate their new environment to approximate their previous family unit.

d. Enlist the help of the custodial parent in interpreting stepparent's behavior for the children.

ANSWER

b. Research shows that discipline of children is a major problem in integration of the blended family unit. Children who have not yet learned to trust a new stepparent respond with shock, resentment, and resistance if forced to comply with discipline from a stepparent.

CHAPTER 13

ITEM 1 Cognitive Type: Interpretation

The nurse is collecting a health history from a parent with a child who has diabetes mellitus. Which of the following questions incorporates interviewing principles?

a. "How much regular and NPH insulin did the child receive this morning and what site was used?"

b. "Has the child had any vomiting, diarrhea, or abdominal pain recently?"

c. "Tell me what you do when your child is having a low blood sugar reaction."

d. "Did you check his blood sugar today?"

ANSWER

c. Open-ended questions such as this allow the interviewee the opportunity to express themselves.

ITEM 2 Cognitive Type: Interpretation

Which of the following should be included as part of the family profile in a child's health history?

a. The maternal grandfather has insulin-dependent diabetes.

b. The child has had a 3-day history of nasal congestion and temperature elevation to 102°F rectally.

c. The adolescent was attentive while the mother provided interview information.

d. The 15-month-old has a history of multiple ear infections "just like his brother."

ANSWER

a. The family profile includes documentation of existing or past conditions that are familial or hereditary.

ITEM 3 Cognitive Type: Application

Jeremy, age 4 years, appears apprehensive as his annual physical examination begins. Which of the following questions is best for the nurse to ask when attempting to gain his cooperation?

a. "Do you like to come to the clinic for your check-up?"

b. "Are you always this shy and quiet?"

c. "Would you like to listen to your heart with the stethoscope?"

d. "I know this must be scary, but I'll be finished very soon."

ANSWER

c. Many children like to be involved in the health examination. In addition to verbal explanations, a child may be more cooperative if allowed to handle the equipment that will be used by the examiner.

ITEM 4 Cognitive Type: Interpretation

The nurse assigned to a 1-year-old child would measure the child's vital signs in which sequence?

a. Temperature, pulse, respirations, blood pressure

b. Pulse, respirations, blood pressure, temperature

c. Blood pressure, temperature, pulse, respirations

d. Respirations, temperature, blood pressure, pulse

ANSWER

b. To increase cooperation and produce accurate results with very young children, vital signs should be taken in the following order: pulse and respirations, blood pressure, and temperature.

ITEM 5 Cognitive Type: Interpretation

Which assessment approach provides the best information about a preschool age child's physical growth pattern?

a. Measure the height, weight, and head circumference.

b. Request comparative information about sibling growth patterns from a parent.

c. Plot the height and weight measurements on a standardized percentile growth grid.

d. Observe the child's general appearance, coordination, and posture.

ANSWER

c. Measurements of height and weight should be obtained and plotted on a standardized anthropometric chart to determine the relationship between them and to identify progress in growth.

ITEM 6 Cognitive Type: Knowledge

Which finding would the nurse recognize as normal when measuring the vital signs of an 8-year-old boy?

a. Pulse rate is 90 beats per minute.

b. Temperature is 100.8°F taken orally.

c. Respiratory rate is 28 breaths per minute.

d. Blood pressure is 130/80 mmHg.

ANSWER

a. This pulse rate is a normal vital sign for an 8-year-old child, while the others are not.

ITEM 7 Cognitive Type: Application

Which of the following techniques should follow inspection during physical assessment of the abdomen?

a. Superficial palpation

b. Percussion

c. Auscultation

d. Deep palpation

ANSWER

c. The nurse should always inspect and auscultate the abdomen prior to percussion or palpation to avoid altering internal structures.

ITEM 8 Cognitive Type: Application

Which is the best method for the nurse to assess visual acuity in a 7-year-old non-English-speaking child?

a. STYCAR chart

b. Allen cards

c. Snellen E chart

d. Snellen Alphabet chart

ANSWER

c. The Snellen E chart can be used when the child is not familiar with the alphabet. The E can be described as a table and the child is asked which direction the table legs point.

ITEM 9 Cognitive Type: Knowledge

Assessment of hearing ability in a 1-year-old child can be accomplished by

a. performing a Weber test.

b. using play audiometry.

c. eliciting the startle reflex.

d. observing for localization of sound.

ANSWER

d. The 12-month-old can localize a sound source from above and below and will automatically respond to sound rapidly.

ITEM 10 Cognitive Type: Application

On auscultation of 5-year-old Janie's lung fields, the nurse notes inspiratory breath sounds that are louder, longer, and higher pitched than the sounds heard on expiration. This type of breath sounds, heard all over the chest except over the sternum and scapula, are called

a. vesicular.

b. bronchial.

c. bronchovesicular.

d. adventitious.

ANSWER

a. The nurse applies knowledge of respiratory assessment to a clinical situation and correctly identifies the type of breath sound.

ITEM 11 Cognitive Type: Knowledge

When assessing the intensity of the first heart sound (S1), the nurse should auscultate over which area of the heart?

a. Near the base

b. Lateral to Erbs point

c. At the apex

d. Along the sternal border

ANSWER

c. The intensity of a heart sound refers to where it is heard the best. S1 should be heard best at the apex; if this is not the case, further evaluation is warranted.

ITEM 12 Cognitive Type: Interpretation

When assessing cranial nerve function in young children, the nurse should

a. enlist the help of a family member in clarifying the child's response.

b. modify examination techniques according to the child's developmental level.

c. expect deviations from normal in cortical sensory interpretations.

d. defer motor nerve function tests until the age of 3 years.

ANSWER

b. Difficulties encountered in the assessment of cranial nerves in young children resulting from developmental level can be addressed by modifying examination techniques to match the developmental capabilities of the child.

ITEM 13 Cognitive Type: Interpretation

Which nursing actions reduce anxiety in the child and family when assessing the genitalia as part of the physical examination?

a. Perform this part of the examination first after explaining the procedure.

b. Encourage the family to leave the room during this part of the examination.

c. Approach this part of the examination in a matter-of-fact manner while exposing only the area to be examined.

d. Deemphasize the importance of this part of the examination since most children have normal genitalia.

ANSWER

c. A matter-of-fact approach and limited body exposure will help put a child and family at ease during genital assessment.

ITEM 14 Cognitive Type: Application

Janice Roth wants to know the purpose of the Denver II which is given as part of her 4-month-old daughter's health examination. How would the nurse respond to Janice's question?

a. "The Denver II will show how your child's intelligence level changes up to 6 years of age."

b. "This test will show us developmental delays so the child can receive necessary services."

c. "The purpose is to evaluate the child's cognitive and psychosocial development."

d. "This test is used to assess the personal/social, fine motor adaptive, language, and gross motor development of your child."

ANSWER

d. The Denver II is a developmental screening test used to assess children from birth to 6 years of age in personal/social, fine motor adaptive, language, and gross motor development. It is not an intelligence test.

CHAPTER 14

ITEM 1 Cognitive Type: Knowledge

Which of the following contributes to the child's development of a self-system?

a. Smooth acquisition of personality traits along a prescribed continuum

b. Genetically inherited traits

c. Financial resources and cultural mobility

d. Significant other and social role expectations

ANSWER

d. Children are not born with a self-system. It is developed over time and includes experiences associated with developmental psychosocial crisis, significant other and social role expectations, health status, and temperament style.

ITEM 2 Cognitive Type: Knowledge

Which of the following poses a threat to the development of the school age child's self-system?

a. Delayed parental response to expressed needs

b. Sexual role confusion when relating to the opposite sex

c. Daily confrontation with teachers' and peers' evaluations of physical, social, and intellectual performance

d. Acceptance of subordination to authority figures outside of the family

ANSWER

c. The nurse recognizes that early childhood is a crucial time for health development of the core components of the self-system. The onslaught of daily evaluations from teachers and peers during the school years is identified as a particular threat to the child's self-esteem.

ITEM 3 Cognitive Type: Interpretation

A family environment that is most likely to foster the development of healthy self-system in children is one in which

a. the children are allowed to establish behavioral direction, are not punished, and are reasoned with if they misbehave.

b. the parenting style is autocratic, obedience is stressed, and children are punished when noncompliant with rules.

c. the children are accepted, respected, and expected to function within clearly defined limits.

d. the parents distance themselves from the children, acknowledge their limitations frequently, and are honest about behavioral expectations.

ANSWER

c. The three elements of the home environment that appear to be critical to the development of a healthy self-system are acceptance of the child, clearly defined limits, and respectful treatment.

ITEM 4 Cognitive Type: Application

Which of the following assessment tools is most appropriate for measuring self-concept in early school age children?

a. Verbal self-rating

b. Draw-a-person test

c. Self-esteem inventory

d. Carey temperament scale

ANSWER

b. Observational scales and draw-a-person tests are preferred for estimating the self-concept of preschool and primary grade children to circumvent the social desirability response bias found in verbal self-ratings.

ITEM 5 Cognitive Type: Knowledge

Which of the following nursing strategies can help a family to build and maintain a healthy self-system in each of its members?

a. Role modeling and friendship

b. Sympathy and empathy

c. Positive feedback, counseling, and education

d. Fostering routines and dependence behaviors

ANSWER

c. The nurse can assess and teach the child and family self-concept building behaviors and can support their efforts through frequent positive feedback, counseling, and broadened education.

ITEM 6 Cognitive Type: Interpretation

To foster a sense of security and belonging in their children, parents should be encouraged to

a. love and respect their children.

b. expose their children to new experiences.

c. provide opportunities for their children to experience success.

d. establish and adhere to clear, reasonable limits.

ANSWER

d. Setting clear, reasonable limits provides an environment that facilitates a child's development of a sense of security and belonging. The child knows what behavior is acceptable and they learn that they are like everyone else.

CHAPTER 15

ITEM 1 Cognitive Type: Application

Which of the following children is at greatest risk for accidental injury?

a. A 2-month-old infant is secured in a car seat that faces toward the rear of the car.

b. A 14-month-old child plays with plastic measuring cups while sitting on the floor in the kitchen.

c. A 9-year-old boy rides a bike in the same direction as traffic on the side of the road.

d. A 2-year-old girl is secured in a high chair while eating a carrot.

ANSWER

d. Hard foods are commonly aspirated by 2- to 4-year-olds. Even though a toddler has some molars, the ability to thoroughly chew hard foods is not mastered until the preschool years.

ITEM 2 Cognitive Type: Knowledge

Which of the following is the leading cause of accidental death in children and adolescents?

a. Burn injuries

b. Motor vehicle accidents

c. Poisonings and ingestions

d. Homicide

ANSWER

b. Motor vehicle accidents are the leading cause of death in children despite legislation and information related to the reduced probability of death when a child is properly secured in a car seat.

ITEM 3 Cognitive Type: Knowledge

The factor that most affects the types of injuries that occur in children is

a. the child's age.

b. the number of children in the home.

c. the child's overall health.

d. the parent's knowledge of safety.

ANSWER

a. Most injuries occur as a result of a complex interaction of a host, an agent, and the environment. A major determinant in the type of injury that occurs is the child's age.

ITEM 4 Cognitive Type: Interpretation

Which of the following is an example of an *active* approach to injury prevention?

a. Installed driver-side airbags in automobiles

b. Recalled infant car seats for defective buckles

c. Seat belt used only for long distance trips

d. Locks placed on all low cabinets in the kitchen

ANSWER

d. An active approach to injury prevention is one in which the individual initiates specific behaviors or adheres to laws and regulations.

ITEM 5 Cognitive Type: Knowledge

Nursing strategies to prevent water-related accidents should include

a. encouraging parents to provide for organized swimming instruction for infants and toddlers.

b. promoting infant aquatic education programs as an effective strategy to prevent drowning.

c. stressing the importance of putting life jackets on all nonswimmers and children under 3 years of age when they are near water.

d. counseling parents about water safety and supervision during routine health visits at 6 months of age.

ANSWER

c. Life jackets should be worn by all children under the age of 3 years and by all children who cannot swim.

ITEM 6 Cognitive Type: Knowledge

Which of the following actions taken by the mother of a 14-month-old toddler indicates that the nurse's teaching about poisoning prevention has been successful?

a. She instructs the child not to chew on her jade plant.

b. She discards all outdated medicine in the bathroom waste basket.

c. She hides caustic cleaning fluids at the back of the refrigerator.

d. She purchases a 30-mL bottle of syrup of Ipecac.

ANSWER

d. Basic objectives in poison prevention include reducing the number of poisonings and reducing the severity of the effects of poisoning should it occur. Syrup of Ipecac is recognized as an agent to induce vomiting in the event of an accidental ingestion.

ITEM 7 Cognitive Type: Application

The initial nursing intervention for a school-age child who has a foreign body lodged in his larynx should be to

a. sweep the finger into the larynx to attempt to remove the object.

b. turn the child face down and pounding him on the back.

c. apply the Heimlich maneuver after establishing that the airway is obstructed.

d. seek the assistance of another adult to begin cardiopulmonary resuscitation.

ANSWER

c. The Heimlich maneuver has been successful in all ages and should be the first choice of emergency treatment for a life-threatening situation caused by aspiration of a foreign body.

ITEM 8 Cognitive Type: Interpretation

To meet the safety needs of young school age children in a community setting, the nurse develops a series of "streetproofing" programs. Which of the following represents the goal of such a program?

a. To create suspicion and fear in a child to prevent abusive overtures from adults

b. To assist a child in acquiring skills to detect danger and cope with threatening situations

c. To organize neighborhood parents in establishing watch patrols to reduce the risk of violence against their children

d. To provide information for parents and children about areas in the community that are safe and friendly for children

ANSWER

b. *Streetproofing* is the term used to describe the process of preparing children for the potential dangers that threaten children when they embark "on the street."

ITEM 9 Cognitive Type: Knowledge

Which of the following poses a risk of suffocation to an 8-month-old infant?

a. A small stuffed animal is placed in the crib for the child to hold.

b. The slats on the crib are 2-3/8 inches apart.

c. The crib is next to a window with draperies that open and close with a cord.

d. The hanging mobile was removed from the crib.

ANSWER

c. Infants can get caught in cords on draperies or on mobiles.

CHAPTER 16

ITEM 1 Cognitive Type: Knowledge

Research supports that existing nutritional problems in children in the United States are related to

a. improper selection of nutrient intake.

b. thiamine and riboflavin deficiencies.

c. inadequate total energy intake.

d. excessive intake of carbohydrates and fats.

ANSWER

c. Cross-sectional surveys of the nutritional status of children in the United States show that nutritional problems are related to inadequate total energy intake rather than improper selection of nutrient intake.

ITEM 2 Cognitive Type: Knowledge

Which statement reflects the relationship between oral gratification in infancy and personality development?

a. Caregivers who are not sensitive to infant cues produce synchrony with the infant.

b. Maladaptive responses to infant feeding are the cause of long-standing nutritional problems.

c. Attachment in infancy is fostered by rhythmic give and take between mother and infant during the feeding process.

d. Satisfaction of an infant's oral needs has no relationship to later eating practices.

ANSWER

c. Through the feeding process, attachment in infancy is fostered by a rhythmic giving and taking between the caregiver and the infant.

ITEM 3 Cognitive Type: Knowledge

Teresa is pregnant for the first time and asks what effect her diet will have on her baby. The nurse should explain that

a. poor nutrition is associated with low birth weight infants.

b. infant obesity is related to excess dietary intake during pregnancy.

c. brain growth will be severely retarded unless the mother's diet meets the daily dietary requirements.

d. excessive weight gain will adversely affect fetal growth.

ANSWER

a. Poor nutrition of the mother during pregnancy (especially during the last trimester) is associated with low birth weight infants.

ITEM 4 Cognitive Type: Knowledge

Which of the following factors affects the development of children's food habits?

a. Cultural preference

b. Temperament

c. Physical stature

d. Blood cholesterol levels

ANSWER

a. Cultural differences, family relationships, life style, peer and social influences (including television), and economic status are some of the nonphysiological variants that affect the development of food habits.

ITEM 5 Cognitive Type: Knowledge

Nutritional counseling is indicated for a child whose

a. family incorporates cultural food preferences into their diet.

b. growth is below the 20th percentile or over the 75th percentile.

c. growth occurs in spurts rather than on a continuum.

d. growth is below the 10th percentile or over the 90th percentile.

ANSWER

d. Conditions indicating that nutritional counseling may be necessary are if the child's growth is below the 10th percentile or greater than the 90th percentile.

ITEM 6 Cognitive Type: Knowledge

Foods sweetened with Aspartame should not be given to children who

a. have phenylketonuria.

b. are hyperactive.

c. have a family history of cancer.

d. have hypercholesterolemia.

ANSWER

a. Aspartame is an acceptable sweetener that was approved by the FDA in 1981. It should not be used, however, by someone with phenylketonuria because it is made from the amino acid phenylalanine.

ITEM 7 Cognitive Type: Interpretation

The nurse conducts a nutritional assessment interview with Tommy, age 7 years, and his mother. Analysis of the data collected suggests the following nursing diagnosis: *Alteration in nutrition: Less than body requirements related to maturational changes that diminish appetite.* Which intervention should the nurse recommend to Tommy's mother?

a. Allow Tommy to eat dessert first to ensure adequate calorie intake.

b. Avoid purchasing junk foods and sweets for snacks so as to enhance Tommy's appetite at mealtimes.

c. Control portion sizes and insist Tommy empty his plate.

d. Encourage Tommy to eat desired foods first and least desired foods last.

ANSWER

b. It should be stressed that if sweets are curtailed and excessive milk intake not permitted, a healthy child will eat when hungry without coercion.

ITEM 8 Cognitive Type: Interpretation

Anne, age 14 years, has decided to become a vegetarian. She refuses to eat meat or eggs in spite of her mother's admonitions. When counseling Anne and her mother, the nurse should

a. suggest that Anne postpone becoming a vegetarian until she is at least 16 years old.

b. explain that vegetarian diets are linked to a decreased cholesterol level and increased risk for cancer.

c. suggest that Anne and her mother jointly plan a diet that ensures adequate dietary protein.

d. explain that adolescents on vegetarian diets are at risk for anorexia.

ANSWER

c. Poorly planned vegetarian diets can increase the risk of diet-related nutritional disorders, especially during the growing years. The best way to ensure a well-planned diet is to encourage the mother's involvement.

ITEM 9 Cognitive Type: Knowledge

Strategies to prevent infant obesity include

a. introduction of solid foods no earlier than 4 to 6 months of age.

b. use of skim milk from 6 to 12 months of age.

c. breastfeeding rather than using iron-fortified formula.

d. maintaining a strict feeding schedule for infants.

ANSWER

a. Introduction of solid foods before 4 to 6 months of age adds extra, unnecessary calories.

ITEM 10 Cognitive Type: Knowledge

Kwashiorkor is a serious form of malnutrition related to

a. a deficiency of calcium and phosphorus.

b. a deficiency of protein resulting in severe muscle wasting.

c. a grossly inadequate caloric intake resulting in gradual wasting.

d. a deficiency of Vitamin C resulting in severe infantile diarrhea.

ANSWER

b. Kwashiorkor is primarily a deficiency of protein resulting in severe muscle wasting.

ITEM 11 Cognitive Type: Knowledge

Therapeutic management of infants with severe nutritional imbalances related to grossly inadequate protein and calorie intake would *not* include

a. antibiotic therapy.

b. gradual dietary rehabilitation.

c. administration of fluids and electrolytes.

d. exercise to reverse muscle wasting.

ANSWER

d. Treatment consists of administration of fluids and electrolytes, antibiotic therapy to treat infections, and a gradual dietary rehabilitation.

ITEM 12 Cognitive Type: Knowledge

Premature infants are at risk for disturbances in vitamin D metabolism because they

a. lack sufficient phosphate and calcium to mineralize rapidly growing bones.

b. usually have hepatic disease from uncontrolled jaundice.

c. are predisposed to familial rickets with hypophosphatemia.

d. get inadequate penetration of sunlight.

ANSWER

a. During the last trimester of pregnancy, significant amounts of calcium phosphate are transferred daily to the fetus. Even with fortified formula, the premature infant receives much less calcium and phosphate than is adequate.

ITEM 13 Cognitive Type: Knowledge

Which of the following signs might be observed in a 15-month-old child with nonorganic failure to thrive?

a. Is soothed gradually when picked up

b. Rocking and clapping to music

c. Puts arms out to be held by nurse

d. Sits in crib and stares intensely at people

ANSWER

d. Intense watchfulness is a behavioral indicator of potential failure to thrive.

ITEM 14 Cognitive Type: Knowledge

Obtaining assessment information about a possible failure-to-thrive infant can be gained through

a. observing the mother and child during feeding.

b. having the mother keep a written record of the child's food intake.

c. periodically calling the mother to ask what the child has had to eat on a particular day.

d. asking the mother to have someone else feed the child for a week and notice if there is any difference in weight gain.

ANSWER

a. The nurse knows that accurate assessment of failure to thrive is based on observation of infant and caretaker in feeding situations.

ITEM 15 Cognitive Type: Application

Which nursing action should be included in the plan of care for a child who is receiving parenteral nutrition?

a. Change tubing by using sterile technique every 8 hours.

b. Check urine glucose, acetone, and specific gravity levels every 6 to 8 hours.

c. Adjust the infusion rate when necessary to ensure administration of the prescribed 24-hour total.

d. Monitor vital signs, blood pressure, and weight daily.

ANSWER

b. Careful monitoring of the child receiving parenteral nutrition includes assessment of metabolic complications. Vital signs should be checked every 4 hours, not just daily,

ITEM 16 Cognitive Type: Knowledge

The best description of a complete formula used for enteral feedings is one that

a. contains sufficient nutrients used as a supplement to oral intake.

b. contains whole molecules of carbohydrates, proteins, and fats.

c. is hydrolyzed or predigested and contains partial molecules of essential nutrients.

d. provides the necessary nutrients to meet the client's needs.

ANSWER

d. Enteral formulas can be classified as complete or incomplete, intact or hydrolyzed. A complete formula provides all of the nutrients necessary to meet the individual's needs when given in sufficient quantities.

CHAPTER 17

ITEM 1 Cognitive Type: Knowledge

Which of the following is a characteristic of play?

a. Goal oriented

b. Reality based

c. Flexible

d. Repetitive

ANSWER

c. For an activity to be characterized as play, there must be flexibility. The child shifts among themes and materials easily.

ITEM 2 Cognitive Type: Interpretation

Which of the following activities helps to foster social interaction *and* reasoning abilities in an 8-year-old child?

a. Practicing piano lessons after school

b. Going to the video arcade after school with friends

c. Playing gin rummy with grandparents

d. Visiting a museum with family members

ANSWER

c. The nurse is able to recognize activities that contribute to the development of cognitive competence in the school age child.

ITEM 3 Cognitive Type: Knowledge

The nurse would expect to observe a group of toddler age children playing

a. with one another but without organization or purpose.

b. next to one another while sharing and trading toys.

c. beside one another with similar toys but without social interaction.

d. close to one another while reenacting a previously observed event.

ANSWER

c. Toddler age children characteristically engage in parallel play.

ITEM 4 Cognitive Type: Interpretation

The nurse is teaching a group of nursery school assistants about promoting growth and development through play. Which materials are appropriate for 2- and 3-year-old children and thus should be included in the nurse's instructions?

a. Push–pull and rocking toys

b. Large beads and sturdy string

c. Table and board games

d. Art supplies with scissors

ANSWER

b. Stringing beads is an activity that promotes fine motor development and imaginative play for this age group and is safe.

ITEM 5 Cognitive Type: Application

At a well child visit, a mother tells the nurse that her only child, 2-year-old Alyssa, plays very nicely by herself and that she makes time to play with Alyssa everyday. Which of the following should the nurse suggest to her to encourage sociodramatic play?

a. Involve Alyssa in a playgroup.

b. Have Alyssa play with another 2-year-old girl.

c. Enroll Alyssa in a dance class.

d. Take Alyssa to a playground.

ANSWER

a. By the time children are toddlers, they need friends to play with. Parents should foster cross-gender play experiences.

ITEM 6 Cognitive Type: Knowledge

When the nurse is assessing the play of a child who has been physically abused or neglected, she might expect to observe

a. aggressive behavior in associative play.

b. initially hesitant play, followed by exploratory play.

c. randomly moving from one play activity to another.

d. noninteractive constructive play.

ANSWER

c. Children who have been abused or neglected may lack energy for play. Kempe and Kempe describe the frozen watchfulness of abused children who expect punishment, are unable to play or explore, and move from one activity to another in a haphazard, impulsive manner.

ITEM 7 Cognitive Type: Application

Five-year-old Katie has acute lymphoblastic leukemia and is scheduled for placement of a broviac catheter for chemotherapy. To use preparation play with Katie, the nurse would

a. show Katie a Mr. Rogers videotape about having an operation.

b. allow Katie to see and handle a broviac catheter, syringe, and dressings.

c. draw pictures with Katie about the broviac catheter.

d. have Katie use a doll to demonstrate what the nurse talked about.

ANSWER

d. If the preparation only involves a demonstration of equipment by the nurse, it is not play. Preparation play involves the child in a play rehearsal with actual medical equipment and dolls or puppets.

CHAPTER 18

ITEM 1 Cognitive Type: Knowledge

During the stress response, perception of the stressor occurs within the

a. cerebral cortex.

b. hypothalamus.

c. pituitary gland.

d. autonomic nervous system.

ANSWER

a. As part of the body's response to stress, the stimulus is perceived and interpreted within the cerebral cortex.

ITEM 2 Cognitive Type: Knowledge

Whether or not a life event is going to be stressful for a child depends primarily on

a. the age at which the event occurs.

b. the child's temperament.

c. the child's perception of the event.

d. the child's developmental level.

ANSWER

c. A variety of factors influences the impact of life events on children. Most important in determining the amount of stress experienced is the child's perception of the particular event.

ITEM 3 Cognitive Type: Application

Which statement is most appropriate for the nurse to make during the assessment phase of crisis intervention with a family?

a. "Let's consider what all of your feelings might mean."

b. "Tell me when you began feeling this way."

c. "Help me to understand why you might be feeling this way."

d. "Let's talk about what you can do about these feelings."

ANSWER

b. The nurse understands that the assessment phase of crisis intervention includes determining the precipitating event and when the feelings of stress began. Other responses are geared more toward the intervention phase.

ITEM 4 Cognitive Type: Application

A nursing assessment of the Walker family revealed that they were all anxious about Mr. Walker's job transfer. Which of the following statements made by the nurse reflects understanding of the intervention strategies for this family?

a. "Johnny really shouldn't be taken out of school in the middle of the year."

b. "What will you do if Mr. Walker doesn't like his new job?"

c. "Let's talk about your feelings about the move."

d. "Let's talk about how you have dealt with new situations before."

ANSWER

d. The nurse understands that during the intervention phase of crisis intervention, the family's previously successful coping mechanisms assist them in developing coping strategies for dealing with the current crisis.

ITEM 5 Cognitive Type: Knowledge

Anticipatory guidance can be most therapeutic during which phase of crisis intervention?

a. Assessment

b. Planning

c. Intervention

d. Evaluation

ANSWER

d. The nurse knows that during the evaluation phase of crisis intervention, the present management of the crisis is used to focus on ways of managing future crises.

ITEM 6 Cognitive Type: Interpretation

The Allens have two children, Melissa, age 14 years, and Steven, age 8 years. Which of the following represents a potential situational crisis for the members of this family?

a. Melissa does not have a date for the freshman dance at school.

b. Mrs. Allen's car was vandalized in the mall parking lot.

c. Steven cannot go on his class trip because he has chickenpox.

d. Mr. Allen received notice that his company was closing.

ANSWER

d. Examples of situational crisis include illness, failure at school, loss of a parent's job, death of a loved one, and divorce of parents.

ITEM 7 Cognitive Type: Application

Three-year-old Michael began kicking and screaming violently when the nurse entered the room with his injection. The nurse should respond by saying

a. "This medicine will help you feel better."

b. "There is no reason to be so upset."

c. "I understand that you are upset, but I need to give you this medicine."

d. "Be a big, brave boy for me."

ANSWER

c. The nurse understands that the young child's cognitive development does not allow him to understand the relationship between medicine and cure. His response should not be ignored. Validating the child's feelings while maintaining control helps the child to cope with stress.

ITEM 8 Cognitive Type: Knowledge

The nurse would expect a toddler to cope with the stress of separation from her parents during hospitalization by

a. regressing.

b. repressing.

c. projecting.

d. rationalizing.

ANSWER

a. The nurse identifies regression as being an age-appropriate ego defense mechanism for the toddler.

ITEM 9 Cognitive Type: Knowledge

Coping strategies for the parents of an ill child can be promoted by the nurse who

a. suggests that the family try not to worry so much.

b. assists the parents in identifying resources to help them deal with day to day tasks.

c. offers to help them as much as possible.

d. allows the family to deny the seriousness of the situation until the crisis has been resolved.

ANSWER

b. The nurse knows that helping parents to identify resources is a strategy that promotes coping.

CHAPTER 19

ITEM 1 Cognitive Type: Application

Which of the following actions taken by a child with a chronic condition is indicative of wellness behavior?

a. An adolescent who has diabetes admonishes her mother for baking a layer cake for her sister's birthday.

b. A third grader who has asthma delays using his inhalant medication until he is finished with an important project.

c. On the first day of kindergarten, a 6-year-old who has cystic fibrosis tells his teacher not to worry if she hears him coughing and spitting into a tissue because he can breathe better when he gets the mucous out.

d. A 14-year-old girl with chronic inflammatory bowel disease takes an elective library studies course during her lunch hour to avoid having an episode of diarrhea in school.

ANSWER

c. Children with chronic illnesses exhibit wellness behavior by assuming direct responsibility for personal needs that reflect sound health practices.

ITEM 2 Cognitive Type: Interpretation

When helping a family to reduce risk and vulnerability in their child who has a chronic illness, the nurse should consider which goal to be most important?

a. Maintaining control of the symptoms of the illness

b. Organizing a support group for families with children who have similar conditions

c. Restricting the child's physical environment to eliminate exposure to pollution, bacteria, and viruses

d. Providing instruction in reducing constitutional factors that impact on the child's response to stressor

ANSWER

a. The nurse recognizes that maintenance of control of symptoms reduces risk and vulnerability in children who have chronic conditions.

ITEM 3 Page 9 Cognitive Type: Interpretation

Children with chronic conditions whose behaviors reflect sick role functioning are at risk for

a. exacerbation of illness.

b. social isolation.

c. noncompliance with treatment regimes.

d. bacterial and viral infections.

ANSWER

b. The nurse recognizes that the sick role frees an individual from certain social responsibilities and obligations and that children with chronic conditions must resume part or all of these responsibilities or be excluded from interactions with others and eventually suffer social isolation.

ITEM 4 Cognitive Type: Interpretation

An 8-year-old child with asthma whose cognitive development reflects concrete operational thought would most likely perceive his chronic condition as

a. a personal challenge to develop independence and control over episodes of bronchospasm.

b. coming from dust and germs in the air that make it hard to breathe.

c. being caused by internal or external environmental factors that initiate episodes of wheezing and coughing.

d. the result of having kissed a grandparent who was sick.

ANSWER

b. The child whose thinking is concrete does not differentiate between mind and body and sees the source of illness as external.

ITEM 5 Cognitive Type: Knowledge

The nurse assigned to a Native American child would incorporate which of the following cultural knowledge into the plan of care?

a. It is disrespectful to make eye contact with the child and family.

b. Illness is perceived as God's will.

c. It is common to be very tactile with family and friends.

d. Touching the person is considered a loss of self-control.

ANSWER

a. Many Native Americans consider making eye contact with another person to be a sign of disrespect.

ITEM 6 Cognitive Type: Application

Which of the following nursing interventions is designed to promote healthy relationships among siblings when one of them has a chronic illness?

a. Encourage parents to involve well siblings in increased domestic responsibilities to provide for more quality time for all family members.

b. Arrange for sibling hospital visitation and elective participation in therapy sessions with the child who is chronically ill.

c. Suggest that parents withhold frightening information about the ill child's condition from siblings to reduce anxiety.

d. Help well children to understand the importance of protecting their ill sibling from the insensitivities of others to help alleviate feelings of anger.

ANSWER

b. Siblings of children with chronic conditions can be supported by nurses who act as advocates for them while promoting activities that encourage a supportive relationship between the children.

ITEM 7 Cognitive Type: Interpretation

A 6-year-old child who has diabetes insists that his nurses cover his injection site with a Superman bandage from the box in his bedside table every time he receives insulin. This child is using which of the following adaptive defenses?

a. Intellectualization

b. Regression

c. Humor

d. Ritualization

ANSWER

d. The nurse recognizes ritualistic behavior as an adaptive defense that can assist children in coping with anxiety in situations where they feel they have little or no control.

ITEM 8 Cognitive Type: Application

Which of the following nursing interventions helps to promote adjustment of a child with a chronic condition who thinks of herself as unable to accomplish anything as a result of her family's well-intended overprotection?

a. Provide the family with literature that describes the long-term consequences of maladaptive coping in chronic illnesses.

b. Explain to the family that they must stop shielding the child from failure if they want her to be accepted by others.

c. Encourage the family to reinforce the child's abilities and praise both the child and family for their efforts in trying.

d. Advise the family to arrange for the child to enter a pediatric chronic care facility until they are able to confront and deal with their feelings of guilt.

ANSWER

c. The nurse applies knowledge of family coping strategies to the promotion of psychosocial adaptation and adjustment of children and families.

ITEM 9 Cognitive Type: Application

Fifteen-year-old Andrea is hospitalized for an exacerbation of cystic fibrosis. An appropriate nursing intervention to help Andrea cope with chronic illness is to

a. talk to Andrea about how cystic fibrosis limits her activities.

b. encourage Andrea to participate in a teen support group.

c. arrange for counseling with a psychologist.

d. suggest Andrea to try out for as many school sports as she can.

ANSWER

b. Adolescent support groups have been established for hospitalized teens. An adolescent with a chronic illness should be encouraged to focus on what they can do versus what they cannot do.

ITEM 10 Cognitive Type: Application

Which of the following nursing actions helps to promote attachment behavior in the parents of a baby born with a chronic condition?

a. Separate the mother and baby from healthy mothers and babies to ensure privacy.

b. Reassure the parents that they will eventually adapt to the baby's handicapping condition.

c. Distract the parents from their grief by initiating conversational topics unrelated to the baby's condition.

d. Emphasize to the parents the baby's normal characteristics while cuddling and making eye contact with the infant.

ANSWER

d. The nurse recognizes positive role modeling actions as a way to promote parent–infant bonding. Emphasizing areas of normal development helps parents to see the child's positive attributes.

ITEM 11 Cognitive Type: Application

The community nurse's role as case manager for a child who has a chronic condition includes

a. assisting the family in organizing and coordinating their child's health care.

b. monitoring the child's physical and psychosocial adaptation to illness.

c. educating the family in promoting self-care activities in the child.

d. measuring the parents' perceptions of the relationships among family members and their functioning in times of crisis.

ANSWER

a. The role of the case manager is one that includes assisting families to manage the many conflicting demands of their child's various health care needs.

CHAPTER 20

ITEM 1 Cognitive Type: Knowledge

According to Kubler-Ross, when parents are confronted with the crisis of impending childhood death, their *first* reaction is

a. isolation and depression.

b. guilt and anger.

c. bargaining and anger.

d. denial and isolation.

ANSWER

d. Five stages have been identified by Kubler-Ross in parents facing a life-threatening illness in their child: denial and isolation, anger, bargaining, and finally, depression and acceptance.

ITEM 2 Cognitive Type: Knowledge

Five-year-old Kevin is hospitalized because of a terminal illness. His parents shout at the nurse when she is 5 minutes late in administering Kevin's pain medication. The nurse recognizes the parents' behavior as

a. a maladaptive coping response to the stress of their son's illness.

b. an expression of the anger they feel because of their son's illness.

c. a reaction that will prevent effective nurse–family communication.

d. a type of coping response that the nurse should immediately report to Kevin's physician.

ANSWER

b. Anger is a typical reaction of parents when their child is dying. Anger is often directed at health professionals. The nurse should respect the parents' feelings and allow expressions of anger without compounding guilt.

ITEM 3 Cognitive Type: Knowledge

Which of the following theorists felt that grief is not a normal psychological functioning and considered it to be a pathological condition?

a. Engel

b. Freud

c. Kubler-Ross

d. Lindemann

ANSWER

b. According to Freud, grief is a departure from normal psychological functioning and he labeled it a pathological condition.

ITEM 4 Cognitive Type: Application

For the past month, the parents of 3-year-old Susan have been anticipating their daughter's death. The nurse can help Susan's parents cope with their anticipatory grief by

a. attempting to lighten their mood and cheer them up.

b. reassuring them that their feelings will pass and they will feel better soon.

c. being physically present with them and encouraging them to participate in Susan's care.

d. suggesting activities that will take their minds off Susan's condition.

ANSWER

c. Anticipatory grief occurs prior to the actual loss and increases in intensity until death. The nurse can help by finding specific ways that parents can maintain a bond with and provide comfort for their child.

ITEM 5 Cognitive Type: Application

Four-year-old Sammy dug up a pet goldfish that he and his father recently buried in the backyard. Which of the following statements should the nurse use to explain Sammy's behavior?

a. Sammy is responding poorly to death, and the parents should seek professional counseling.

b. Sammy is checking to see if the fish went to heaven.

c. Sammy thinks he can bring the goldfish back to life if he digs it up.

d. Sammy needs reassurance that the fish is still dead and that it can be found where it was buried.

ANSWER

d. Children aged 3 to 5 years are unable to distinguish living from nonliving. Children this age think the dead live on under new circumstances.

ITEM 6 Cognitive Type: Knowledge

Which of the following statements is true concerning an 8-year-old child's concept of death?

a. Death is seen as temporary and reversible.

b. Death is seen as possible for the old and ill and often personified as scary, dangerous, and mean.

c. Death is viewed as departure and is associated with a lack of movement.

d. Death is seen as universal and a phenomenon that is inevitable and final for all living things.

ANSWER

b. For children aged 5 to 9 years, death is associated with the old and ill. Children this age also attribute specific characteristics to death, such as scary, dangerous, and mean. Children between 3 and 5 years of age understand death as a departure, believe it to be temporary, reversible, and associated with a lack of movement. By 10 to 12 years of age, children see death as inevitable, universal, and final.

ITEM 7 Cognitive Type: Application

The father of critically ill Joey has begun to shower presents on his son. Joey's mother tells the nurse that her husband has also begun to ignore the other children in the family and insists on spending all of his free time with Joey. The nurse recognizes the father's response as an indication of

a. anger at his wife for allowing Joey to become ill.

b. guilt feelings for not spending more time with Joey.

c. positive coping mechanisms.

d. understandable feelings of resentment toward the other children.

ANSWER

b. Guilt is a common feeling experienced by parents of dying children and may result in overindulging the ill child. Parents may experience guilt if they feel they have not given enough of themselves to the dying child.

ITEM 8 Cognitive Type: Application

The mother of a hospitalized terminally ill child tells the nurse that Alicia, an 8-year-old sibling of the ill child, has been "acting out" in school and having nightmares for the past week. The nurse should respond by telling Alicia's mother to

a. not worry about Alicia's behavior, as it is typical for many 8-year-old children.

b. reassure Alicia that she is loved and encourage her to express her fears and concerns.

c. stop talking about the terminally ill child in front of Alicia, as such discussions are upsetting her.

d. ask the grandparents to spend more time with Alicia while her mother is at the hospital.

ANSWER

b. Siblings of dying children may exhibit behavioral problems such as crying, school difficulties, nightmares, and enuresis. To help siblings cope with life-threatening illness, parents should be honest and open with them, reassuring them of their love.

ITEM 9 Cognitive Type: Application

Which of the following interventions is most helpful in supporting a dying child's family as they cope with the various decision-making periods of a lengthy terminal illness?

a. Encourage the parents to take their child home to die, as this is usually best.

b. Encourage the parents to go through all of the Kubler-Ross stages of facing death in a child as quickly as possible.

c. Refer the child's family to the hospital clergy service as soon as possible.

d. Use active listening to identify specific fears and concerns of the child's family members.

ANSWER

d. Parents of the dying child must make many difficult decisions. The nurse can be supportive to the family during this difficult decision-making time by using active listening and by helping family members to clarify their own thoughts and feel comfortable in their decisions.

ITEM 10 Cognitive Type: Knowledge

Which of the following nursing interventions can be used to help the dying child cope with nausea and vomiting?

a. Offer high fat foods such as french fries and potato chips frequently.

b. Provide dry foods such as crackers, plain cookies, and toast in the morning.

c. Encourage a generous intake of fluids with each meal.

d. Offer frequent servings of hot tea and hot cocoa.

ANSWER

b. Nausea and vomiting are frequently associated with terminal process and can be treated in part by diet. Dry foods such as crackers, plain cookies, and toast decrease nausea, especially in the morning.

ITEM 11 Cognitive Type: Knowledge

Which of the following statements is an accurate description of the physical signs of imminent death in the terminally ill child?

a. The child's muscle tone increases.

b. The child's skin becomes warm, moist, and less mottled.

c. Respirations become irregular and resemble a Cheyne–Stokes pattern.

d. Periods of wakefulness increase and the child becomes more alert.

ANSWER

c. Certain signs usually precede death, such as a change in normal respirations to a Cheyne–Stokes pattern, a decrease in periods of wakefulness and alertness, skin that is mottled and cool to the touch, and a decrease in muscle tone.

ITEM 12 Cognitive Type: Knowledge

Nurses who care for dying children should prepare themselves professionally by

a. concentrating on the physical aspects of nursing a dying child.

b. avoid discussing their work outside of the hospital environment.

c. talking about death in professional support groups that include nurses, physicians, and clergy.

d. maintaining a "professional" attitude by pushing aside their own mood changes and feelings of anger.

ANSWER

c. Nurses who care for dying children must acknowledge that some days they will feel unable to cope with a dying child and family. Nurses must seek support from other professionals and support systems to help them deal with their own expressions of grief.

CHAPTER 21

ITEM 1 Cognitive Type: Interpretation

When planning a hospital tour for a group of preschool-age children, the nurse should

a. arrange for the group to observe children undergoing venipuncture or medication administration.

b. restrict the size of the group to no more than five children.

c. provide for a supervised needle play experience.

d. organize activities to allow for a brief question and answer period.

ANSWER

d. Preparation of well children by means of a hospital tour can be accomplished in groups of ten, should be totally non-threatening, and should provide for explanation and clarification of misconceptions.

ITEM 2 Cognitive Type: Interpretation

Preparation of toddlers for a planned hospitalization should include

a. honest explanations about painful events the child will experience.

b. encouraging parents to plan a pleasant outing for the child and to compare this event to the experience of hospitalization.

c. simple, repetitive discussions about the upcoming hospitalization over a period of several weeks.

d. reading picture books about hospitalization to the child a few days before admission.

ANSWER

d. Toddlers should be prepared for hospitalization within the confines of their mental ability. Explanations should be given two to three days in advance and should not include descriptions of threatening procedures.

ITEM 3 Cognitive Type: Knowledge

Which nursing action should be implemented prior to the arrival of a child for admission to the pediatric unit?

a. Provide children in the room selected for admission with information about their new roommate's condition.

b. Take age-appropriate play materials to the room selected for admission.

c. Obtain information about the child's nutrition and elimination needs from the admissions office.

d. Clean the bed and equipment cabinet selected for admission with disinfectant.

ANSWER

b. Nursing actions prior to the arrival of a child are designed to ease the admission process and to initiate a sense of security in the child.

ITEM 4 Cognitive Type: Knowledge

Children between the ages of 6 months and 4 years experience which of the following as a major stressor during hospitalization?

a. Disruption of routine

b. Separation anxiety

c. Fear of bodily injury

d. Loss of control

ANSWER

b. Separation from parents is the most important stressor associated with hospitalization from middle infancy through the preschool years.

ITEM 5 Cognitive Type: Application

Jenny, age 3 years, has been hospitalized for the past 10 days. Her primary nurse notes that she no longer cries or resists when her incisional wound is irrigated and redressed. Jenny does, however, have a temper tantrum every evening when her parents visit. The nurse concludes that Jenny's behavior

a. is a sign of adaptation to the hospital environment.

b. reflects despair associated with separation from her parents.

c. is associated with her parents' inability to set limits.

d. may have long-term effects on her development unless her parents are encouraged to visit less frequently during this "settling in" phase.

ANSWER

b. A young child experiences a continuing conscious need for parents during the despair stage of reaction to hospitalization.

ITEM 6 Cognitive Type: Application

The initial nursing intervention for a 3-year-old child who is experiencing a sleep pattern disturbance while hospitalized should be aimed at

a. identifying the child's usual bedtime routines or rituals.

b. minimizing the child's age-related fear of the dark by leaving a light on over the bed.

c. determining the source of the child's separation anxiety by observing play behaviors.

d. enforcing naptime and bedtime limits to provide the child with a sense of security and control.

ANSWER

a. Usual sleep pattern, including bed and naptime rituals, must be identified, as these routines are important for promoting sleep in the young child.

ITEM 7 Cognitive Type: Application

To promote adequate caloric intake in a 5-year-old boy who is in the hospital for treatment of a fractured femur, the nurse would

a. allow the child to assist in selecting foods from a printed menu.

b. provide the child with a star chart and stickers to be placed on the chart each time he finishes a meal.

c. explain, in simple terms, the relationship between nutrition and bone healing.

d. arrange for the dietitian to see the child to facilitate his understanding of the importance of eating.

ANSWER

a. The preschool age child is motivated to cooperate if provided with opportunities to practice new skills such as beginning recognition of words.

ITEM 8 Cognitive Type: Application

Keith, age 3-1/2 years, is hospitalized following emergency surgery for an incarcerated hernia. The nurse observes Keith's mother scolding him for voiding in the bed. How should the nurse intervene?

a. Explain to the mother that incontinence is expected after this type of surgery.

b. Teach the mother how to use a social reward approach to get him to use the urinal rather than scolding him.

c. Reassure the mother that temporary loss of elimination control is common when a young child is in the hospital.

d. Take a supply of diapers to Keith's room for him to wear while he is confined to bed.

ANSWER

c. Parents should be reassured that regressive toileting behavior commonly results from the stress of hospitalization and that it is temporary.

ITEM 9 Cognitive Type: Application

To promote a sense of security in the hospitalized infant, the nurse should

a. provide clean toys that can be mouthed.

b. ensure that side rails are locked securely.

c. respond to infant cues indicating fatigue, hunger, or need to be held.

d. schedule intrusive treatments when parents can be present.

ANSWER

c. Nursing intervention to meet the emotional and social needs of hospitalized infants should center around nurturing behaviors.

ITEM 10 Cognitive Type: Application

Which activity would best foster the development of conservation and classification skills in the hospitalized school age child?

a. Give the child a list of rules to follow while in the hospital.

b. Enlist the child's participation in keeping her own intake and output records.

c. Provide the child with crayons and paper and encourage her to draw pictures of hospital equipment.

d. Ask the child to gather equipment necessary to complete a familiar procedure.

ANSWER

b. Activities that provide for intellectual stimulation and that appeal to the school age child's sense of industry will help to promote growth and development during hospitalization.

ITEM 11 Cognitive Type: Application

Which of the following teaching strategies facilitates coping in the preschool age child who is hospitalized for a planned surgical procedure?

a. Explain how pain will not be a problem after surgery since special medicine is available.

b. Limit preparatory activities to those that address information requested by the child.

c. Allow play experiences with a doll that has a wound dressing and intravenous tubing.

d. Describe the operation as a small cut that may hurt and will be covered with a big bandage.

ANSWER

c. Preschoolers need explanations that are neutral in vocabulary and accompanied by play experiences that portray realistic bodily changes that may occur.

ITEM 12 Cognitive Type: Application

Which response is best when the single parent of a hospitalized toddler says, "I'm afraid I will only be able to visit for a few hours in the morning. I live 50 miles away and I have to be home when the other children get out of school."

a. "Please try to arrange for someone else to be here in the evening since most of the other children have visitors then and your son will probably be lonely for you."

b. "Mornings are a good time for you to be here. We're so busy then it will be a real help for you to feed and bathe your son."

c. "You should try to arrange for a babysitter at home since your son's treatments are scheduled for the afternoon and he will need your support."

d. "Breakfast is served early so I'll help your son with his meal and make sure he has toys to play with until you arrive, then you can bathe and dress him if you like."

ANSWER

d. The nurse's sensitivity to the special needs of single parents is an important link in the effective adaptation of the child and family.

ITEM 13 Cognitive Type: Application

Five-year-old Sally has been hospitalized for one week after a motor vehicle accident. Her mother asks the nurse if her 10-year-old son could visit Sally on the weekend. How would the nurse respond?

a. "Sally and her brother can speak to each other on the telephone, but siblings under 12 years of age are not permitted in patient areas."

b. "Yes, he can visit Sally but the visit must be limited to 30 minutes in the evening."

c. "Siblings may visit, but it is the parent's responsibility to prepare the child psychologically for the visit."

d. "You might plan to bring your son in at lunchtime so he could help Sally with her meal."

ANSWER

d. Proponents of sibling visits suggest sibling rivalry can be alleviated by increasing the sibling's active involvement in the care of the hospitalized child.

ITEM 14 Cognitive Type: Application

When preparing a child for discharge from the hospital, the primary nurse should

a. counsel parents to be patient with the child at home since most hospitalized children experience regressions in behavior.

b. provide the child and family with instructions about resuming the usual activities of daily living.

c. encourage parents to provide for a period of recuperation at home during which they should assume temporary responsibility for all aspects of the child's care.

d. conduct a home visit to assess the physical environment and capabilities of the family to care for the child at home.

ANSWER

b. The nurse plays a major role in discharging a child from the hospital. Instructions given to the parents should address physical care, activities of daily living (ADLs), medications, and follow-up appointments.

CHAPTER 22

ITEM 1 Cognitive Type: Knowledge

Pediatric home care is considered to be cost effective if it

a. alleviates the financial responsibilities of insurance carriers and health care institutions.

b. entails technological support services provided by a licensed community agency.

c. minimizes the psychosocial impact of illness by maintaining a more normal environment.

d. increases the number of paid professionals who interact with the child in a therapeutic manner.

ANSWER

c. Home health care is cost effective if it provides high quality services to the most people at the most reasonable price. Normalization of a child's environment promotes recovery.

ITEM 2 Cognitive Type: Knowledge

Nursing assessment of family readiness for home care of an ill child includes

a. advising the family whose resources are inadequate for home care to place their child in an extended care facility.

b. assisting parents in changing cultural values and beliefs that are in conflict with the treatment plan designed by the health care staff.

c. stressing to the family that anxieties associated with home care treatments will eventually subside.

d. gathering information about physical and emotional support resources available to the family.

ANSWER

d. Gathering information about family resources is an essential part of the assessment of a family's readiness to care for a child at home.

ITEM 3 Cognitive Type: Knowledge

Which of the following is an essential component of home health nursing practice?

a. Fluency in a foreign language

b. Expertise in ventilator management

c. Acceptance of various lifestyles and cultures

d. Physical and occupational therapy skills

ANSWER

c. The effective nurse in a home care setting is nonjudgmental about a family's lifestyle and cultural practices and makes judgments according to identified outcomes for the treatment plan rather than on the basis of differences or similarities in values.

ITEM 4 Cognitive Type: Interpretation

A home health nurse is observing the mother of a 3-year-old while she correctly cleanses and redresses her son's burn wound. The child is crying and kicking. The mother tells the nurse that doing this three times a day is wearing her out. Which of the following nursing diagnoses represents appropriate analysis of this situation?

a. Altered family processes are related to incomplete adjustment to the physical and emotional stress of home care.

b. Knowledge deficit is related to burn care procedures and developmental response to pain.

c. Ineffective individual coping is related to unavailability of support resources.

d. Impaired home maintenance management is related to lack of preparation for home care services.

ANSWER

a. The nurse recognizes the defining characteristics associated with altered family processes and selects the appropriate nursing diagnosis.

ITEM 5 Cognitive Type: Interpretation

The community health nurse is referred to a 10-year-old child with cystic fibrosis continuing intravenous antibiotic therapy at home following discharge from the hospital. When planning for the first phase of interaction with the family, the nurse would

a. Telephone the family to let them know when to expect the first home visit.

b. Review the child's hospital discharge plan and identify areas of family strength and potential for effective coping.

c. Plan extra time to spend with the child during the first visit.

d. Clarify the family's perceptions of the child's illness and their expectations regarding home health care.

ANSWER

c. The nurse recognizes an appropriate strategy for gaining the trust and cooperation of a child and family during the engagement phase of interactions in home care management.

ITEM 6 Cognitive Type: Interpretation

Termination of services for home care management of children occurs

a. at the time of a terminally ill child's death.

b. when a child experiences an exacerbation of disease requiring hospitalization for treatment.

c. after evaluation of the child's and family's progress toward desired outcomes has been determined.

d. as soon as the family is ready to assume full responsibility for the child's care.

ANSWER

d. Termination of home care services occurs when the child's condition no longer warrants professional involvement in the home, either because of improvement in health care status or because the family is able to assume full responsibility for the treatment plan. After the death of a child, one or more follow-up visits should be made to the home.

ITEM 7 Cognitive Type: Knowledge

Which of the following statements addresses an important difference between pediatric and adult home care?

a. The focus of pediatric home care is teaching the child to function independently.

b. Pediatric home care is less likely to require social services.

c. The length of service is generally shorter in pediatric home care.

d. The need for support services is greater in pediatric home care.

ANSWER

d. There is an increased need for specially trained home health aides and volunteers who deal with the child's personal care needs and psychological and social development.

ITEM 8 Cognitive Type: Interpretation

The future effectiveness of home health care for children will be based on

a. advances in technology.

b. the basic needs of children and families involved.

c. computerization of record keeping.

d. availability of highly specialized health care professionals.

ANSWER

b. The effectiveness of home care will continue to be dependent on the nurse's ability to provide for the needs of children and families who experience illness and require support in the adjustment process.

CHAPTER 23

ITEM 1 Cognitive Type: Knowledge

When parents or legal guardians cannot be reached in life-threatening situations, consent for emergency care may be given by

a. grandparents or other relatives.

b. school officials.

c. day care administrators.

d. babysitters.

ANSWER

a. The nurse knows that only grandparents or relatives may give consent for treatment in the absence of parents or legal guardians. The other persons listed must have written permission from the parents to be considered in giving consent.

ITEM 2 Cognitive Type: Knowledge

Research studies conducted on pediatric patients over the age of 7 years

a. require only that the parents or legal guardians give informed consent for participation.

b. are limited to those children who are able to understand the purpose of the research project.

c. require the assent of the child and the child's parents.

d. includes obtaining informed consent for participation from all immediate and extended family members.

ANSWER

c. The nurse knows the stipulations placed on research with pediatric patients from the U.S. Department of Health and Human Services.

ITEM 3 Cognitive Type: Knowledge

When a parent gives informed consent for a child's treatment, it implies he or she has full knowledge of

a. the medical personnel who will be treating the child.

b. the length of the treatment.

c. the risks and benefits of the treatment.

d. the success rate of the treatment.

ANSWER

c. Informed consent implies knowledge of the risks and benefits of the intervention as well as the consequences of alternative interventions.

ITEM 4 Cognitive Type: Application

Which assessment approach is likely to provide the most useful information about the learning needs of parents and children in a health care setting?

a. Refer the family to social services for assistance in obtaining financial resources.

b. Ask the parent and child to describe what they know about a particular event while observing their behavior for incongruities.

c. Encourage the parent to be honest with their child when explaining a painful procedure.

d. Inform the parent and child about coping strategies known to be useful in relieving anxiety associated with illness.

ANSWER

b. The nurse recognizes assessment strategies important to the teaching process. Referral, encouragement, and information are intervention strategies.

ITEM 5 Cognitive Type: Application

Educational strategies to address a knowledge deficit in the 10-year-old child should include

a. visual aids and simple explanations given just prior to an event or procedure.

b. scientific diagrams and literature that describe symptoms and potential problems associated with an illness or event.

c. games or paper and pencil activities that contain content to be learned.

d. doll play and equipment for manipulation in short teaching sessions with peers who are experiencing similar events or procedures.

ANSWER

c. In this case, the appropriate educational strategy to facilitate learning is through games and drawing activities that appeal to the school age child.

ITEM 6 Cognitive Type: Application

When caring for the infant or child who is in a crib, the nurse should always

a. ensure that the siderails remain at the halfway position.

b. keep one hand securely on the child.

c. position the child at the farthest point from a lower siderail.

d. assess the child's ability to roll over or stand prior to turning around to obtain equipment from the bedside table.

ANSWER

b. The nurse recognizes that the most important action to take to prevent injury associated with falling out of a crib is to keep one hand on the child at all times.

ITEM 7 Cognitive Type: Application

Which of the following behaviors observed by the nurse in a pediatric hospital unit necessitates intervention?

a. The father of a 12-year-old girl stands outside the bathroom while she takes a shower.

b. A 3-year-old child's aunt restrains him in a highchair and assists him with his lunch.

c. The mother of an infant places her baby on his back to change his diaper.

d. Grandparents bring colorful balloons when they visit their young grandchild.

ANSWER

d. Balloons pose a threat to young children because of the risk of aspiration of small fragments if balloons break.

ITEM 8 Cognitive Type: Application

During an admission interview, the mother of a 2-month-old asks if she can bathe her baby while she is in the hospital. The nurse should

a. ask the mother to demonstrate her ability to bathe the baby safely before granting her request.

b. support the mother's desire to participate in her infant's care and give her clear instructions about any bathing restrictions.

c. explain that bathing children in the hospital is a nursing responsibility, but that she would be allowed to feed the infant.

d. suggest to the mother that she direct her energies toward comforting the infant and getting her own rest since the nursing staff is more experienced.

ANSWER

b. The nurse recognizes that meeting the hygienic needs of their children provides parents with an opportunity to participate and feel useful when their child is hospitalized.

ITEM 9 Cognitive Type: Interpretation

Which of the following is an appropriate nursing diagnosis for the convalescing 15-year-old teen who refuses to go to his physical therapy session during visiting hours?

a. Fear related to potential for pain

b. Powerlessness related to lack of consultation regarding decision

c. Ineffective individual coping related to separation from support systems

d. Anxiety related to perceived threat to biological integrity

ANSWER

b. This nursing diagnosis statement reflects the most likely analysis of the problem based on the nurse's knowledge of adolescent developmental needs.

ITEM 10 Cognitive Type: Knowledge

The nurse is assigned to care for a 6-month-old infant. The best site to assess this infant's pulse is

a. apical.

b. radial.

c. brachial.

d. femoral.

ANSWER

a. The apical pulse rather than the peripheral pulse is usually assessed in young children.

ITEM 11 Cognitive Type: Knowledge

Which of the following is the *most* important factor in obtaining an accurate blood pressure reading in an infant or child?

a. Availability of an electronic doppler device

b. Preprocedural preparation to decrease anxiety and encourage relaxation

c. Selection of a cuff that covers two-thirds of the upper arm and is 1-1/2 times larger than the arm circumference

d. Inflation of the cuff until the pulse is no longer felt

ANSWER

c. The nurse recognizes that using a cuff that is correctly sized to the infant's or child's arm is most important in obtaining an accurate blood pressure reading.

ITEM 12 Cognitive Type: Application

Which nursing intervention will facilitate the collection of a urine specimen from an infant or very young child who has an adhesive plastic urine bag in place?

a. Increase oral fluid intake to enhance urine production.

b. Restrain the child in a prone position to prevent loosening of the bag.

c. Check the urine bag after 2 to 3 hours to ensure ample amounts of urine.

d. Place the child in a semi-Fowler's position to enhance flow of urine by gravity into the bag.

ANSWER

d. When a urine bag has been adequately secured and properly placed, the semi-Fowler's position helps to prevent loosening of the bag and facilitates flow of urine by gravity into the bag.

ITEM 13 Cognitive Type: Knowledge

When is the best time for the nurse to obtain a sputum specimen from an 18-month-old toddler?

a. Soon after she awakens in the morning.

b. Immediately after her noon meal.

c. During the evening when her mother can be present to assist in restraining her.

d. After teaching her to cough and expectorate into a cup.

ANSWER

a. The best time to collect a sputum specimen is when a patient awakens in the morning.

ITEM 14 Cognitive Type: Application

The nurse explains that a stat hemoglobin level has been ordered for 5-year-old Brian. The child cries, "Mommy, stay with me!" His mother asks the nurse if she can stay during this procedure. How would the nurse respond?

a. "I'm sorry. Hospital policy is that parents must leave the room when procedures are performed."

b. "Yes, but please stand by the window and do not speak to Brian until I have finished."

c. "I won't need your help. Another nurse is going to come in soon."

d. "Yes, you can talk to Michael while I collect this blood specimen."

ANSWER

d. The nurse should agree with the child's and parent's preferences if they are within hospital policy.

ITEM 15 Cognitive Type: Application

Which type of restraint is necessary to prevent 6-month-old Kristen from touching her cleft lip repair incision?

a. Modified mummy restraint

b. Jacket restraint

c. Alternate arm restraints

d. Elbow restraints

ANSWER

d. Flexion of the elbows must be prevented to ensure that children will not be able to reach their face or head while those areas are in need of protection from manipulation.

ITEM 16 Cognitive Type: Application

When caring for the child in need of restraint to meet therapeutic goals, the nurse can reduce feelings of powerlessness by

a. ensuring that the child is released from the restraint for short periods.

b. inspecting the child's skin for signs of impairment.

c. assuring the child that the restraint will be removed as soon as someone is available to stay at the bedside.

d. enlisting the help of a psychiatric nurse specialist to assist the child in developing coping strategies.

ANSWER

a. Immobility imposed by restraints results in feelings of powerlessness. The nurse is responsible for providing opportunities for freedom of movement to facilitate expression and coping strategies in the child who requires restraint.

ITEM 17 Cognitive Type: Knowledge

When caring for a child who requires short-term isolation for an infectious disease, the nurse can best reduce the potential for transmission of organisms by

a. stressing proper handwashing with everyone who enters the child's room.

b. restricting the child's visitors to the immediate family during the isolation period.

c. providing for an adequate supply of gowns and masks at the entrance to the child's room.

d. teaching the child basic principles of hygienic care and how to avoid contaminating equipment placed in the isolation room.

ANSWER

a. Proper handwashing is the most important precaution to take to prevent the transmission of organisms when caring for children in isolation.

ITEM 18 Cognitive Type: Application

The mother of a 1-month-old newborn calls the clinic nurse to inquire about how to treat her baby's fever, which has been elevated to 102°F for the past 24 hours. The nurse should

a. explain to the mother how to give a tepid water sponge bath to bring the baby's fever down.

b. tell the mother to give the baby acetaminophen infant drops every 4 hours based on the baby's weight.

c. advise the mother to bring the baby to the clinic today to be examined by the physician.

d. recommend to the mother that she increase the baby's fluid intake, watch for any changes in behavior, and call back tomorrow if the baby is still feverish.

ANSWER

c. The nurse recognizes that fever in any child under 6 months of age is likely to be caused by serious illness and that a febrile neonate should be seen promptly by a physician.

ITEM 19 Cognitive Type: Knowledge

Home management of children with fever includes antipyretic therapy. Safe acetaminophen dosage is based on which of the following formulas?

a. 10–20 mg/kg/dose, every 4–6 hours, as necessary

b. 80 mg/ml/year of age, every 4–6 hours, prn

c. 20–30 mg/kg/dose, as necessary

d. 50–65 mg/kg daily, in divided doses every 4 hours, prn

ANSWER

a. The nurse recognizes the formula for calculating safe acetaminophen dosage based on a child's weight.

ITEM 20 Cognitive Type: Interpretation

The nursing management of children in the preoperative period should include

a. distracting the child from fears associated with surgery by providing age-appropriate unrelated play activities.

b. limiting an apprehensive parent's involvement in the teaching process to reduce transfer of anxiety to the child.

c. explaining all expected events in accordance with the child's cognitive level.

d. respecting a parent's request that the child not be informed about possible pain until after surgery.

ANSWER

c. Honesty in preparing children of all ages is mandatory to foster coping and cooperation.

ITEM 21 Cognitive Type: Application

When a child returns to the pediatric unit following a surgical procedure, the nurse should first

a. review the postoperative orders with the recovery room nurse just outside the child's room.

b. administer pain medication to enhance the child's ability to cooperate with transferring from the stretcher to the bed.

c. complete a general assessment of the child's physical condition.

d. assess the intravenous site and add potassium to the unit to promote urination.

ANSWER

c. When attending to the postoperative child, the nurse immediately performs a general assessment of the child's condition.

CHAPTER 24

ITEM 1 Cognitive Type: Knowledge

The nurse administering oral prednisone to a child should be aware that the undesirable effects of glucocorticoids are the result of

a. identical drug receptors located in many different cell types in the body.

b. the same drug receptors through extension of the therapeutic action.

c. different types of drug receptors throughout the body.

d. interactions with other drugs the child is receiving.

ANSWER

a. Glucocorticoid receptors are found on the surface of a wide variety of cell types in the body with which they can interact.

ITEM 2 Cognitive Type: Knowledge

Elimination of drugs occurs primarily through the

a. gastrointestinal tract.

b. kidneys.

c. respiratory tract.

d. liver.

ANSWER

b. Elimination of drugs from the body occurs primarily through the renal system.

ITEM 3 Cognitive Type: Knowledge

Which of the following age-related differences causes delayed absorption of orally administered drugs in neonates and young infants?

a. Highly acidic gastric pH

b. Immature blood flow to muscles and tissues

c. Larger proportion of body water

d. Reduced gastric motility and irregular peristalsis

ANSWER

d. Gastric emptying time does not reach the adult level of 2 hours until 6 to 8 months of age. Prolonged exposure of certain drugs to gastric contents can increase destruction of the drug, and reduced gastric motility delays entry of orally administered drugs into the lower intestinal tract where most absorption takes place.

ITEM 4 Cognitive Type: Interpretation

To obtain information about the best approach to take when administering medication to children, the nurse should

a. ask the child to decide when and where the medication should be given.

b. consult a pharmacology textbook that includes age-related strategies for giving drugs to children.

c. ask the child's parent how medications are given at home or how they have been given by other nurses.

d. place the child in several different restraining positions to select one that is least traumatic.

ANSWER

c. The nurse recognizes that parents can offer important information about their child's needs and that the best approach when administering medication to children is to involve parents.

ITEM 5 Cognitive Type: Interpretation

Which of the following nursing interventions is directed toward the prevention of injury when administering medication to a child?

a. Check the child's bedside name card.

b. Firmly stabilize the body part involved.

c. Restrain the child with a blanket secured over the trunk and extremities.

d. Use the dorsogluteal site for injections with young children.

ANSWER

b. In all instances of medication administration, firm stabilization of the body part involved is necessary to avoid injury to the child.

ITEM 6 Cognitive Type: Application

The recommended dose of a drug is 60–90 mg/kg daily in five or six divided doses. You have an order to administer 120 mg of the drug every 4 hours to a child who weighs 10 kg. Your *first* action would be to

a. look at the drug container to determine how many milligrams are contained in each milliliter.

b. check whether the dose exceeds the maximum allowed in 24 hours.

c. locate the correct drug in the correct preparation.

d. perform the necessary calculations to obtain the amount desired in equivalent cubic centimeter dosage.

ANSWER

b. The nurse recognizes that the first step to take to ensure safe administration of medications to children is to check that the dose does not exceed the maximum daily allowable dose.

ITEM 7 Cognitive Type: Knowledge

To facilitate the administration of oral medication to a preschool-age child, the nurse should

a. dilute the medication in a favorite liquid and allow the child to hold the cup.

b. mix the medication in a small amount of ice cream and watch to see that the child swallows all of the medication.

c. explain the purpose of the medication and allow the child time to express resistance before giving the medication.

d. set limits about the need to take medication and offer praise immediately after the task is accomplished.

ANSWER

d. Preschool age children need assistance to achieve control and will feel better once a task has been successfully accomplished. Prolonged reasoning and arguing should be avoided.

ITEM 8 Cognitive Type: Application

Ramona, age 8 years, has an infection in her external ear canal. When teaching Ramona and her mother how to administer ear drops, the nurse should

a. demonstrate for the mother how to pull the pinna of Ramona's ear up and back while instilling the ear drops.

b. instruct them to keep the medication in the refrigerator until just before administration.

c. explain to Ramona that she should remain seated with her head tilted back for several minutes after receiving the ear drops.

d. show the mother how to place and secure a cotton ball into Ramona's ear canal using nonallergic tape after administration of the ear drops.

ANSWER

a. For a child over 3 years of age, the pinna is gently pulled up and back to straighten the ear canal.

ITEM 9 Cognitive Type: Knowledge

Which of the following is the recommended site for safe administration of an intramuscular injection to a child who is 2-1/2 years old?

a. Dorsogluteal

b. Deltoid

c. Ventrogluteal

d. Vastus lateralis

ANSWER

d. The vastus lateralis muscle remains the only recommended site for intramuscular injections until the age of 3 years.

ITEM 10 Cognitive Type: Interpretation

Douglas, age 16 years, is to receive an intramuscular injection. To facilitate his cooperation with the administration of this medication, the nurse's initial intervention would be to

a. tell him what he will feel.

b. explain the purpose of the medication.

c. offer him a choice of injection sites.

d. describe the steps in the procedure.

ANSWER

b. The adolescent should first be given a clear explanation of the purpose of an intramuscular injection since understanding the reason for the medication is more likely to facilitate participation in the procedure.

CHAPTER 25

ITEM 1 Cognitive Type: Knowledge

An example of a recurrent acute pain is the pain from

a. the metastasis of osteosarcoma.

b. an appendectomy.

c. juvenile rheumatoid arthritis.

d. an open reduction of a fractured tibia.

ANSWER

c. Long-term pain described as recurrent acute is pain from underlying continued nociceptive input and is characterized by sudden onset, limited duration, and periods of comfort between recurrences, which in this case, describes juvenile rheumatoid arthritis.

ITEM 2 Cognitive Type: Knowledge

A factor that would *not* affect a child's tolerance for pain is

a. his pain threshold.

b. the method by which narcotics are administered.

c. his cultural values and beliefs.

d. the pain duration.

ANSWER

a. *Pain threshold* is when the child first experiences the discomfort, while *pain tolerance* is the time when the child can no longer stand the discomfort.

ITEM 3 Cognitive Type: Knowledge

The most important factor affecting a child's perception and expression of pain is

a. previous pain experiences.

b. her developmental stage.

c. cultural influences.

d. her coping strategies.

ANSWER

b. Application of the Gate Control Theory to pain in children requires an understanding of those factors that modulate the child's ability to perceive and express the pain experienced. The most important of these factors is the child's stage of development.

ITEM 4 Cognitive Type: Knowledge

Which of the following statements about pain in children is true?

a. The immaturity of the nervous system in young children provides them with increased thresholds for pain.

b. Recovery from pain experience occurs at a faster rate in children than in adults.

c. Narcotic use in children is dangerous because of the increased risk of addiction and respiratory depression.

d. Infants have the capacity to respond to a painful stimulus.

ANSWER

d. Evidence firmly supports the infant's capacity for response to a painful stimulus and pain perception.

ITEM 5 Cognitive Type: Knowledge

Research indicates that a physiological response to pain in children under 1 year of age includes

a. increased oxygen saturation.

b. decreased respiratory rate.

c. increased heart rate.

d. increased vagal tone.

ANSWER

c. Physiological responses to a noxious stimulus include increased heart rate, increased respiratory rate, palmar sweating, intracranial pressure, decreased vagal tone, and decreased oxygen saturation.

ITEM 6 Cognitive Type: Knowledge

Four-year-old Sarah has been diagnosed with Wilm's tumor and is scheduled for a nephrectomy tomorrow. To establish a baseline about Sarah's pain-related behaviors, the nurse asks Sarah's parents which of the following questions?

a. "How would you describe your child's tolerance to pain?"

b. "Describe how your child reacts to pain."

c. "Could you estimate how much pain your child is presently feeling?"

d. "How does your child respond to acetaminophen?"

ANSWER

b. The Pain Experience History is helpful in establishing a child's previous experiences with and responses to pain. One of the questions the nurse would ask the parent(s) is "How does your child usually react to pain?"

ITEM 7 Cognitive Type: Application

Sarah returned from surgery 1 hour ago. What should the nurse know about the Poker Chip Tool if she is planning to use it to assess Sarah's postoperative pain?

a. Since the Poker Chip Tool rates intensity of pain, the nurse will want to ask Sarah additional questions about her pain.

b. Children need to be able to count to 100 to use this assessment tool.

c. The scoring system transforms the child's numeric rating into categories of pain intensity.

d. Best results are obtained with older children who can conceptualize pain abstractly.

ANSWER

a. The Poker Chip Tool conveys only the intensity of pain so the nurse will need to question the child further.

ITEM 8 Cognitive Type: Knowledge

An appropriate plan for pain relief for the child experiencing continuous moderate to severe pain is to

a. administer narcotic analgesia on an as-needed basis.

b. use nonsteroidal antiinflammatory drugs (NSAIDS).

c. give around-the-clock analgesia.

d. give the maximum dosage of narcotic at less frequent intervals.

ANSWER

c. Continuous pain requires a constant blood level of analgesic achieved through around-the-clock administration or through continuous administration.

ITEM 9 Cognitive Type: Application

Tierra, a 2-year-old girl admitted with lead poisoning, has been receiving calcium disodium edetate injections. Which of the following nursing interventions would be implemented for its potential as a source of comfort for Tierra?

a. Prepare Tierra several hours before the injection is given and allow her to stay with the nursing staff.

b. Allow Tierra to watch a younger child receive an injection.

c. Encourage Tierra to draw a picture of the pain experienced when an injection is given.

d. Hold Tierra while rocking in a chair after each injection.

ANSWER

d. Holding and rocking are potential sources of comfort for children of toddler age.

ITEM 10 Cognitive Type: Knowledge

A common fear shared by many parents regarding the administration of morphine to a child is the fear of

a. respiratory depression.

b. psychological dependence.

c. a medication error.

d. injury due to drowsiness.

ANSWER

b. Research has found that many parents fear that their child will become addicted to narcotics that are ordered for pain relief.

ITEM 11 Cognitive Type: Knowledge

Which of the following nonpharmacological interventions used to help ease pain involves teaching children to use their imagination to create pleasant images?

a. Distraction

b. Guided imagery

c. Relaxation

d. Hypnosis

ANSWER

b. Children who are capable of some degree of abstract thinking can be assisted in selecting and concentrating on sensual images that are pleasant and feel good as a means of gaining mastery over their pain.

ITEM 12 Cognitive Type: Knowledge

The use of distraction to interrupt a child's perception of pain can be evaluated as effective if the child

a. reports that pain has decreased.

b. ceases to request analgesic medication.

c. is able to focus on something other than pain.

d. asks to go to the playroom with other children.

ANSWER

c. Distraction can interrupt the perception of pain during the distracting activity, but it has no action beyond that period. When the activity ends, pain returns.

CHAPTER 26

ITEM 1 Cognitive Type: Knowledge

Infants and young children are especially vulnerable to fluid and electrolyte imbalances. One factor that contributes to this vulnerability is

a. decreased body water content.

b. lowered metabolic care.

c. increased extracellular fluid volume.

d. decreased body surface area.

ANSWER

c. In infants and young children, a greater proportion of fluid is in the extracellular space. This places the infant at risk for imbalances since extracellular fluid is lost first when a condition predisposing to fluid loss occurs.

ITEM 2 Cognitive Type: Knowledge

Which of the following factors is responsible for the edema that accompanies an allergic reaction?

a. Increased capillary hydrostatic pressure

b. Lymphatic obstruction

c. Increased capillary permeability

d. Decreased plasma oncotic pressure

ANSWER

c. Increased interstitial fluid volume occurs when the integrity of the capillary membrane is altered, as in an allergic reaction.

ITEM 3 Cognitive Type: Knowledge

A 2-month-old is admitted to the pediatric intensive care unit for treatment of hyponatremia. The mother reports feeding the baby only plain water for the last 24 hours because his formula was making him vomit. This baby's electrolyte imbalance was caused by

a. isotonic dehydration.

b. excessive intake of electrolyte-free fluid.

c. parental neglect.

d. fluid shifts from intracellular to extracellular spaces.

ANSWER

b. Disproportionately large amounts of electrolyte-free solutions (water) result in hyponatremia. Insufficient sodium to keep water from entering the cells results in a shift of water from the extracellular spaces to the intracellular spaces where sodium concentration is higher.

ITEM 4 Cognitive Type: Knowledge

Which symptom should the nurse expect to find in a child with hypercalcemia associated with prolonged immobilization?

a. Muscle cramps

b. Excessive thirst

c. Tremors

d. Muscle hypotonicity

ANSWER

d. Lack of postural changes to the skeleton results in loss of calcium from bone. Developmental differences in children may cause increased plasma levels of calcium when the kidney is unable to excrete calcium quickly enough.

ITEM 5 Cognitive Type: Knowledge

Which of the following laboratory values reflects acid–base balance in the body?

a. Arterial blood pH is 7.40.

b. Hydrogen ion concentration is 30 nanoequivalents.

c. Bicarbonate is 30 mmol/L.

d. Partial pressure of carbon dioxide is 25 mm/Hg.

ANSWER

a. Normal arterial blood pH is 7.40. pH and hydrogen ion concentration are inversely related; as H ion concentration rises, pH falls and vice versa.

ITEM 6 Cognitive Type: Knowledge

The most common cause of metabolic acidosis in children is

a. diarrhea.

b. pyloric stenosis.

c. head trauma.

d. cardiac failure.

ANSWER

a. Excessive loss of bicarbonate ions in the stool when diarrhea is present results in primary metabolic acidosis.

ITEM 7 Cognitive Type: Interpretation

To obtain relevant information from the mother of a toddler who has had severe diarrhea over the last 24 hours, the nurse should ask which question?

a. "How much does your child weigh?"

b. "Have you taken your child's temperature during this illness?"

c. "What do you give your child to eat and drink when he has loose stools?"

d. "Have you noticed any change in how often or how much your child has been urinating?"

ANSWER

d. Questions in the nursing history that are pertinent when fluid or electrolyte imbalance is suspected should concern changes in a child's usual state of health.

ITEM 8 Cognitive Type: Knowledge

Clinical findings that the nurse should expect when assessing a 3-year-old who is moderately dehydrated include

a. decreased urine output, mottled skin color, and elevated temperature.

b. tachycardia, 10% loss of body weight, and gray skin color.

c. oliguria, bulging fontanel, and decreased blood pressure.

d. 5% loss of body weight, tachycardia, and increased blood pressure.

ANSWER

b. The moderately dehydrated child exhibits a 10% loss of body weight, gray skin color, oliguria normal blood pressure, and tachycardia.

ITEM 9 Cognitive Type: Application

Maintenance fluid requirements for an infant who weighs 10 kg are

a. 400 mL/8 hours.

b. 1000 mL/day.

c. 1200 mL/day.

d. 100 mL/hour.

ANSWER

b. Calculation of maintenance fluid requirements is based on caloric expenditure. An infant weighing 3–10 kg expends 100 cal/kg/day of fluid to maintain homeostasis (see Table 26-6).

ITEM 10 Cognitive Type: Knowledge

When administering potassium chloride to an infant, the nurse should

a. monitor vital signs every 15 minutes for 2 hours after giving the drug.

b. add the drug to a soluset with 15 mL of D 5/0.2 NS and drip over 20 minutes.

c. withhold the drug in the presence of anuria or oliguria.

d. give the drug IV push over 15 minutes after checking the IV site for signs of infiltration.

ANSWER

c. Potassium chloride is added to the IV fluid only after urinary flow has been established.

ITEM 11 Cognitive Type: Application

The mother of 4-year-old Keith calls the nurse to ask for advice. Her son awakened this morning with fever of 101°F, vomited his breakfast, and now refuses to eat anything. The nurse should

a. reassure the mother that Keith does not need to eat as long as he drinks large amounts of water.

b. advise the mother to give Keith skim milk and low fat ice cream to prevent dehydration.

c. urge the mother to take him to the clinic to be examined by a physician.

d. recommend a variety of clear fluids that the mother should offer Keith in frequent, small amounts.

ANSWER

d. Parents should be advised to give clear liquids in the event of fever or vomiting. Water and skim milk should not be given, as both can contribute to dehydration if given in large amounts.

ITEM 12 Cognitive Type: Application

The plan of care for an 8-year-old child who requires intravenous fluid therapy should include

a. teaching the child how to safely manipulate the IV when getting out of bed and ambulating.

b. releasing the restraining extremity hourly to assess the IV site and perform range of motion (ROM) exercises.

c. providing a variety of play activities that can be accomplished in bed or in a wheelchair.

d. arranging for constant parental or nursing supervision for all out-of-bed activities.

ANSWER

a. The school age child can be expected to cooperate with IV therapy and should be provided with instructions for protecting the integrity of an IV while out of bed or walking.

ITEM 13 Cognitive Type: Interpretation

One sign that should alert the nurse to a potential problem in an infant who has a peripheral vein IV line is

a. a lack of blood return when assessing the IV line for potency.

b. a urine specific gravity of 1.020.

c. cool, taut skin and blanching at the venipuncture site.

d. a serum sodium level of 142 mEq/L.

ANSWER

c. Signs of infiltration of IV infusions include pain, swelling, tenderness, cool skin, and blanching of the insertion site.

ITEM 14 Cognitive Type: Knowledge

Headache, shallow respirations, and restlessness noted in an adolescent following excessive ingestion of alcohol are clinical manifestations of

a. respiratory alkalosis.

b. hyperkalemia.

c. compensatory metabolic acidosis.

d. respiratory acidosis.

ANSWER

d. Excessive alcohol ingestion may depress respiration causing retention of carbon dioxide and the development of respiratory acidosis. Neurologic alterations associated with carbon dioxide retention may be exhibited with respiratory acidosis.

CHAPTER 27

ITEM 1 Cognitive Type: Knowledge

A major responsibility of the nurse in helping a family who has a child with developmental disabilities is

a. supervising the interdisciplinary team that decides the care of the child.

b. identifying problem areas and aiding family decision making.

c. assessing the degree of the child's handicap and providing treatment.

d. developing an educational plan for the child.

ANSWER

b. The nurse's role is to identify, prevent, and reduce problems the family faces when there is a child with a disability in the home.

ITEM 2 Cognitive Type: Application

An 8-month-old child is brought to the clinic for a routine health checkup. During the physical examination, the nurse practitioner suspects that the child may have some developmental delays and decides to do a screening test. The nurse explains to the mother that the purpose of the developmental screening test is to

a. measure the child's intelligence.

b. diagnose the child's disability.

c. determine if the child has age-appropriate behavior.

d. determine the child's future developmental potential.

ANSWER

c. The purpose of the developmental screening test is to define a potential problem or find any deviation in growth patterns. If found, then the child can be referred for further diagnostic testing.

ITEM 3 Cognitive Type: Knowledge

One factor that makes early intervention programs for children with multiple handicaps successful is

a. the parents being active participants.

b. a child developmental specialist coordinating the health care team.

c. the child having no mental or speech impairment.

d. the family living near a medical center that provides such a service.

ANSWER

a. Parents must be active participants, as they have the day-to-day responsibility for the care and nurturing of the handicapped child.

ITEM 4 Cognitive Type: Interpretation

A community health nurse visits a family who has a 2-week-old infant with a brain injury from a difficult birth. When the nurse inquires about the mother's health, the mother states she cries frequently and lacks energy to do simple tasks. The nurse attributes this to the initial emotional response of parents who learn that their child has a disability, a reaction described as

a. mourning the loss of the "expected healthy child."

b. fearing to face friends and family.

c. total rejection of the injured child.

d. lack of knowledge about the child's condition.

ANSWER

a. Mourning for the lost healthy child is a common initial emotional reaction when a parent learns that the child is disabled.

ITEM 5 Cognitive Type: Application

The nurse becomes an advocate for people with developmental disabilities by

a. favoring separate but equal services for handicapped persons.

b. asking these clients to come to the clinic only at special times.

c. supporting and working for additional human rights legislation.

d. approving of the institutionalization of clients with disabilities.

ANSWER

c. The role of advocate fosters independence in the client. The role also means that the nurse treats these clients in a similar manner as other people.

ITEM 6 Cognitive Type: Application

A 7-year-old girl is having difficulty with reading and spelling and has been determined to have developmental dyslexia. The nurse counsels the parents that they can help the child by

a. placing her in a special school.

b. restricting her physical activities.

c. maintaining her on a low sugar and low fat diet.

d. setting aside time daily to read to her.

ANSWER

d. Children with dyslexia need to be part of their peer group and attend regular school. Parents can help the child by reading to her and encouraging her in physical activities that promote eye to hand coordination.

ITEM 7 Cognitive Type: Application

Cerebral palsy is a disorder in which individuals have difficulty with voluntary muscle control. In describing the disorder to parents, the nurse states that cerebral palsy

a. is an intellectual disorder.

b. originates in the prenatal period and early years of life.

c. is manifested by peculiar behaviors and mannerisms.

d. is progressive, causing the child to become very dependent.

ANSWER

b. Cerebral palsy originates during the prenatal period through the early years of life. Brain damage is permanent and not progressive. Intelligence may or may not be affected and must be assessed at periodic intervals.

ITEM 8 Cognitive Type: Application

A 4-year-old boy with spastic cerebral palsy is in the hospital for assessment of his physical condition. In writing the nursing care plan, the nurse includes play activities that will

a. lessen the physical efforts of the child to promote rest.

b. minimize speaking because the child has speech difficulties.

c. help the child relax muscles that are usually tense.

d. be solitary in nature to decrease competing with the other children.

ANSWER

c. Children with spastic cerebral palsy are recognizable by their tense muscles. All play activities should take this in consideration. All other aspects of the child's development should be considered on any nursing care plan, such as interaction with peers and speech development.

ITEM 9 Cognitive Type: Knowledge

The three defining characteristics of the term *mental retardation* are

a. reading difficulties, subnormal intelligence, and inability to live independently.

b. subaverage intellectual functioning, impaired social adaptation, and age of onset.

c. IQ below 50, need for special education, and reliance on social services.

d. high or low intellectual functioning, mainstreaming, and poor social support.

ANSWER

b. The three characteristics that define mental retardation are subnormal intellectual functioning, impaired social adaptation, and occurrence before 18 years of age.

ITEM 10 Cognitive Type: Knowledge

A major responsibility of the nurse in helping families who have a child with mental retardation is

a. teaching about the child's disabilities.

b. recognizing that each family has unique methods of coping.

c. arranging for home tutorial assistance for the child's education.

d. having the entire family participate in genetic screening.

ANSWER

b. Every family who has a child with mental retardation responds to its situation in a unique way. The nurse must understand how the family is adapting so they can be given the appropriate assistance.

ITEM 11 Cognitive Type: Interpretation

A priority focus of the nurse's health teaching for parents who have a preadolescent girl with mental retardation is

a. dietary control to prevent obesity.

b. helping her learn to manage money.

c. self-protection and self-care through sex education.

d. self-care abilities and career planning.

ANSWER

c. Adolescent girls are at risk for sexual abuse, and parents need to know how to protect them.

ITEM 12 Cognitive Type: Knowledge

When a child with mental retardation is hospitalized, the nurse must

a. know the child's chronological age to plan appropriate play activities.

b. assess the child's developmental level and level of understanding.

c. explain all procedures that will be done to avoid frightening the child.

d. ask the mother if the child can read, write, or spell.

ANSWER

b. Children with mental retardation differ in what they understand. Nursing care and explanations must be geared toward the child's developmental level and ability to comprehend.

ITEM 13 Cognitive Type: Application

The community health nurse visits a family who has a 10-year-old boy with moderate mental retardation but no physical disabilities. The family is planning a vacation that includes overnight camping. The family wonders if this is an appropriate activity for the child. The nurse should

a. discuss the many dangers that this experience would pose for the child.

b. state that the child has little ability to comprehend such an activity.

c. recognize that the whole family will benefit from this normalizing activity.

d. suggest alternative activities for the family vacation.

ANSWER

c. The family should participate in as many activities as possible in accordance with the normalization process that is advocated for people with mental retardation.

ITEM 14 Cognitive Type: Knowledge

The development of children with Down syndrome is enhanced when they

a. are exposed to as many normal experiences as possible.

b. have more contact with other children with mental retardation.

c. are placed in behavior modification programs with food rewards.

d. are taught academic skills in the home setting.

ANSWER

a. Children with Down syndrome need to be with peers and have as many normal life experiences as possible.

ITEM 15 Cognitive Type: Knowledge

The nurse caring for a 15-month-old toddler with fetal alcohol syndrome would expect this child to exhibit

a. hydrocephalus.

b. a thin upper lip.

c. low set ears.

d. a prominent maxilla.

ANSWER

b. For a diagnosis of fetal alcohol syndrome, the infant or young child must have signs from each of three categories: growth retardation, central nervous system involvement, and deformities of the head and face.

CHAPTER 28

ITEM 1 Cognitive Type: Application

While making a home visit to the Ford family, the nurse notes several bruises and burns on their 8-month-old son. The nurse should

a. call the child protection services to report possible abuse.

b. discuss the family with the physician at the next team meeting.

c. tell the mother that child protection services will be notified if bruises are found during the next home visit.

d. note the observation in the record for further follow up.

ANSWER

a. The nurse recognizes mandatory responsibility for reporting possible child abuse and acts accordingly.

ITEM 2 Cognitive Type: Knowledge

Based on research findings, one might expect a child who has been physically abused to

a. ask help from their teachers more than other children.

b. have close friendships as they seek companionship outside their family.

c. be more verbally aggressive toward their peers than other children.

d. try harder to succeed in school as an attempt to gain recognition.

ANSWER

c. The nurse knows that abused children are more verbally aggressive toward peers and teachers, as evidenced through research studies.

ITEM 3 Cognitive Type: Knowledge

Which theoretical perspective on child abuse incorporates the view that parents who were abused as children are at risk for abusing their children?

a. Mental illness model

b. Human ecological model

c. Social learning theory model

d. Psychological–sociological model

ANSWER

c. The social learning theory reflects the view that human behaviors are learned through observation.

ITEM 4 Cognitive Type: Knowledge

The most important characteristic of nurses who provide effective care to abused children and their families is

a. theoretical knowledge of the field.

b. the ability to clarify their own attitudes and feelings about abuse.

c. physical assessment skills.

d. experience in working with families from a variety of socioeconomic backgrounds.

ANSWER

b. The nurse recognizes that personal attitudes can influence interactional skills with abusive families and will override any other skills or knowledge.

ITEM 5 Cognitive Type: Application

During her son's 6-month check up, a mother says to the nurse, "My husband seems so jealous of the time I spend with the baby." The nurse's most appropriate comment would be

a. "Most dads are."

b. "Tell me more about this."

c. "You probably just think he feels that way."

d. "Has he abused the baby in any way?"

ANSWER

b. The nurse knows that jealousy exhibited by fathers is a possible risk factor in abuse. Further assessment is needed, which requires gathering more information through an open-ended question.

ITEM 6 Cognitive Type: Application

When interviewing parents who abuse their children, the nurse could promote rapport by saying

a. "Why did you do such a thing?"

b. "I can understand how frustrating young children can be, but to hit him like that is difficult for me to comprehend."

c. "All parents get angry at their children, but most don't hit their children so hard."

d. "All parents get angry at their children and sometimes they might feel like hitting them."

ANSWER

d. The nurse knows that remaining nonjudgmental and accepting of parents helps to establish rapport. Only the last statement is nonjudgmental.

ITEM 7 Cognitive Type: Application

During a visit to the pediatric clinic, the nurse notes that Susie, age 4 years, is wary of adults, withdrawn, and unexpressive. She also seems to seek little support from her mother. Based on these behaviors, the nurse suspects abuse. Her initial action should be to

a. call child protection services.

b. ask Susie's mother if she abuses her.

c. further assess Susie and her family.

d. contact Susie's nursery school teacher for her impressions.

ANSWER

c. The nurse recognizes that the child's behaviors are indicators of possible abuse. The nurse also recognizes that further assessment of the child and family is necessary to make such a diagnosis.

ITEM 8 Cognitive Type: Application

Which of the following is appropriate nursing documentation of assessment data on possible physical abuse?

a. Johnny's left buttock is severely bruised and there is a welt on the back of his left upper thigh.

b. Johnny has several dime-sized bruises on his left buttock and a 2-inch welt on the back of his left upper thigh.

c. Johnny's buttocks and thighs appear to be very sensitive to touch evidenced by bruising.

d. Buttocks reveal bruising and upper thigh reveals welts from apparent bruising.

ANSWER

b. The best documentation of data on possible abuse is the one that is the most objective, clear, and concise.

ITEM 9 Cognitive Type: Knowledge

The most appropriate role for the nurse to assume in child abuse situations is

a. child advocate.

b. surrogate parent.

c. authority figure.

d. best friend.

ANSWER

a. The nursing role in abuse situations is to act as a parent and child advocate.

ITEM 10 Cognitive Type: Knowledge

When hospitalized, physically abused children often

a. feel relieved to be separated from their parents.

b. respond to the staff in the same ways as nonabused children.

c. are glad to be with other children because of previous family isolation.

d. are upset, as are other children, about being separated from their parents.

ANSWER

d. The nurse knows that although children may have been abused, being separated from parents is still a severe loss.

ITEM 11 Cognitive Type: Application

The nurse's initial response to a parent who brings his abused child to the emergency room for treatment should be

a. "It's about time you brought him here."

b. "It's good that you brought him here."

c. "Why didn't you bring him sooner?"

d. "You should have called the child abuse hot line before you hit him."

ANSWER

b. The nurse must convey to the parent that bringing an abused child for treatment is a responsible act that indicates their concern for the child.

ITEM 12 Cognitive Type: Application

Which question is most appropriate for the nurse to ask when assessing a family for suspected nutritional neglect?

a. "How is Scott's appetite?"

b. "What did Scott have to eat today for breakfast?"

c. "Is Scott a fussy eater?"

d. "Do you think that Scott gets enough to eat?"

ANSWER

b. To intervene effectively with neglectful parents, the nurse must use simple, specific, concrete questions to collect data about the child's eating habits.

ITEM 13 Cognitive Type: Knowledge

Adult perpetrators of child sexual abuse are usually

a. strangers to the child.

b. known to the child.

c. unable to relate sexually to adult partners.

d. dependent on alcohol or other drugs.

ANSWER

b. The nurse is aware that the child usually knows the perpetrator. There is no definite evidence that most perpetrators demonstrate the latter two choices.

ITEM 14 Cognitive Type: Knowledge

One of the more common responses to sexual abuse in female adolescents is

a. running away.

b. fantasizing.

c. regression.

d. development of unusual fears.

ANSWER

a. While the nurse knows that fantasizing, regression, and the development of fears are possible responses to sexual abuse, running away is the most common response for female adolescents.

ITEM 15 Cognitive Type: Application

Which comment made by the nurse during an initial interview with a sexually abused child is most appropriate?

a. "Tell me everything that happened. I'm very interested."

b. "I understand that you are upset, but don't worry. We will help you."

c. "Are you sure that this is exactly what happened?"

d. "I have talked with other children who have had the same thing happen to them."

ANSWER

d. The nurse knows that it is reassuring for sexually abused children to know that other children have been in the same situation.

ITEM 16 Cognitive Type: Knowledge

In incest, mothers are often

a. unaware of the incestuous relationship.

b. aware of the incestuous relationship.

c. very assertive with their husbands.

d. emotionally dependent on their daughters.

ANSWER

b. The nurse knows that mothers are usually aware of incestuous father–daughter relationships, but often feel unable to do anything about them.

ITEM 17 Cognitive Type: Knowledge

The immediate treatment goal for the sexually abused child in an incestuous family focuses on

a. allowing the child victim to express feelings.

b. stopping the abuse.

c. promoting the positive aspects of the marital relationship.

d. alerting other siblings of the ongoing situation.

ANSWER

b. The nurse knows that the immediate treatment focuses on stopping the abuse. Other options are important to consider, but not until the child is safe.

CHAPTER 29

ITEM 1 Cognitive Type: Interpretation

A child with a slow-to-warm temperament born into a family who values routine and moderation presents a phenomenon known as

a. synchrony.

b. goodness of fit.

c. self-fulfilling prophecy.

d. adaptive syndrome.

ANSWER

b. The nurse knows that a goodness of fit exists when the properties of a child's environment and expectations are in harmony with the child's own capacities. A child with initial hesitancies will fit well into a family who values routine and moderation of activities.

ITEM 2 Cognitive Type: Interpretation

A 7-year-old girl is brought to the clinic because she is complaining of a stomachache. The clinic nurse notes that the child was examined for the same problem the previous week. Suspecting that the child may have school phobia, the nurse should ask the mother if the child

a. is afraid to go to school.

b. misses school frequently because of the pain.

c. has nightmares or other psychological problems.

d. has a poor academic record.

ANSWER

b. School phobia often presents with somatic complaints first. The nurse must seek a pattern about school attendance before conclusions are made about the child having school phobia.

ITEM 3 Cognitive Type: Application

To facilitate the return to school of a child with school phobia, the nurse would

a. tell the child to return to school as soon as possible.

b. discuss the child's problems with his immediate peer group.

c. refer parents to mental health and school counselors.

d. tell the parents to ignore the child's physical complaints.

ANSWER

c. Children with school phobia need to attend school, but parents must work with school authorities and others to eliminate the causes of the child's fears.

ITEM 4 Cognitive Type: Application

An 8-year-old boy is hospitalized and evaluated for encopresis. His nursing care plan should include

a. dietary management with low fiber foods.

b. restrictions in fluid intake.

c. daily discussions with the child about his "soiling behavior."

d. a schedule for toileting at regular intervals.

ANSWER

d. A child with encopresis is treated with a high fiber diet, increase in fluids, laxatives, and regular toileting. If necessary, family therapy can be done.

ITEM 5 Cognitive Type: Interpretation

A 10-year-old boy is brought in the clinic for a physical examination. His mother says she is worried because he tells lies and she thinks he is stealing money from his older brother. To gain further information, the nurse should ask,

a. "Do you want to talk to the doctor about this?"

b. "Do you scold him when he does these things?"

c. "Does he know right from wrong?"

d. "Can you describe when these things happen?"

ANSWER

d. The nurse needs to know the developmental stage and age of the child, duration and frequency of the behavior, and whether there is actual intent to distort truth before any parental counseling can be done.

ITEM 6 Cognitive Type: Application

The parents of 9-year-old Jenny are concerned about her aggressive behavior. The nurse suggests that they implement which of the following strategies to deal with their daughter's behavior?

a. Help Jenny to express her feelings of anger and frustration.

b. Use physical punishment when aggressive behavior occurs.

c. Develop a high-control parenting style.

d. Give three warnings to Jenny when she is misbehaving before taking any disciplinary action.

ANSWER

a. Nurses can counsel parents to handle the child's aggressive behavior by setting consistent limits, showing affection, rewarding social acts with expressions of approval, and assisting the child with verbalization of frustration and anger.

ITEM 7 Cognitive Type: Application

During a well child examination, a mother tells the nurse that her 5-year-old son is prone to temper tantrums. How would the nurse counsel her to deal with this behavior?

a. Give the child something he likes if he will stop the tantrum.

b. Make sure the mother points out the behavior when it occurs.

c. Take away privileges when the child has a temper tantrum.

d. Explain age-appropriate behaviors and parent's expectations to the child.

ANSWER

d. When a child displays infantile behavioral patterns, management includes clearly communicating age-appropriate behaviors and expectations to the child.

ITEM 8 Cognitive Type: Application

Five-year-old Joey has had a history of nighttime bedwetting for the past 2 months. How would the nurse explain the etiology of enuresis to Joey's parents?

a. "The most common cause of bedwetting is urinary tract infection."

b. "Your expectations of Joey are too high. Most children do not develop nighttime bladder control until school age."

c. "Some children have a smaller functional bladder capacity."

d. "Excessive fluid intake in the evening has been associated with enuresis."

ANSWER

c. If the child has a smaller functional bladder capacity, he is not physically ready for full control of urinary function.

ITEM 9 Cognitive Type: Application

Rachel, age 4-1/2 years, has been bedwetting on and off since she stopped using diapers. What is the nurse's best response to her parent's question, "What can we do to help her?"

a. "Most children outgrow this problem by age 6. It would be helpful for you to note any patterns that develop."

b. "We can teach Rachel to stretch her bladder by giving fluids and asking her to hold her urine as long as she can."

c. "A signal alarm attached to the pajamas has been very effective with children between the ages of 4 and 6 years."

d. "A combination of medication and waking Rachel every 2 hours during the night to void would be the best plan."

ANSWER

b. The therapeutic management of enuresis includes retention control training. Conditioning treatments such as the signal alarm device is not recommended for children less than 8 years of age.

ITEM 10 Cognitive Type: Interpretation

Manda, a 13-year-old girl, comes to the office of the school nurse. Manda is obese and states she wants to lose weight. In addition to assessing Manda's dietary intake and physical activity, the nurse needs information about

a. her metabolic rate.

b. whether she was breast or bottle fed in infancy.

c. the eating habits of her family.

d. number of siblings living in the home.

ANSWER

c. Although there are various theories about the cause of obesity in children, the dietary practices of the family usually influence how much and what a child eats.

ITEM 11 Cognitive Type: Knowledge

When an adolescent is hospitalized for the treatment of anorexia nervosa, the responsibility of the nurse is to

a. teach the adolescent about proper nutrition.

b. place limits on the amount of time the parents can visit.

c. acknowledge the adolescent's right to have feelings of anger and sadness.

d. weigh the adolescent every 8 hours on the same scale.

ANSWER

c. Adolescents with anorexia nervosa may have feelings about meeting treatment goals. Encourage the adolescent to take responsibility for those feelings.

ITEM 12 Cognitive Type: Knowledge

A developmental factor, as opposed to familial or social factors, responsible for substance abuse in teenagers is

a. rebellion against adult authority.

b. escape from family conflicts.

c. television advertising that glamorizes drugs or alcohol.

d. physical abuse of the child at an early age by the parents.

ANSWER

a. Adolescents developmentally want to be independent and different from parents. Rebelling may be a motive for substance abuse.

ITEM 13 Cognitive Type: Knowledge

The *intensive* pattern of substance abuse by an adolescent is characterized by

a. a need to satisfy a curiosity.

b. occasional use of the substance, such as at a party.

c. use of the drug to stay awake to study for a final examination.

d. use of the drug on a daily or more often basis.

ANSWER

d. Intensive use involves daily substance abuse. The nurse can differentiate this type of abuse from experimental, recreational, or dependent types.

ITEM 14 Cognitive Type: Application

A school nurse speaking to a group of adolescents about preventing substance abuse should teach them

a. the motor vehicle laws that prohibit driving while intoxicated.

b. problem-solving skills and ways to bolster their self-esteem.

c. the principles of adolescent development and the need to rebel against authority.

d. how to manage the drug emergencies of their friends.

ANSWER

b. In the prevention of substance abuse, the nurse uses a positive approach. Problem-solving skills, resistance to social pressure, and increased self-esteem are methods for teaching prevention.

ITEM 15 Cognitive Type: Interpretation

Profound depression in childhood may be characterized by the child's

a. crying and withdrawal when parents discipline them for undesirable behavior.

b. refusal to play a new board game with a peer.

c. diminished interest in play activities for longer than a 2-week period.

d. transitory decrease in appetite in response to the birth of a sibling.

ANSWER

c. Profound depression is characterized by changes in the child's usual behavior that continue for a prolonged period of time.

ITEM 16 Cognitive Type: Application

During routine health care visits, when adolescents state that they are sad and would be better off dead, the nurse should respond,

a. "Everyone feels sad now and then."

b. "Suicide never solved anyone's problems."

c. "I'm going to refer you to our mental health nurse."

d. "Please sit down so we can talk about this."

ANSWER

d. All threats or thoughts of suicide or death should be taken seriously by parents and nurses. The nurse can then ask specific questions about when and how often such thoughts occur.

ITEM 17 Cognitive Type: Knowledge

The objective of a therapeutic management program for children with autism is to help the child

a. become person oriented rather than object oriented.

b. be more concerned about her own achievements.

c. avoid situations that cause parents to show their displeasure.

d. learn new skills to compete with peers.

ANSWER

a. The autistic child fails to develop normal social skills. The therapeutic management of children with autism involves helping them relate to others.

ITEM 18 Cognitive Type: Interpretation

A weight-loss program for an obese adolescent would include

a. a steady weight loss of 1–2 pounds per week.

b. 2–3 hours of aerobic exercise daily.

c. eating a high-protein diet.

d. family counseling to deal with conflicts caused by the obesity.

ANSWER

a. It is essential to work with adolescents to achieve a slow, consistent weight loss of 1–2 pounds per week.

CHAPTER 30

ITEM 1 Cognitive Type: Knowledge

The crucial difference between viability and nonviability in preterm infants is

a. neurological development.

b. respiratory development.

c. gastrointestinal development.

d. cardiovascular function.

ANSWER

b. Adequate development of the alveoli is the most significant factor determining the ability of the premature to survive extrauterine life.

ITEM 2 Cognitive Type: Knowledge

A physiological factor contributing to greater risk for alteration in skin integrity in the preterm infant is

a. an immature immunological system.

b. malfunction of regulatory organs such as kidneys and respiratory tract.

c. decreased lanugo on the infant's body.

d. diminished cohesion between the dermis and epidermis.

ANSWER

d. Diminished cohesion between the dermis and epidermis and immaturity of the stratum corneum put the perterm infant at greater risk for skin damage.

ITEM 3 Cognitive Type: Interpretation

A baby girl born at 35 weeks gestation with a birth weight of 2000 g would be considered

a. small for gestational age and low birth weight.

b. appropriate for gestational age and very low birth weight.

c. preterm and large for gestational age.

d. preterm and low birth weight.

ANSWER

d. Infants born before 38 weeks gestation are considered preterm. Infants are assessed as low birth weight if they weigh less than 2500 g.

ITEM 4 Cognitive Type: Knowledge

When assessing an infant born at 29 weeks gestation, the nurse would expect the infant's physical appearance to include

a. thick, soft strands of hair on the head.

b. maintaining an overall posture of flexion.

c. no blood vessels visible through pale, translucent skin.

d. large head in proportion to the body.

ANSWER

d. Because of the cephalocaudal progression of development, the younger the gestational age, the larger the head will appear in proportion to the body.

ITEM 5 Cognitive Type: Knowledge

To conserve the preterm infant's energy during feeding, the nurse would

a. feed larger amounts less frequently.

b. use a softer nipple for formula feeding.

c. use a higher calorie formula.

d. give one-half of the feeding orally and gavage the rest.

ANSWER

b. A softer preemie nipple delivers formula with less sucking effort.

ITEM 6 Cognitive Type: Knowledge

Nursing interventions to minimize the risk of retinopathy of prematurity include

a. careful assessment of the infant receiving oxygen therapy.

b. a daily ophthalmological exam to evaluate the retina.

c. protecting the infant's eyes when receiving phototherapy.

d. placing black and white objects in the isolette.

ANSWER

a. The nurse is in a key position to recommend decreases in oxygen therapy as the infant's condition improves.

ITEM 7 Cognitive Type: Knowledge

A behavior suggestive of a neonatal seizure is

a. jitteriness of legs, which stops when touched.

b. twitching on one side of the face.

c. clonic movements of extremities.

d. fluttering eyelids.

ANSWER

d. Seizures in the preterm infant are difficult to diagnose. Blinking or fluttering eyelids is associated with a subtle seizure.

ITEM 8 Cognitive Type: Knowledge

The nurse is evaluating a preterm infant for sensory alterations. An indication that the infant is overstimulated might include

a. arching of trunk.

b. clenching fists.

c. wide eyes.

d. tachycardia.

ANSWER

a. The nurse must assess the infant for avoidance behaviors associated with overstimulation, which include arching of the trunk, gaze aversion, finger splaying, crying, and yawning.

ITEM 9 Cognitive Type: Knowledge

Hyperbilirubinemia is a special concern in a preterm infant because of its

a. immature liver function.

b. poor vascular system.

c. decreased respiratory function.

d. immature endocrine system.

ANSWER

a. Because of the immaturity of a preterm infant's liver, the potential for hyperbilirubinemia is increased compared to the full-term newborn.

ITEM 10 Cognitive Type: Application

Which of the following nursing actions decreases the risk of injury to the infant undergoing phototherapy for hyperbilirubinemia?

a. Giving small, frequent feedings of glucose water.

b. Covering the eyes with opaque patches.

c. Keeping the infant's torso and extremities lightly protected with a thin blanket.

d. Cleansing the infant's diaper area with alcohol three times a day.

ANSWER

b. Protecting the infant's eyes from the ultraviolet lights used for phototherapy is necessary to prevent injury to the retina.

ITEM 11 Cognitive Type: Knowledge

Gavage feedings are frequently needed to meet the nutritional needs of infants because

a. lactose enzyme activity is not adequate.

b. suck and swallow reflexes are uncoordinated.

c. renal solute load must be considered.

d. hyperbilirubinemia is likely.

ANSWER

b. Recognition of developmental differences of each system in the preterm infant is important when developing care plans.

ITEM 12 Cognitive Type: Knowledge

Immediate nursing care for the preterm infant experiencing an episode of apnea should be

a. cutaneous stimulation.

b. bag and mask ventilation.

c. a pulsating waterbed.

d. supplemental oxygen.

ANSWER

a. The nurse is able to apply knowledge of the causes of apnea to nursing care of patients.

ITEM 13 Cognitive Type: Application

Ultrasonography performed on a premature infant reveals the presence of a periventricular–intraventricular hemorrhage. The baby's parents ask the nurse about the long-term effects of this problem. Which of the following is the most appropriate response to their question?

a. "Most babies with this complication develop hydrocephalus and require surgery to decrease the water on the brain."

b. "Most babies with this problem do not experience any long-term effects since the hemorrhage resolves itself over time."

c. "It is difficult to answer your question at this time; your baby will be carefully monitored for any signs of neurological impairment."

d. "Try to concentrate on dealing with this crisis; we can talk about long-term effects at a later time."

ANSWER

c. The nurse understands that the outcome for infants with cerebral bleeding is highly variable depending on the location and extent of damage.

ITEM 14 Cognitive Type: Knowledge

The etiology of respiratory distress syndrome in preterm infants has been identified as

a. insufficient amount of surfactant.

b. pulmonary hypoperfusion.

c. alveolar overinflation.

d. persistent fetal circulation.

ANSWER

a. Respiratory distress syndrome occurs in preterm infants because of insufficient surfactant.

ITEM 15 Cognitive Type: Application

A nursing diagnosis for the preterm infant is the following: *Potential for inadequate gas exchange between the pulmonary and vascular systems.* Nursing interventions to maintain adequate gas exchange would include

a. providing for increased fluid intake.

b. organizing care to minimize handling.

c. giving frequent cutaneous stimulation.

d. maintaining a low-humidity environment.

ANSWER

b. Excessive handling will agitate the infant and increase metabolism and energy expenditure. This in turn increases oxygen needs and further compromises gas exchange.

CHAPTER 31

ITEM 1 Cognitive Type: Knowledge

Genetic information for transmission of traits from parents to children is contained in

a. chromosomes.

b. nucleosomes.

c. DNA.

d. chromatic.

ANSWER

c. Genomic information is housed on linear strands of DNA.

ITEM 2 Cognitive Type: Knowledge

Every organism has a definite number of chromosomes that are specific to that species in number, size, and shape. The human has

a. 22 autosomes and one sex chromosome.

b. 46 pairs of chromosomes.

c. 23 pairs of chromosomes.

d. autosomal trisomy.

ANSWER

c. There are 23 pairs of human chromosomes, 22 autosomes (those common to both sexes), and one pair of sex chromosomes (XX in females and XY in males).

ITEM 3 Cognitive Type: Knowledge

Through genetic counseling of the parents of a baby with Down syndrome, the mother has been identified as a balanced translocation carrier. The risk of this couple conceiving another child with trisomy 21

a. is 5–15%.

b. is 1–2%.

c. increases with maternal age.

d. is 4%.

ANSWER

a. If the mother is the translocation carrier, there is a 5–15% chance that any child she conceives will have Down syndrome. This type of Down syndrome is not influenced by maternal age.

ITEM 4 Cognitive Type: Knowledge

A child born to an individual who has an autosomal dominant genetic disorder

a. will be a genetic carrier of the disorder.

b. has a 50% chance of inheriting the same disorder.

c. is not at risk for inheriting the disorder.

d. inherits the same disorder but may have variable symptomatology.

ANSWER

b. Individuals with a disease caused by one abnormal dominant gene have a 50% risk of passing it to their offspring.

ITEM 5 Cognitive Type: Knowledge

The child with a recessive disorder inherited the abnormal gene from

a. the father.

b. both parents.

c. the mother.

d. neither parent, since it is a mutation.

ANSWER

b. It is necessary for both parents to carry the same abnormal gene to have a child with a recessive disorder.

ITEM 6 Cognitive Type: Interpretation

A 20-year-old female who has a sex-linked recessive disorder may not show any evidence of disease because

a. she has one normal sex chromosome.

b. she is protected by 44 normal autosomes.

c. the disorder will appear later in life.

d. the disorder skips a generation.

ANSWER

a. A female who has an abnormal recessive gene on the X chromosome will not show any evidence of the disorder since she has another X chromosome with a normal dominant gene that provides for normal function.

ITEM 7 Cognitive Type: Knowledge

An X-linked recessive disorder affecting males is

a. Huntington disease.

b. Marfan syndrome.

c. Duchenne muscular dystrophy.

d. cystic fibrosis.

ANSWER

c. In X-linked disorders, females are carriers and usually affected. Duchenne muscular dystrophy is an example of such a disorder.

ITEM 8 Cognitive Type: Knowledge

What is meant by *threshold effect* in multifactorial inheritance?

a. The threshold can be raised by altering environmental influences.

b. It is the point at which the combination of genetic and environmental influences exceeds the body's ability to adapt.

c. Individuals with a lowered threshold will exhibit disease symptoms.

d. Multiple factors contribute to variation in the manifestations of certain diseases.

ANSWER

b. The threshold effect is the point at which the additive effects of genetic and environmental influences exceeds the ability of the body to adapt and malformations or diseases are expressed.

ITEM 9 Cognitive Type: Application

In performing a newborn assessment, one observation that would alert the nurse to the possibility of Down syndrome is

a. hypotonia.

b. a heart murmur.

c. a small, round head.

d. webbed fourth and fifth fingers.

ANSWER

a. Hypotonia is a significant finding in almost all Down syndrome infants.

ITEM 10 Cognitive Type: Knowledge

The genetic counseling process includes diagramming the data gathered from a family on the medical, health, social, and ethnic backgrounds of their first- and second-degree relatives. This genetic assessment tool is called

a. the family karyotype.

b. a genetic health survey.

c. the generational genogram.

d. the family pedigree.

ANSWER

d. The family pedigree represents a family's multigenerational health history in the form of a diagram that outlines patterns of inherited disorders.

ITEM 11 Cognitive Type: Interpretation

A finding noted on physical assessment that alerts the nurse to the possibility of genetic disease is

a. epicanthal folds in a 2-year-old girl.

b. asymmetry of the nose in a 13-year-old boy.

c. closure of the anterior fontanel in a 15-month-old child.

d. height and weight under the third percentile in a 1-year-old baby.

ANSWER

d. The nurse should be alert to a variety of genetic causes of failure to thrive, such as later onset metabolic diseases. Accurate measurements of height, weight, and head circumference are critical.

ITEM 12 Cognitive Type: Interpretation

The nurse would be alerted to the need for genetic evaluation in a 3-day-old infant if the infant exhibited

a. the top of ears aligning with the eyes.

b. two horizontal and one vertical palmar creases.

c. a hairy patch at the base of the spine.

d. a head circumference measurement of 35 cm.

ANSWER

c. Subtle signs such as a hairy patch at the base of the spine should alert the nurse to request further evaluation.

ITEM 13 Cognitive Type: Interpretation

The genetic counseling process is designed to provide the family with

a. advice that directs their choice of options.

b. medical treatment and follow-up care for an identified anomaly.

c. medical data, recurrence risk, options, support, and referral.

d. early childhood education and habilitation resources.

ANSWER

c. The nurse prepared as a genetic counselor practices prevention, counseling, and education as well as intervention in a supportive manner.

ITEM 14 Cognitive Type: Application

The mother of a newborn, diagnosed with a genetic defect, cries and asks, "What did I do wrong?" The best response by the nurse is

a. "Perhaps you did something you are not aware of. Let's talk about it."

b. "I understand how you are feeling. It must be difficult for you to understand why this happened to your baby."

c. "You should not feel badly about this. Genetic defects are an act of nature and you should not blame yourself."

d. "Why are you feeling upset? Would you like to talk about it?"

ANSWER

b. The skilled and caring nurse can make a difference in the family's ability to work through these initial feelings by empathizing and being nonjudgmental.

CHAPTER 32

ITEM 1 Cognitive Type: Knowledge

Infants and young children are more vulnerable to respiratory alterations than adults are because

a. oxygen consumption in children is lower in proportion to body surface area.

b. cilia lining the lungs are nonfunctional during early childhood.

c. children have fewer accessory muscles for respiration.

d. cartilaginous airways in children are underdeveloped and smaller in diameter.

ANSWER

d. Airway diameter in absolute terms is smaller in the infant or young child than in the adult. The potential for edema and obstruction of the airway is further enhanced due to underdeveloped cartilage in the trachea and bronchi.

ITEM 2 Cognitive Type: Knowledge

Pulmonary function tests may be performed on a child who is experiencing an alteration in respiratory function to

a. determine the etiology of the alteration.

b. assess the degree of pulmonary disease.

c. identify the location of respiratory obstruction.

d. define lesions in the chest wall.

ANSWER

b. Pulmonary function tests are used to assess the degree of pulmonary disease and the response to therapy and to help distinguish between restrictive and obstructive disease.

ITEM 3 Cognitive Type: Knowledge

To meet the safety needs of a child who has a nasal cannula in place for oxygen therapy, the nurse should

a. ensure that the flow does not exceed 6 L/minute.

b. measure oxygen concentration with an analyzer to determine flow rate.

c. change the tubing every 8 hours.

d. secure the cannula in place over the nasal bridge with adhesive tape.

ANSWER

a. Oxygen flow rates when using a nasal cannula should not exceed 6 L/minute because gastric distention, regurgitation, and sinus headache can occur with higher flow rates.

ITEM 4 Cognitive Type: Knowledge

When caring for a child in a mist tent that is being used to deliver oxygen therapy, the nurse should instruct family members to

a. take the child out of the tent for brief periods of comforting whenever the child cries.

b. leave one side rail down with the canopy tucked tightly under the mattress for easy access in an emergency.

c. use the side zippers or lean into the tent with the canopy in place when feeding or playing with the child.

d. turn the cooling unit down and cover the child with extra blankets if the child's temperature drops.

ANSWER

c. The level of oxygen concentration in a mist tent that can be maintained is directly related to the number and length of times that a tent is opened. Parents should be taught how to assist in preventing escape of large amounts of oxygen.

ITEM 5 Cognitive Type: Knowledge

Chest physical therapy is often used in the pulmonary care of children. The primary purpose of this intervention is to

a. effect maximal inspiration, resulting in optimal lung inflation.

b. clear excess or abnormal secretions from the lungs.

c. promote a normal pattern of breathing through correct use of the diaphragm.

d. stimulate deep breathing and coughing.

ANSWER

b. When pulmonary secretions cannot be removed by normal processes, chest physical therapy is performed to assist the child in clearing excess or abnormal secretions from the lungs.

ITEM 6 Cognitive Type: Knowledge

A nursing action that should be included in the plan of care for a child who has a tracheostomy is

a. enlisting the assistance of another nurse when changing the tracheostomy ties.

b. cleaning the skin around the tracheostomy with betadine swabs.

c. changing the tracheostomy tube biweekly.

d. placing a gauze pad between the skin and the tracheostomy tube.

ANSWER

a. Two people are required to change the ties that secure a tracheostomy tube in place to prevent decannulation.

ITEM 7 Cognitive Type: Application

The nursing management of a child with nasopharyngitis (common cold) is primarily directed toward

a. ensuring compliance with antibiotic therapy to prevent complications.

b. relieving discomfort associated with nasal obstruction and fever.

c. maintaining nutritional intake to prevent dehydration.

d. preventing thermal injuries associated with steam vaporizers.

ANSWER

b. The common cold is self-limiting and treatment should focus on supportive measures to relieve related discomforts.

ITEM 8 Cognitive Type: Application

The nursing plan of care for a child who has acute otitis media should include

a. teaching parents how to administer ear drops.

b. promoting compliance with antibiotic therapy.

c. preparing the child for myringotomy and insertion of a tympanostomy tube.

d. assisting parents to identify and eliminate environmental allergens.

ANSWER

b. To promote resolution of middle ear infection, the nurse must emphasize to the parents the importance of completing the full course of antibiotic therapy even though the child seems completely well.

ITEM 9 Cognitive Type: Application

Nursing care of the child who has had a tonsillectomy should include

a. applying warm compresses to the neck.

b. watching for excessive swallowing.

c. keeping the child in a supine position.

d. offering small amounts of liquids through a straw.

ANSWER

b. Following tonsillectomy, the nurse should watch for signs of hemorrhage. Excessive swallowing indicates that blood is trickling down the child's throat.

ITEM 10 Cognitive Type: Knowledge

A pathophysiological mechanism responsible for symptoms associated with croup syndromes is

a. inflammation of the bronchiole smooth muscle associated with bronchospasms.

b. obstruction of respiratory passages by edema and laryngospasm.

c. narrowing of the respiratory airway associated with an allergic reaction.

d. destruction of laryngeal tissues by thick, tenacious mucous.

ANSWER

b. The laryngeal airway in a young child is relatively smaller and mucous membrane is more loosely attached, resulting in rapid compromise (obstruction) by edema and spasm.

ITEM 11 Cognitive Type: Knowledge

Kathy, age 18 months, is admitted to the hospital with acute laryngotracheobronchitis. In assessing her respiratory status, the nurse should expect to note

a. an inspiratory stridor and barking cough.

b. a prolonged expiration and productive cough.

c. severe retractions and nasal flaring.

d tachypnea and paroxysmal cough.

ANSWER

a. Croup is characterized by a brassy, barking, nonproductive cough, inspiratory stridor, and varying degrees of respiratory distress. These symptoms occur because of inflammation and edema of the upper airway resulting in narrowing of the air passages (see Table 38-13).

ITEM 12 Cognitive Type: Application

A child with acute laryngotracheobronchitis is placed in a cool, high-humidity tent connected to room air. The primary reason for using this tent is to

a. decrease insensible water loss.

b. provide a moist environment with oxygen at 30%.

c. prevent dehydration and reduce fever.

d. liquify secretions and relieve laryngeal spasm.

ANSWER

d. The use of cool mist relieves some of the distress of croup by decreasing laryngeal edema and liquefying secretions.

ITEM 13 Cognitive Type: Interpretation

Your neighbor calls you over to her home because Susie, her 4-year-old daughter, has a temperature of 103°F, a severe sore throat, and is drooling while leaning forward with her mouth open. Your action would be to

a. recommend encouraging fluids, giving acetaminophen, and putting Susie to bed.

b. inspect Susie's throat and tonsils using a spoon handle as a tongue blade.

c. suggest that you drive them both to the nearest emergency room.

d. advise Susie's mother to call her pediatrician's office to arrange for Susie to be examined today.

ANSWER

c. The nurse recognizes the symptoms of acute epiglottis, which warrants immediate medical attention.

ITEM 14 Cognitive Type: Application

Brian is a 3-month-old infant admitted to the pediatric unit for treatment of bronchiolitis. Brian's vital signs are temperature 101.6°F (rectally), pulse 160 (apical), and respirations 70. He is irritable, fussy, and coughs frequently. Oxygen therapy is ordered for Brian primarily to

a. reduce fever.

b. allay anxiety and restlessness.

c. liquify secretions.

d. relieve dyspnea and hypoxemia.

ANSWER

d. The nurse recognizes that oxygen therapy alleviates dyspnea and hypoxia. A respiratory rate of 70 breaths per minute in a 3-month-old indicates distress.

ITEM 15 Cognitive Type: Knowledge

A nursing intervention that should be included in a plan of care for a child with pneumonia is

a. strict isolation procedures.

b. frequent assessment of vital signs and auscultation of breath sounds.

c. administration of cough suppressant medication.

d. position changes every 3–4 hours.

ANSWER

b. To promote adequate oxygenation, the nurse checks vital signs and breath sounds frequently when caring for the child with pneumonia.

ITEM 16 Cognitive Type: Knowledge

Airway narrowing characteristic of an asthma episode is caused by

a. laryngeal edema, dehydration, and anxiety.

b. bronchospasm, respiratory mucosal edema, and increased production and accumulation of mucous.

c. increased negative pleural pressure, laryngospasm, and mucous plugging.

d. carbon dioxide retention, pharyngeal hyperemia, and alveolar collapse.

ANSWER

b. The nurse recognizes the pathophysiological mechanisms responsible for airway narrowing in asthma.

ITEM 17 Cognitive Type: Interpretation

John, age 10 years, is admitted to the hospital for treatment of an acute asthma attack. When assessing his respiratory status, the nurse should expect to note

a. accessory muscles of respiration in use as a factor contributing to inspiratory stridor.

b. mild inspiratory stridor with audible wheezing on inspiration.

c. intercostal retractions on inspiration and expiratory wheezing.

d. rapid, shallow respiration markedly increased in rate and a hoarse cough.

ANSWER

c. Clinical manifestations of acute narrowing of the lower airway (asthma) include prolonged expiration, wheezing on expiration, and intercostal retractions.

ITEM 18 Cognitive Type: Interpretation

Becky's father expresses concern about his daughter's asthma. In counseling him about the disease, which of the following statements is most appropriate?

a. Becky's illness is chronic and requires that she be limited to quiet play activity.

b. Becky will outgrow her asthma, so her father does not have to worry about her future.

c. Becky's asthma can be controlled and she can participate in usual childhood activities.

d. Becky is likely to develop chronic obstruction pulmonary disease as she gets older.

ANSWER

c. Parents should be assisted in helping a child with asthma to achieve optimal growth and development while being aware of its chronicity and measures to control exacerbations.

ITEM 19 Cognitive Type: Knowledge

Joshua, who has asthma, is receiving intravenous aminophylline to relieve bronchospasm. Side effects indicating toxicity for which the nurse should observe are

a. tachycardia, agitation, and vomiting.

b. bradycardia, fatigue, and increased blood pressure.

c. tachypnea, drowsiness, and increased pulse.

d. fluid retention, ataxia, and decreased blood pressure.

ANSWER

a. Classic manifestations of aminophylline toxicity are irritability, marked restlessness, tachycardia, and vomiting.

ITEM 20 Cognitive Type: Interpretation

Which observation indicates that the nurse's teaching about activity tolerance for a 17-year-old boy with exercise-induced bronchospasm has been successful?

a. He joins the swimming team.

b. He enters a 10-km road race.

c. He takes a summer job as assistant coach for Little League.

d. He performs relaxation and breathing exercises after basketball practice.

ANSWER

a. The child with exercise-induced asthma should participate in sports and exercise activities that do not require sustained effort, which include swimming, tennis, and baseball.

ITEM 21 Cognitive Type: Knowledge

One laboratory result found in children who have cystic fibrosis is

a. gluten substrates extracted from the stool.

b. increased sodium chloride content in sweat.

c. elevated plasma proteins.

d. presence of small rectal polyps.

ANSWER

b. Elevated sodium and chloride in the sweat occurs in 98–99% of children who have cystic fibrosis.

ITEM 22 Cognitive Type: Knowledge

A pathophysiological mechanism responsible for respiratory alterations seen in children with cystic fibrosis is

a. decreased ciliary action causing stasis of mucous in lungs.

b. edema of the epiglottis causing upper airway occlusion.

c. excessive production of thick mucous leading to obstruction.

d. laryngeal stricture leading to bronchospasm.

ANSWER

c. The primary pathophysiology of cystic fibrosis is abnormal secreting and accumulation of viscous mucous.

ITEM 23 Cognitive Type: Interpretation

Kelly is an 11-year-old child with cystic fibrosis who was admitted to the hospital for treatment of a respiratory infection. Aerosol treatments, chest percussion, and postural drainage are ordered for Kelly. The goal that rationalizes these procedures is to

a. decrease respiratory effort and mucous production.

b. dilate the bronchiolus and clear secretions.

c. increase efficiency of the diaphragm and gas exchange.

d. stimulate coughing and arterial oxygen consumption.

ANSWER

b. Inhalation therapy promotes bronchodilation, and chest physical therapy clears the airway of excessive mucous secretions.

ITEM 24 Cognitive Type: Knowledge

The purpose of a child with cystic fibrosis taking pancreatic enzymes is to facilitate

a. absorption of vitamins A, C, and K.

b. increased carbohydrate metabolism for growth.

c. digestion and absorption of fats.

d. sodium excretion and electrolyte balance.

ANSWER

c. Obstruction of the pancreatic ducts causes trypsin, lipase, and amylase enzyme deficiencies. These enzymes are necessary for digestion and absorption of fats and must be replaced orally.

ITEM 25 Cognitive Type: Application

Dietary therapy for children with cystic fibrosis should include a

a. low fat, low protein diet, with added salt and fat-soluble vitamins.

b. high protein, moderate fat, high caloric diet, with free use of salt and fat-soluble vitamins.

c. low protein, low fat diet, with no added salt and no fat-soluble vitamins.

d. high fat, high protein diet, with 2 grams of additional salt daily.

ANSWER

b. Malabsorption is due to obstruction of the pancreatic ducts and absence of digestive enzymes. A diet high in calories, protein, vitamins, and salt provides essentials needed for growth that may be lost through the stool.

ITEM 26 Cognitive Type: Application

When teaching parents of an infant who has bronchopulmonary dysplasia (BPD), the nurse should provide information about how to

a. encourage additional fluids to help liquify secretions.

b. decrease environmental stimuli to promote rest.

c. reduce caloric intake to prevent pulmonary edema.

d. perform chest physical therapy to maintain adequate oxygenation.

ANSWER

d. Parents should be taught about chest physical therapy and should practice the techniques because this intervention is important in maintaining oxygenation and preventing lower airway infection in the infant who has BPD.

ITEM 27 Cognitive Type: Application

A nursing action that should be included in the care plan for an infant who has apnea episodes is

a. positioning the infant in an elevated seat with the neck hyperflexed.

b. feeding the infant through a gastrostomy tube.

c. teaching the infant's family how to perform cardiopulmonary resuscitation.

d. organizing assessment and intervention activities to provide for minimal stimulation.

ANSWER

c. Parents of infants with apnea are taught to use a monitor, how to respond to an alarm, and how to perform cardiopulmonary resuscitation.

ITEM 28 Cognitive Type: Knowledge

Which of the following criteria should be met prior to discontinuation of apnea monitoring?

a. Infant must have experienced an illness or an immunization without a recurrence of apnea.

b. Infant has only one minor alteration in cardiac function noted on an electrocardiogram.

c. Infant has not experienced an apneic episode for 6 weeks.

d. Infant has experienced only one event requiring vigorous stimulation in a 2-month period.

ANSWER

a. Each of several criteria for monitor discontinuation in apnea must be met, including that the infant must have had an upper respiratory infection, a DPT immunization, or another illness without recurrence of apnea.

ITEM 29 Cognitive Type: Interpretation

When a family experiences the death of an infant from sudden infant death syndrome (SIDS), the emergency room nurse should

a. allow individual family members to be alone to regain their composure.

b. provide the family with an opportunity to see and hold the dead infant.

c. distract the family from the initial shock by asking about the child's previous health history.

d. explain to the family that the death was probably not preventable.

ANSWER

b. During the critical period after a SIDS death, parents of the infant should not be left alone, should be allowed to express their grief rather than be distracted from it, and should be informed that the death was not preventable. The opportunity to see or hold the infant facilitates the family's acceptance of the death.

ITEM 30 Cognitive Type: Interpretation

At 1 minute of age, the nurse suctions the nares of a neonate and notes cyanosis and respiratory distress during the procedure. This neonate's symptoms are most likely due to

a. laryngomalacia.

b. tracheoesophageal fistula.

c. choanal atresia.

d. bronchopulmonary dysplasia.

ANSWER

c. Choanal atresia should be suspected if, during suctioning of the nares, the nurse observes respiratory difficulty and cyanosis.

CHAPTER 33

ITEM 1 Cognitive Type: Knowledge

The vulnerable period for cardiac malformation is during the

a. 2nd to 9th week of gestation.

b. 12th to 14th week of gestation.

c. 16th to 18th week of gestation.

d. 20th to 24th week of gestation.

ANSWER

a. The nurse recognizes that the critical period of gestation for cardiac development is well before the mother may know she is pregnant. This information has implications in terms of reassurance of the parents and decreasing their sense of guilt when they question events that occur later in the pregnancy.

ITEM 2 Cognitive Type: Knowledge

All of the following symptoms should alert the nurse to the possibility of congenital heart disease in an infant *except*

a. difficulty and fatigue during feedings.

b. frequent respiratory infections and dyspnea.

c. nasal breathing.

d. activity intolerance.

ANSWER

c. Nasal breathing is normal for infants, as they are obligate nose breathers.

ITEM 3 Cognitive Type: Interpretation

Diagnostic assessment of the infant with a possible congenital heart defect includes blood pressure measurements taken in

a. the right arm preductally.

b. the left arm postductally.

c. one leg and one arm.

d. all four extremities.

ANSWER

d. Pulse pressure difference either between the two upper extremities or between the upper and lower extremities assist in determining the presence of a congenital heart defect and may also indicate the type of defect.

ITEM 4 Cognitive Type: Interpretation

A complete blood count is ordered for a child with a congenital heart defect. The results are an elevated hemoglobin and hematocrit. Which of the following statements reflect the correct interpretation of this information?

a. The child is not anemic since the hemoglobin and hematocrit are elevated.

b. The body is compensating for tissue hypoxia by increasing red blood cell production.

c. The child is severely dehydrated, and the loss of vascular fluid has elevated the hematocrit.

d. The child is hyperoxic due to the increased oxygen-carrying capacity of the blood.

ANSWER

b. The body compensates for the tissue hypoxia by stimulating the bone marrow to produce increased red blood cells.

ITEM 5 Cognitive Type: Application

Two-year-old Jason is to undergo a cardiac catheterization. Which of the following are appropriate preparatory nursing orders?

a. Bring a doll in the evening before the procedure and show Jason where the catheter will be inserted.

b. Explain the procedure to Jason in simple sentences just before giving the preoperative sedation.

c. Give the preoperative sedation but do not cover the injection site with a bandage, as this will only frighten him.

d. Ask parents to leave the room while the preoperative instructions and medications are given.

ANSWER

b. The nurse recognizes the developmental stage of the toddler. Body intactness, short attention spans, and need for parental support are concerns in preparing a child for a frightening procedure.

ITEM 6 Cognitive Type: Interpretation

A toddler has just returned from her cardiac catheterization. Which of the following objective assessment data noted in the immediate postcardiac catheterization period are indicative of serious complications?

a. Rapid capillary refill and ability to wiggle toes

b. Temperature of 98.8°F and pulse 110

c. Weak pedal pulse and foot cool

d. Blood pressure of 80/50 and dressing dry

ANSWER

c. Arterial thrombosis and spasm of the vessels, which are indicated by a weak pedal pulse and a cool foot, are complications of cardiac catherization.

ITEM 7 Cognitive Type: Knowledge

Instructions for home care of the child following cardiac catheterization include

a. giving a liquid diet every 3–4 hours for 24 hours at home.

b. maintaining a dry, clean dressing over the catheterization site for 1 to 2 days.

c. reporting slight discoloration at the catheter site to the physician.

d. giving only sponge baths for the first 24 hours at home.

ANSWER

d. The child's nutritional status is important to promote wound healing, but diet usually need not be altered once the child is home. The nurse recognizes that the catheterization site is a potential source for infection and must be kept clean, dry, and open to air.

ITEM 8 Cognitive Type: Application

Parent care for the family of a child with congenital heart disease includes

a. acknowledgment of the fears and anxiety surrounding their child's health.

b. reassurance that nurses and physicians will provide all the child's care and relieve them of the burden.

c. explanations that outbursts of anger are inappropriate and unnecessary in a hospital setting.

d. reassurance that once the surgery is over and successful, feelings of anticipatory grief will subside.

ANSWER

a. Anticipatory grief before and after surgery is normal. Parents often feel powerless and angry when confronted with congenital heart disease. It is up to the nurse to recognize and acknowledge these feelings, then give the parents a role in the child's care when they are ready to assume such responsibility.

ITEM 9 Cognitive Type: Knowledge

A congenital heart defect resulting in increased pulmonary blood flow is

a. ventricular septal defect.

b. coarctaction of the aorta.

c. tetralogy of Fallot.

d. pulmonary stenosis.

ANSWER

a. Ventricular septal defect causes a left-to-right shunting of blood, thus increasing pulmonary blood flow.

ITEM 10 Cognitive Type: Knowledge

The four components of Tetralogy of Fallot are

a. tricuspid atresia, atrial septal defect, pulmonary stenosis, and left ventricular hypertrophy.

b. pulmonary stenosis, ventricular septal defect, right ventricular hypertrophy, and overriding aorta.

c. dextroposition of the aorta, aortic stenosis, patent ductus arteriosus, and ventricular septal defect.

d. atrial septal defect, ventricular septal defect, pulmonary atresia, and aorta arising from the right ventricle.

ANSWER

b. Tetralogy of Fallot is defined as a disorder that includes these four components.

ITEM 11 Cognitive Type: Application

A child with tetralogy of Fallot, scheduled for a cardiac catheterization, becomes cyanotic when crying for his mother. An appropriate nursing action at this time is to

a. have the child ambulate to increase oxygenation.

b. assess the child for thrombus formation.

c. draw arterial blood gases.

d. place the child in a knee-chest position.

ANSWER

d. The knee-chest position enhances systemic venous return, which helps to dilate the right ventricle.

ITEM 12 Cognitive Type: Knowledge

A child is diagnosed with tricuspid atresia. Prostaglandin E_1 is given intravenously. The parents ask how long the child will remain on the prostaglandin E_1. The nurse's response is that prostaglandin E_1 will be given

a. intermittently until corrective surgery is performed.

b. continuously throughout the preoperative and postoperative periods until the child is stable.

c. continuously until corrective surgery is performed.

d. intermittently throughout the preoperative and postoperative periods until the child is stable.

ANSWER

c. The nurse recognizes that prostaglandin E_1 is given continuously to maintain patency of the ductus arteriosus until corrective surgery is performed. This drug facilitates pulmonary blood flow that would otherwise be absent.

ITEM 13 Cognitive Type: Knowledge

In preparing a family for seeing their child immediately postcardiac surgery, the nurse should explain and show a picture of the many tubes that will be present. To facilitate the family's understanding of the need for chest tubes, the nurse should explain that

a. chest tubes remove air and blood that may have accumulated during surgery.

b. the lungs have small tears in them due to the surgery and the tubes equalize the pressure in the chest.

c. reestablishment of negative pressure in the pleural space is essential to proper lung ventilation.

d. chest tubes provide a way in which medication can be instilled directly into the chest cavity.

ANSWER

a. The nurse understands the need for the removal of air and blood from the thoracic cavity in the immediate postoperative period.

ITEM 14 Cognitive Type: Knowledge

A mother expresses concern about what activities her 10-year-old son will be able to do once at home following his recent cardiac surgery. The most appropriate response by the nurse is,

a. "Your son will have to be told what he cannot do so he understands his limitations."

b. "Your son will have to limit his activities to quiet games."

c. "Your son will be able to exercise and play as long as he is not fatigued."

d. "Your son will need to understand that he cannot be involved in athletics."

ANSWER

c. Children with congenital heart disease usually are not restricted in their activities. It is better to emphasize what they *can* do than to point out limitations.

ITEM 15 Cognitive Type: Knowledge

Which of the following home instructions for parents of children taking digoxin is most correct?

a. Mix medication with a small amount of formula or food to ease acceptance by the child.

b. If vomiting occurs a short time after the medication has been given, repeat the dose immediately.

c. If a dose is forgotten for more than 6 hours, the medication should be staggered to get it back on schedule.

d. If the child experiences nausea, vomiting, listlessness, or anorexia, the physician must be notified.

ANSWER

d. The nurse recognizes that digoxin is a potent medication and must be administered with caution. Signs of digoxicity such as nausea, vomiting, listlessness, anorexia, bradycardia, and dysthymias, warrant immediate medical attention.

ITEM 16 Cognitive Type: Knowledge

A child with congestive heart failure has a low serum potassium level. This is most likely due to

a. digoxin therapy, which promotes potassium excretion.

b. spironolactone (aldactone) therapy, which promotes potassium excretion.

c. fluid retention, which dilutes the serum concentration of potassium.

d. furosemide (Lasix) therapy, which promotes potassium excretion.

ANSWER

d. Potassium losses are generally due to diuretic therapeutic drugs such as furosemide (Lasix), chlorthiazide (Diuril), and ethacrynic acid (Edecrin).

ITEM 17 Cognitive Type: Knowledge

Nursing actions to help a child and family live with a life-long problem of hypertension are primarily directed toward

a. ongoing physical assessment.

b. screening for complications.

c. teaching healthy patterns of living.

d. collaboration with physical and occupational therapists.

ANSWER

c. Extensive teaching is necessary for the child and family with hypertension. Life-long health attitudes must be established through early education.

ITEM 18 Cognitive Type: Knowledge

Parent education for the child with infective endocarditis should include

a. maintaining strict bedrest for up to 6 weeks.

b. antibiotic prophylaxis for dental procedures.

c. administration of anticoagulant medications.

d. need for future cardiac catheterization to remove vegetations.

ANSWER

b. Antibiotic prophylaxis for at-risk procedures is used to prevent recurrences of infective endocarditis.

CHAPTER 34

ITEM 1 Cognitive Type: Knowledge

The major physiologic component of red cells is

a. hemoglobin.

b. plasma.

c. erythropoietin.

d. hematocrit.

ANSWER

a. Hemoglobin, the major component of red cells, is responsible for oxygen and carbon dioxide transport.

ITEM 2 Cognitive Type: Knowledge

A toddler is brought to the hospital with a suspected bacterial infection. A complete blood count with differential is drawn, which describes

a. red blood cells.

b. hematocrit.

c. white blood cells.

d. platelets.

ANSWER

c. The nurse recognizes that the differential count refers to the type of white blood cells present and gives an indication of the type of infection present.

ITEM 3 Cognitive Type: Knowledge

A child with sickle cell anemia presents with a history of sudden onset of rapid breathing, faintness, and pallor. Physical examination reveals an enlarged spleen and tender abdomen. The child is most likely experiencing

a. aplastic crisis.

b. dactylitis crisis.

c. sequestration crisis.

d. vaso-occlusive crisis.

ANSWER

c. Sequestration crisis is characterized by sudden pallor, faintness, and rapid breathing. These are signs of shock or deficient intravascular blood volume resulting from sudden pooling of large volumes of blood within the spleen.

ITEM 4 Cognitive Type: Knowledge

Nursing intervention for the child in sickle cell crisis is primarily directed toward

a. pain relief.

b. oxygen therapy.

c. administration of blood.

d. maintaining adequate hydration.

ANSWER

d. Maintaining adequate hydration is a primary nursing responsibility since dehydration enhances the sickling process, which in turn increases pain and gas exchange impairment.

ITEM 5 Cognitive Type: Knowledge

Mary is to begin therapy for β-thalassemia. Which of the following would be the most appropriate teaching instructions for her parents?

a. Routine immunizations should be avoided. Blood transfusions will be given on an outpatient basis. Hard lumps may form at the desferal infusion site.

b. Routine immunizations should be given. Blood transfusions will be given on an outpatient basis. Hard lumps may form at the desferal infusion site.

c. Routine immunizations should be avoided. Blood transfusions will be given during overnight hospital stays. Hard lumps should be reported immediately if noted at the desferal infusion site.

d. Routine immunizations should be given. Blood transfusions will be given during overnight hospital stays. Hard lumps should be reported immediately if noted at the desferal infusion site.

ANSWER

b. Routine immunizations are necessary since the β-thalassemia child is at risk for infections. Blood transfusions will be given on an out-patient basis to disrupt the child's routine as little as possible. Desferal infusions often result in hard lumps at the infusion site.

ITEM 6 Cognitive Type: Knowledge

If a transfusion reaction occurs, the most appropriate nursing intervention is to

a. slow the blood and saline infusion rates down and call the physician immediately.

b. stop the blood, keep the IV open with normal saline, and call the physician immediately.

c. monitor the vital signs closely and slow the blood down, maintaining a normal saline infusion.

d. stop the blood and saline infusions and monitor the vital signs closely for the next 15 minutes.

ANSWER

b. Blood transfusion reactions are medical emergencies. Blood must be stopped immediately, IV lines kept open with normal saline for venous access, and the physician should be notified immediately.

ITEM 7 Cognitive Type: Knowledge

To administer blood safely, the nurse must

a. double check patient and blood information with another qualified health care professional.

b. prepare to hang blood within two hours of receiving it from the blood bank.

c. monitor vital signs hourly during the entire blood administration procedure.

d. adjust the drip rate to ensure infusion over a 6-hour period.

ANSWER

a. Blood products must always be checked by two people for proper patient and product identification. Hospital policy dictates the appropriate personnel. Blood should be hung immediately upon receipt, finished within 4 hours of the transfusion's starting time, and vital signs are taken every 15–30 minutes during the procedure.

ITEM 8 Cognitive Type: Application

Heparin therapy may be part of the therapeutic management of disseminated intravascular coagulation (DIC). The rationale for this therapy is to

a. increase the bleeding time.

b. decrease the platelet count.

c. decrease fibrinolysis.

d. prolong the coagulation time.

ANSWER

c. Heparin therapy is sometimes used to interfere with the process of coagulation and to decrease the degradation of fibrin and fibrinogen. This therapy then resolves the dissemination of clots by impeding the binding of fibrinogen and fibrin degradation products.

ITEM 9 Cognitive Type: Knowledge

Altered comfort and pain related to hemarthrosis is a common nursing diagnosis for a child with hemophilia. Hemarthrosis is most correctly defined as

a. central nervous system bleeding.

b. bleeding from administration of cryoprecipitate.

c. pain from gastrointestinal bleeding.

d. bleeding into joint spaces.

ANSWER

d. Hemarthrosis refers to bleeding into the joints. It is the most common site of injury in the hemophiliac.

ITEM 10 Cognitive Type: Application

For the female with von Willebrand disease, appropriate health teaching includes

a. explaining the necessity of avoiding all forms of birth control pills.

b. reassurance that pregnancy and childbirth can be successfully achieved.

c. information on the avoidance of cryoprecipitate therapy during menses.

d. reassurance that no special treatment is necessary once menstruation is established.

ANSWER

b. Menstruation poses special problems for the female with von Willebrand disease. Cryoprecipitate therapy during menses and the use of anovulatory birth control pills may be necessary. Pregnancy and childbirth are possible.

ITEM 11 Cognitive Type: Knowledge

The child with a suspected bacterial infection would most likely have a differential count that has a

a. shift to the left–more mature cells present.

b. shift to the left–more immature cells present.

c. shift to the right–more mature cells present.

d. shift to the right–more immature cells present.

ANSWER

b. A child with a bacterial infection will usually have more immature cells present in the differential count. The number of band cells is usually increased significantly, which is referred to as a shift to the left.

ITEM 12 Cognitive Type: Application

Jennifer is a 2-month-old premature infant. A diet and iron supplement that would provide appropriate nutrition for her to prevent iron-deficiency anemia is

a. breast milk without iron supplementation until 6 months of age.

b. commercially prepared formula and supplemental iron at 1 mg/kg/day.

c. commercially prepared formula and supplemental iron at 2 mg/kg/day.

d. fresh milk and supplemental iron at 2 mg/kg/day started at 4 months of age.

ANSWER

c. The nurse recognizes the need to start iron supplementation earlier in the preterm infant than in the full-term infant because iron stores are laid down during the last few weeks of gestation.

ITEM 13 Cognitive Type: Application

The nurse is teaching a mother about foods to be included in a diet for iron-deficiency anemia. The selection offering the best sources of iron is

a. fish fillet sandwich, corn, and apricots.

b. scrambled egg, fried potatoes, and apple.

c. peanut butter and jelly sandwich, carrots, and banana.

d. roast beef sandwich, green beans, and raisins.

ANSWER

d. Iron-rich foods include organ meats, muscle meats, dried legumes, nuts, green vegetables, dried fruits, and whole wheat or iron-enriched flour and bread.

ITEM 14 Cognitive Type: Application

Jonathan, 2 years old, has idiopathic thrombocytopenic purpura. When he is discharged from the hospital with a platelet count of $100,000/mm^3$, the nurse would inform Jonathan's parents that

a. Jonathan should be watched carefully so he does not fall.

b. fever, headaches, or vomiting should be reported to the physician.

c. Jonathan's blood count should be checked in 1 month.

d. brushing teeth should be avoided; teeth can be cleaned with a soft cloth.

ANSWER

b. Symptoms of central nervous system bleeding should be reported immediately.

ITEM 15 Cognitive Type: Knowledge

A laboratory finding suggestive of severe aplastic anemia is

a. neutrophils less than 9500 and reticulocytes less than 1%.

b. platelet count less than 100,000 and increased cellularity in bone marrow.

c. reticulocyte count less than 2% and platelets less than 20,000.

d. hemoglobin less than 10 g/dL and neutrophils less than 5000.

ANSWER

a. By definition, severe aplastic anemia includes two of these three parameters: neutrophils less than 9500, platelets less than 20,000, and reticulocytes less than 1%.

CHAPTER 35

ITEM 1 Cognitive Type: Knowledge

Which nursing action is of primary importance when preparing to administer a nasogastric tube feeding to an infant?

a. Warm and measure the formula to be given.

b. Instill 0.5–5.0 mL of air into the tube while auscultating for a rushing sound over the epigastric area.

c. Place the infant in an upright position.

d. Provide a pacifier for the infant to suck while being fed.

ANSWER

b. Checking for proper placement of a nasogastric tube prior to feeding is essential to prevent possible aspiration of formula.

ITEM 2 Cognitive Type: Knowledge

Which instruction should be given to parents who will be feeding their child through a gastrostomy tube?

a. Formula feedings should be gently pushed in through a syringe.

b. A reddened area around the tube may be observed.

c. Epithelial tissue at the insertion site indicates immunologic rejecting of the tube.

d. A tube that is dislodged requires emergency treatment to prevent excessive blood loss.

ANSWER

b. A reddened area around the insertion site of a gastrostomy tube is normal except in the presence of foul drainage or otherwise unexplained fever.

ITEM 3 Cognitive Type: Knowledge

A safe procedure for enema administration to an infant is

a. 50 mL of warm water given through a small, well-lubricated plastic suction catheter.

b. 200 mL of a warmed normal saline solution given via a No. 10 French rubber catheter.

c. 100 mL of a one part castile soap to one part warm water solution given through a No. 12 French catheter.

d. 300 mL of warmed normal saline gently pushed into the rectum with a rubber-tipped syringe.

ANSWER

b. An isotonic solution (normal saline) of not more than 280 mL should be used when administering an enema to an infant to prevent rapid fluid shifts from the bowel.

ITEM 4 Cognitive Type: Application

A feeding instruction that should be given to the parent of an infant who has a cleft palate is

a. follow a formula feeding with a small amount of glucose water.

b. position the bottle nipple in the cleft and remove it only for burping.

c. hold the baby in an upright position with the nipple placed normally in the mouth.

d. place the baby in a flat, side-lying position after feedings.

ANSWER

c. The baby should be positioned upright at a 60°–80° angle with the head resting in the bend of the parent's elbow. Placing the nipple in the cleft impedes sucking.

ITEM 5 Cognitive Type: Interpretation

Wilma, age 6 weeks, has just returned to the pediatric unit following surgical repair of her cleft lip. The nursing action that *best* protects Wilma's operative site is

a. providing a pacifier to reduce restlessness and crying.

b. cleansing the wound with warm normal saline.

c. applying bilateral elbow restraints.

d. positioning on either side with blanket rolls.

ANSWER

c. Arm restraints and watchfulness are the most effective methods for preventing an infant or child from disturbing the operative site after cleft lip repair.

ITEM 6 Cognitive Type: Knowledge

A symptom that the nurse should expect in an infant who has pyloric stenosis is

a. choking and coughing with feeding.

b. abdominal distention.

c. projectile vomiting after feeding.

d. hematemesis.

ANSWER

c. In pyloric stenosis, the sphincter is hypertrophied, resulting in a narrowed opening that impedes the effectiveness of peristaltic movements in the stomach. Forceful stomach contractions against resistance is responsible for projectile vomiting.

ITEM 7 Cognitive Type: Interpretation

Nursing management of the newborn who has a tracheoesophageal fistula is primarily directed toward

a. preventing respiratory tract injury.

b. fostering parental attachment.

c. limiting environmental stimuli.

d. maintaining fluid balance.

ANSWER

a. The goal of immediate care is to prevent aspiration of secretions and regurgitation of stomach contents through the fistula into the pulmonary structures.

ITEM 8 Cognitive Type: Knowledge

The herniation of abdominal viscera into the base of the umbilical cord is called

a. diaphragmatic hernia.

b. gastroschisis.

c. omphalocele.

d. umbilical hernia.

ANSWER

c. An omphalocele is a herniation of variable amounts of abdominal viscera through the open umbilical ring into the base of the umbilical cord.

ITEM 9 Cognitive Type: Application

Which discharge instruction should be given to the parents of a 6-month-old following outpatient surgery for repair of an inguinal hernia?

a. Maintain the compression dressing for 1 week.

b. Expect edema to decrease after several days.

c. Change diapers more frequently than usual.

d. Remove the protective sealant from the wound with soap and water after 10 days.

ANSWER

c. Changing diapers frequently will decrease the potential for wound contamination with urine or feces.

ITEM 10 Cognitive Type: Interpretation

One-week-old Kyle is admitted to the hospital for emergency surgery to correct malrotation of the bowel. The nurse should expect that Kyle will have a nasogastric tube inserted to

a. lavage the stomach.

b. decompress the abdomen.

c. provide fluid and electrolyte replacement.

d. reduce intestinal peristalsis.

ANSWER

b. Nasogastric tubes are inserted preoperatively to remove air and secretions from the stomach and intestines which decompress the abdomen.

ITEM 11 Cognitive Type: Application

When caring for an infant following reduction of intussusception by barium enema, the nurse should instruct parents to

a. call the physician from home when the baby passes the first stool.

b. feed the baby full-strength formula thickened with rice cereal.

c. dilate the anal sphincter with a rectal thermometer.

d. save all diapers for inspection by the nurse.

ANSWER

d. Following reduction of intussusception by hydrostatic pressure, the infant will be hospitalized. Parents are encouraged to care for the infant, but the nurse should record and describe all stools accurately.

ITEM 12 Cognitive Type: Knowledge

William, age 6 months, is admitted to the hospital for a rectal biopsy to confirm a suspected diagnosis of Hirschsprung disease. Symptoms that the nurse should expect to note when assessing William's health status are

a. rectal bleeding, diarrhea, and weight loss.

b. history of constipation, abdominal distention, and palpable fecal mass.

c. irritability, vomiting, and dehydration.

d. history of colic, bloody diarrhea, and nausea.

ANSWER

b. Beyond the newborn period, Hirschsprung disease is characterized by constipation, abdominal distention, and fecal retention that is palpable as a large mass.

ITEM 13 Cognitive Type: Application

The rectal biopsy of an infant with Hirschsprung disease shows an absence of ganglion cells, and she is scheduled for surgery to create a temporary colostomy. Her postoperative care should include strategies for

a. limiting physical activity.

b. dilating the stoma.

c. assessing bowel function.

d. preventing prolapse of the rectum.

ANSWER

c. Defecation through the colostomy is expected on the third postoperative day. Assessment of bowel status should always be initiated following surgical manipulation of the intestines (see Table 35-9).

ITEM 14 Cognitive Type: Application

A child who has a temporary colostomy is readmitted to the hospital at the age of 1 year for colostomy closure and a corrective pull-through operation. Following this procedure, nursing care would include

a. measuring rectal temperature every 4 hours to detect signs of infection.

b. removing the anal Penrose drain on the second postoperative day.

c. teaching parents how to administer cleansing enemas at home for the first week after discharge.

d. irrigating the nasogastric tube every 4 hours with saline.

ANSWER

d. Following colostomy closure surgery, a nasogastric tube is placed to prevent distention of the abdomen. Irrigation is necessary to ensure potency.

ITEM 15 Cognitive Type: Knowledge

Which of the following statements is most accurate regarding necrotizing enterocolitis?

a. Infants who are breastfed are protected against developing the disease.

b. It is a multifactorial disease that primarily affects low birth weight infants.

c. Infants born to a parent with ulcerative colitis are genetically predisposed to the disease.

d. It is an infectious process that develops as a complication of respiratory distress syndrome.

ANSWER

b. Necrotizing enterocolitis is primarily a disease of low birth weight infants and is believed to be multifactorial in etiology.

ITEM 16 Cognitive Type: Interpretation

Danielle, age 13 years, is seen in the gastrointestinal clinic for evaluation of symptoms characteristic of inflammatory bowel disease. The nurse should plan to prepare Danielle and her parents for diagnostic studies that include

a. flat plate of the abdomen, Meckel scan, and barium enema.

b. cholangiography, abdominal ultrasound, and colonoscopy.

c. barium enema, upper gastrointestinal series with small bowel follow-through, and sigmoidoscopy.

d. upper gastrointestinal radiography, endoscopy, and 24-hour pH monitoring.

ANSWER

c. Assessment of the child who exhibits symptoms of inflammatory bowel disease includes a complete history and physical examination and diagnostic studies listed in choice (c).

ITEM 17 Cognitive Type: Knowledge

Zach is diagnosed as having Crohn disease. Some manifestations that the nurse should expect to find when reviewing his health history assessment are

a. fever, crampy abdominal pain with diarrhea, and growth retardation.

b. bloody diarrhea, vomiting undigested food, and anorexia.

c. abdominal distention, flatus, and watery diarrhea.

d. nausea, abdominal pain, and diarrhea alternating with constipation.

ANSWER

a. Crampy abdominal pain, diarrhea, and constitutional symptoms are characteristic of Crohn disease. Growth retardation is considered a common occurrence in inflammatory bowel disease.

ITEM 18 Cognitive Type: Application

The nursing management of an adolescent with inflammatory bowel disease (IBD) should include strategies for

a. ensuring compliance with antibiotic therapy.

b. eliminating all high fiber and high fat foods from the diet.

c. dealing with the embarrassment and stress of diarrhea.

d. limiting participation in sports and exercise activities.

ANSWER

c. The adolescent with IBD is at risk for school avoidance and increased stress associated with embarrassment and anxiety related to the clinical manifestations of the disease.

ITEM 19 Cognitive Type: Knowledge

Which of the following are given prophylactically to children at risk for the development of peptic ulcers secondary to serious illness or trauma?

a. Sucralfate and antacids

b. Milk and calcium supplements

c. Liquid antacids and cimetidine

d. Corticosteroids and sulfasalazine

ANSWER

c. Liquid antacids are given to keep gastric pH above 5, and histamine H_2 receptor antagonists (cimetidine or rantitidine) are effective in blocking secretion of stomach acid. Both of these medications are given to prevent the development of stress ulcers.

ITEM 20 Cognitive Type: Interpretation

When the school nurse questions a 10-year-old boy about his complaint of abdominal pain, the nurse is alerted to the possibility of appendicitis by

a. right upper quadrant pain and diarrhea.

b. right lower quadrant pain and vomiting.

c. left lower quadrant pain and low grade fever.

d. left upper quadrant pain after eating.

ANSWER

b. The presence of low grade fever, periumbilical or right lower quadrant pain, and vomiting should alert the nurse to seek immediate medical attention for the child.

ITEM 21 Cognitive Type: Application

Which instructions should be given to the parents of a 4-year-old girl who has gastroenteritis?

a. Eliminate bananas, rice, and applesauce from the child's diet.

b. Provide small, frequent amounts of flat soda, jello water, or half-strength apple juice.

c. Give only water for 24 hours followed by small feedings of crackers and soup.

d. Offer skim milk, dry cereal, or fresh fruit when abdominal cramping subsides.

ANSWER

b. Dietary guidelines at home for children with infectious diarrhea should include giving clear liquids in small, frequent amounts.

ITEM 22 Cognitive Type: Application

Nursing interventions for the family who has an infant with colic should be primarily directed toward

a. teaching pharmacological management.

b. providing emotional support.

c. eliminating dietary lactose.

d. promoting correct feeding practices.

ANSWER

b. The family who experiences the daily disruption, frustration, and sense of helplessness associated with the clinical manifestations of colic will require consistent, nonjudgmental, and empathetic emotional support from the nurse.

ITEM 23 Cognitive Type: Application

Jonna, age 4 months, has gastroesophageal reflux (GER). After feeding and burping her, the nurse should

a. secure her in an infant seat.

b. lay her down to change her diaper with a pillow propped under her head.

c. position her on her side with a blanket roll.

d. place her in a prone position with her head and chest elevated to 30°.

ANSWER

d. The prone, 30° slant position is used for infants with GER for one to several hours after feeding. This prevents regurgitation of stomach contents into the esophagus through an incompetent lower esophageal sphincter.

ITEM 24 Cognitive Type: Knowledge

Therapeutic management of the child with celiac disease includes

a. a lifetime gluten-free diet.

b. growth hormone replacement therapy.

c. anticholinergic drugs to decrease diarrhea.

d. vegetable protein supplementation.

ANSWER

a. In celiac disease, there is damage to the mucosa of the small bowel by gluten-containing foods, which results in nutrient malabsorption.

ITEM 25 Cognitive Type: Knowledge

Which of the following statements accurately describes biliary atresia?

a. It results from an acute viral hepatic infection in the newborn period.

b. Infants with this anomaly are born with cystic or absent bile ducts.

c. It is caused by prenatal exposure to carcinogens.

d. Infants with this disease are not candidates for liver transplantation.

ANSWER

b. The cause of biliary atresia is unknown. This congenital defect is characterized by bile duct atresia that may occur in any part or all of the liver duct system.

CHAPTER 36

ITEM 1 Cognitive Type: Application

Preprocedural preparation for the child who is going to have a voiding cystourethrogram (VCUG) should include

a. administering a cleansing enema.

b. explaining discomfort associated with urethral catheterization.

c. assessing allergies to iodine.

d. restricting fluids for 8 hours prior to the procedure.

ANSWER

b. A VCUG involves catheterization and filling of the bladder with contrast medium, and the child should be prepared for the sensations associated with this aspect of the procedure.

ITEM 2 Cognitive Type: Application

Nursing care of the infant with exstrophy of the bladder prior to surgical correction includes

a. keeping vaseline gauze over the bladder area at all times.

b. cleansing the suprapubic area with Phisohex at every diaper change.

c. allowing the infant to sleep in a side-lying or supine position.

d. covering the bladder mucosa with a Silastic shield.

ANSWER

d. Prior to surgery, the bladder mucosa is protected with a Silastic shield or other device that permits drainage but prevents infection.

ITEM 3 Cognitive Type: Application

The nursing intervention that should be included in the plan of care for a male infant following surgical repair of hypospadias is

a. sterile dressing changes every 4 hours.

b. removal of the suprapubic catheter on the second postoperative day.

c. frequent inspection of the tip of the penis.

d. urethral catheterization if voiding does not occur over an 8-hour period.

ANSWER

c. Following hypospadias repair, a pressure dressing is applied to the penis to reduce bleeding and tissue swelling. The penile tip should be assessed frequently for signs of circulatory impairment.

ITEM 4 Cognitive Type: Knowledge

Which of the following statements is accurate regarding cryptorchidism?

a. It is a common anomaly in which the meatal opening is proximal to the glans penis.

b. Infants with this condition require surgery in the newborn period to prevent sterility.

c. It is a condition in which a testicle has not descended into the scrotal sac.

d. Infants born at term are more likely to be affected with this condition than are premature infants.

ANSWER

c. The incidence of undescended testicles is higher in premature infants. Surgical repair is deferred until after the first birthday because of the possibility of spontaneous testicular descent during the first year of life.

ITEM 5 Cognitive Type: Knowledge

Which of the following renal changes are associated with hydronephrosis?

a. The kidney becomes distended with urine and the renal pressure increases.

b. The renal pelvis and calyces are damaged from recurrent urinary tract infection.

c. A defect in the basement membrane allows protein to pass freely into the urine.

d. There is an abnormal backflow of urine from the bladder into the kidneys.

a. Partial or complete obstruction in the urinary tract can cause accumulation of urine in the renal pelvis and calyses.

ITEM 6 Cognitive Type: Knowledge

A result from a clean-voided urine specimen indicative of a urinary tract infection is

a. specific gravity of 1.020.

b. cloudy color.

c. 100,000 bacterial colonies per milliliter.

d. a large amount of casts present.

ANSWER

c. The diagnosis of urinary tract infections rests on the detection of bacteria in the urine. Infected urine usually contains over 100,000 colonies/mL, usually of a single organism.

ITEM 7 Cognitive Type: Knowledge

Which of the following contributes to the increased incidence of urinary tract infection in female children?

a. Girls cannot be protected with circumcision.

b. The urethra is in close proximity to the anal opening.

c. Vaginal secretions are acidic.

d. Toddler age girls touch their genitalia more often than do boys of the same age.

ANSWER

b. Females are especially at risk for bacterial invasion of the urinary tract because of basic anatomical differences.

ITEM 8 Cognitive Type: Application

The nurse should include which information when teaching to support home management of the child who has a urinary tract infection?

a. Follow-up urine cultures are necessary to detect recurrent infections and antibiotic effectiveness.

b. Antibiotics should be discontinued 48 hours after symptoms subside.

c. Recurrent symptoms should be treated by renewing the antibiotic prescription.

d. Complicated urinary tract infections are most often related to poor perineal hygiene practices.

ANSWER

a. A routine follow-up urine specimen is usually obtained 2 or 3 days after the cessation of antibiotic treatment.

ITEM 9 Cognitive Type: Knowledge

The child with vesicoureteral reflux is at risk for

a. hemolytic–uremic syndrome.

b. glomerulonephritis.

c. renal infection.

d. nephrotic syndrome.

ANSWER

c. Residual urine in the bladder predisposes to bacterial growth. Bladder infections lead to renal infections when infected urine refluxes from the bladder into the kidney.

ITEM 10 Cognitive Type: Application

Which nursing action is appropriate when providing pain relief for a child following reimplantation of the ureters to correct vesicoureteral reflux?

a. Administer prescribed narcotic analgesics prior to urination.

b. Differentiate between bladder spasm and general postoperative discomfort.

c. Maintain complete bedrest for the first 48 hours after surgery.

d. Identify developmental abilities and usual routines associated with urinary elimination.

ANSWER

b. Nursing strategies for pain relief following reimplantation of the ureters includes careful assessment of the source and type of pain experienced. Antispasmodics are more effective for pain associated with smooth muscle spasms of the bladder and ureter.

ITEM 11 Cognitive Type: Knowledge

Symptoms characteristic of nephrotic syndrome include

a. hematuria, periorbital edema, and flank pain.

b. proteinuria, generalized edema, and oliguria.

c. oliguria, hypertension, and bruising.

d. colicky pain, tachypnea, and hematuria.

ANSWER

b. Nephrotic syndrome is characterized by massive proteinuria, hypoproteinemia, oliguria, generalized edema, and hyperlipidemia.

ITEM 12 Cognitive Type: Application

An intervention that should be included in the nurse's plan of care for a child with nephrotic syndrome is to

a. restrict oral fluids to half maintenance.

b. encourage complete bedrest.

c. provide a low protein, no salt diet.

d. observe for side effects of corticosteroid medication.

ANSWER

d. Corticosteroids are administered to the child with nephrotic syndrome to induce remission. The nurse should plan to assess for side effects of these steroids.

ITEM 13 Cognitive Type: Knowledge

The major symptoms of acute renal failure is

a. lethargy and malaise.

b. periorbital edema and weight gain.

c. oliguria and anuria.

d. hematuria and proteinuria.

ANSWER

c. The principle manifestations of acute renal failure are oliguria and anuria.

ITEM 14 Cognitive Type: Knowledge

Which of the following signs noted on assessment of a child with acute renal failure should alert the nurse to a complication associated with excess intravascular fluid?

a. Increased urine output, bradycardia, and flank pain

b. Weight loss, pallor, and fever

c. Tachypnea, rales and rhonchi, and tachycardia

d. Hypotension, vomiting, and diarrhea

ANSWER

c. Pulmonary edema, a serious complication of acute renal failure, results when vascular fluid backs up into the lungs because the heart is unable to accommodate the increased vascular load.

ITEM 15 Cognitive Type: Knowledge

Theresa, age 8 years, has acute glomerulonephritis. The nurse should expect her urine to contain

a. streptococcal bacteria.

b. blood.

c. increased water molecules.

d. calcium casts.

ANSWER

b. Urinalysis findings consistent with glomerulonephritis include specific gravity less than 1.030, positive blood and protein, and white and red blood cell casts.

ITEM 16 Cognitive Type: Application

An important nursing intervention to support the therapeutic management of the child with acute glomerulonephritis is

a. measuring weight daily.

b. monitoring for signs of hypokalemia.

c. increasing oral fluids.

d. providing sodium supplements.

ANSWER

a. The child with acute glomerulonephritis should be monitored for fluid imbalance which is done through daily weighings.

ITEM 17 Cognitive Type: Knowledge

Clinical manifestations seen in children during the renal insufficiency phase of chronic renal failure are

a. growth retardation, hypertension, and skin dryness.

b. vomiting, seizures, and cardiac failure.

c. headache, oliguria, and confusion.

d. easy to fatigue, anorexia, and weight loss.

ANSWER

a. During the renal insufficiency phase of chronic renal failure, the child may have nocturia, growth retardation, hypertension, and skin dryness or itching (uremic frost). Seizures, cardiac failure, headache, and confusion are seen in later stages of chronic renal failures.

ITEM 18 Cognitive Type: Knowledge

Which of the following information would the nurse consider significant for a child admitted to the hospital with a diagnosis of hemolytic–uremic syndrome (HUS)?

a. She has a family history of renal disease.

b. She had gastroenteritis 1 week ago.

c. Her usual diet is low in iron-rich foods.

d. Her throat culture was positive for streptococcus.

ANSWER

b. Hemolytic–uremic syndrome usually follows gastroenteritis or viral illness within several days to 2 weeks.

ITEM 19 Cognitive Type: Knowledge

Which statement is true regarding renal transplantation in children?

a. Children with nonrenal systemic disease are not considered for transplantation.

b. Opportunistic infection is the most common cause of transplant failure.

c. Immunosuppressive agents are used to prevent rejection of the transplanted kidney.

d. Pretransplant growth retardation is successfully reversed after transplantation.

ANSWER

c. Immunosuppressant therapy is used to minimize the transplant recipient's immune response.

CHAPTER 37

ITEM 1 Cognitive Type: Knowledge

The primary organs and tissues of the immune system are the

a. spleen, lymph nodules, and nodes.

b. blood- and gut-associated lymphoid tissue.

c. skin- and bronchus-associated lymphoid tissue.

d. thymus and bone marrow.

ANSWER

d. The primary organs and tissues are the thymus and bone marrow. The others are the secondary organs and systems of the immune system.

ITEM 2 Cognitive Type: Knowledge

The child receiving long-term corticosteroid therapy should be monitored for

a. hypoglycemia.

b. growth retardation.

c. hyperkalemia.

d. fluid volume deficits.

ANSWER

b. Protein catabolism and inhibition of growth hormone associated with corticosteroid therapy can lead to linear growth retardation.

ITEM 3 Cognitive Type: Knowledge

The most frequently and severely affected organs in systemic lupus erythematosus are

a. joints and eyes.

b. skin and kidneys.

c. heart and blood.

d. lungs and intestine.

ANSWER

b. Many tissues and organs are affected by inflammatory changes and vasculitis, but the most seriously affected are the skin and kidneys.

ITEM 4 Cognitive Type: Knowledge

Which of the following is an important consideration for the long-term management of systemic lupus erythematosus (SLE)?

a. Pregnancy should be avoided with the use of oral contraceptives.

b. Hearing should be evaluated regularly.

c. Any exposure to sunlight must be avoided.

d. Fatigue, stress, and anxiety can trigger an exacerbation.

ANSWER

d. Rest is a significant component of care for the child with SLE. Increased stress, fatigue, or anxiety can trigger an exacerbation of the disease process.

ITEM 5 Cognitive Type: Interpretation

Home care for the child with juvenile arthritis involves

a. aerobic exercises that actively puts each joint through a full range of motion.

b. activities that maintain mobility and range of motion but do not strain inflamed joints.

c. avoidance of any physical exercise that puts stress on weight-bearing joints.

d. complete rest except when joints are not stiff or painful.

ANSWER

b. A program of activities is selected to maintain mobility and range of motion but not to strain inflamed joints.

ITEM 6 Cognitive Type: Knowledge

Common side effects of antihistamines include

a. agitation, gross motor tremors, and tachycardia.

b. blurred vision, dyspnea, and hypertension.

c. drowsiness, sedation, and headaches.

d. pruritus, hematuria, and dysuria.

ANSWER

c. Side effects of antihistamines are common but differ markedly with the individual. They include drowsiness, sedation, headache, tinnitus, GI complaints, dry mouth, dizziness, blurred vision, depression, nervousness, hypotension, polyuria, and dysuria.

ITEM 7 Cognitive Type: Knowledge

Using Coombes and Gell's classification, a type I immediate hypersensitivity allergy can be differentiated from the other three types because it involves

a. circulating antigen–antibody complexes that release chemical mediators to cause inflammatory response and activate the complement system.

b. interaction of antigen with certain T cell lymphocytes that cause inflammation and tissue injury.

c. antigen interaction with IgE bound to certain cells causing release of chemical mediators and local inflammation.

d. lysis of cell membranes of foreign red blood cells or bacteria.

ANSWER

c. Type I reactions involve the antigen interacting with IgE (and possibly IgM molecules) bound to a mast cell, basophil, macrophage, or lymphocyte. This causes the cell to release chemical mediators, creating a local inflammatory response.

ITEM 8 Cognitive Type: Knowledge

One of the major chemical mediators released by the sensitized cell in type I (immediate hypersensitivity) reactions is

a. histamine.

b. leukophorin.

c. glucocorticosteroids.

d. serolysin.

ANSWER

a. Histamine is one of the major chemical mediators released in a type I allergic reaction. It helps produce the local inflammatory response.

ITEM 9 Cognitive Type: Interpretation

Clinical manifestations of type I allergic disorders caused by chemical mediators include

a. dilation of the smooth muscles of the bronchial tree.

b. increased nasal and airway mucus production.

c. decreased vascular permeability.

d. alternating constriction and relaxation of the smooth muscles of the gastrointestinal system.

ANSWER

b. Histamine release causes contraction of the smooth muscles of the bronchial tree and GI system, increased vascular permeability, and constriction of pulmonary vessels. Histamine increases nasal mucus production, while leukotrienes increase mucus production in the airways.

ITEM 10 Cognitive Type: Interpretation

History taking is particularly important in allergic disorders because

a. times and events associated with the symptoms provides clues to the antigen as well as the diagnosis.

b. a strong family history of allergies is always present in children with delayed hypersensitivity.

c. a history of previous drug or environmental reactions is diagnostic for allergies.

d. few tests are available to actually diagnose allergies so the history is the basis of diagnosis.

ANSWER

a. Valid recall of times and events associated with symptomatology is critical in providing clues to the causal antigen and in establishing the diagnosis. A family history of allergies is usually present in atopic allergic conditions.

ITEM 11 Cognitive Type: Application

The most important nursing action for the child with allergic rhinitis is

a. recognition of side effects from commonly prescribed medications.

b. teaching the child and family to manage symptoms at home.

c. ensuring compliance with immunotherapy regimen.

d. increasing humidification in the home environment.

ANSWER

b. Because allergic rhinitis is a long-term or life-time problem, the most important strategy is to teach the child and family strategies for self-management in the home.

ITEM 12 Cognitive Type: Application

Nursing care of the child with pruritus from atopic dermatitis includes

a. keeping the child's environment warm and dry.

b. bathing several times daily using bacteriostatic soap and bath oils.

c. using cool, wet compresses of Burrow's solution.

d. applying a heavy layer of cortisone ointment to the skin lesions.

ANSWER

c. Heat and dryness increase itching. Bathing is limited, and only mild soaps that do not remove lipids should be used. Burrow's solution soaks dry, weeping lesions, rehydrates the skin, and cools inflammation.

ITEM 13 Cognitive Type: Knowledge

Elimination of identified or common allergies is an approach often used in treating children with atopic dermatitis. Foods commonly implicated are

a. wheat, eggs, and milk.

b. shellfish, orange juice, and rye.

c. rice, pork, and artificial coloring.

d. corn, oats, and tomatoes.

ANSWER

a. Eggs, milk, and wheat are the leading causes of food allergies and ones likely to be introduced early in the child's diet.

ITEM 14 Cognitive Type: Application

One common strategy nurses use to prevent potentially life-threatening episodes of urticaria and angioedema is to

a. control physical factors such as heat and cold in the child's environment.

b. teach parents to prevent children from being stung by insects.

c. carefully assess clients for history of drug allergies or reactions.

d. eliminate foods that cause allergies from children's diets.

ANSWER

c. Common causes of angioedema and urticaria include drugs, foods, and insect stings and bites, among others. Since physical factors, foods, and insect stings cannot be controlled by the nurse, every client can and should be screened for a history of drug reactions and allergies before medications are given.

ITEM 15 Cognitive Type: Interpretation

An emergency kit for the child who has a history of anaphylactic reaction to an insect sting should minimally contain

a. oral antihistamine and epinephrine in a prefilled syringe.

b. oral corticosteroids and an airway.

c. oral and topical antihistamines.

d. oxygen and a tourniquet.

ANSWER

a. Emergency kits should always contain at least an oral antihistamine and epinephrine in a ready-to-administer subcutaneous form. Oral corticosteroid and topical medications may be used but are not a priority in emergency kits.

ITEM 16 Cognitive Type: Interpretation

Which of the following statements about elimination and challenge testing in food allergies is correct?

a. Common allergies such as milk and wheat are removed from the diet for approximately 3 weeks.

b. Several of the suspected foods are reintroduced every 3 days.

c. The amount of food is decreased gradually while monitoring for reactions.

d. A food that causes symptoms is again removed from the diet.

ANSWER

d. Diagnosis of food allergies is confirmed after two or more elimination trials.

ITEM 17 Cognitive Type: Knowledge

Home management of the child with allergic contact dermatitis involves

a. preventive management to maintain skin integrity and treatment of symptoms.

b. desensitization therapy to airborne antigens in the child's environment.

c. oral corticosteroid treatment on a continuing basis to control inflammation.

d. oral analgesics to control pain and itching.

ANSWER

a. Measures to maintain skin integrity and prevent infection and treatment of symptoms are methods to manage allergic contact dermatitis. Contactants rather than inhalants are the allergens, and desensitization is rarely effective.

ITEM 18 Cognitive Type: Knowledge

Infants infected with HIV *in utero* or at birth

a. have a longer incubation period and a slower progression of disease.

b. are susceptible to bacterial and viral infections.

c. usually achieve developmental milestones on schedule.

d. often show evidence of musculoskeletal and renal problems.

ANSWER

b. HIV-infected children are subject to opportunistic infections. Children infected *in utero* have a shorter incubation period and a more rapid progression of the disease.

ITEM 19 Cognitive Type: Application

Peter, a 1-year-old boy who is HIV-positive, will be receiving intravenous gamma globulin. A nursing action involved in the administration of this drug is

a. shake vial vigorously prior to withdrawing gamma globulin.

b. observe child closely for tachycardia and hypotension.

c. administer gamma globulin in a 0.9% saline solution.

d. stop the transfusion if the child develops a fever or dyspnea.

ANSWER

d. The most common side effects of intravenous gamma globulin are skin rash, urticaria, fever, and dyspnea. If any of these signs or symptoms occur, stop the transfusion.

ITEM 20 Cognitive Type: Application

Which statement would the nurse include when educating the foster family of Amy, an HIV-infected infant, about caring for her at home?

a. The virus is not transmitted by casual contact between family members.

b. All family members should receive the live oral polio vaccine.

c. Any household item having contact with the child should be sterilized.

d. A normalizing activity for the child would be cleaning the fish tank.

ANSWER

a. There are no reported cases of transmission of the virus by casual contact between family members.

ITEM 21 Cognitive Type: Application

The nursing action that would best meet the nutritional needs of a child with Stevens–Johnson syndrome is to

a. offer the child foods high in carbohydrates and fat.

b. administer nasogastric feedings as ordered.

c. administer antihistamines before each meal.

d. offer the child liberal quantities of clear liquids.

ANSWER

b. Lesions in the mouth and mucous membranes of the gastrointestinal tract may necessitate nasogastric feedings.

ITEM 22 Cognitive Type: Knowledge

The nurse can best help prevent rheumatic fever by teaching parents to

a. insist that all sore throats be treated with antibiotics.

b. avoid exposure to the streptococcus organism.

c. identify early signs and symptoms of rheumatic fever.

d. recognize streptococcal symptoms and seek appropriate diagnosis and treatment

ANSWER

d. Early recognition of strep symptoms and effective treatment can prevent rheumatic fever. Since most children with acute pharyngitis have viral infections, cultures are important so that bacterial infections can be treated with antibiotics.

ITEM 23 Cognitive Type: Knowledge

Common major manifestations of rheumatic fever include

a. arthritis, carditis, and erythema marginata.

b. fever, arthralgia, and chorea.

c. subcutaneous nodules and maculopapular rash.

d. elevated sedimentation rate and C reactive protein.

ANSWER

a. Jones criteria for major manifestations include carditis, polyarthritis, chorea, erythema margina, and subcutaneous nodules. Both chorea and erythema marginatum are rare manifestations.

ITEM 24 Cognitive Type: Knowledge

What would the nurse teach parents of a child with Kawasaki disease about aspirin therapy?

a. Increase the dosage if the child is exposed to or develops chickenpox.

b. Aspirin therapy can prolong clotting time.

c. Signs of toxicity include fatigue and diarrhea.

d. Live virus immunizations should be delayed for 3 months.

ANSWER

b. Aspirin therapy can decrease the platelet count and alter clotting time.

ITEM 25 Cognitive Type: Knowledge

Manifestations of the acute phase of Kawasaki disease include

a. dry, peeling skin.

b. fever for longer than 5 days.

c. thrombophlebitis.

d. red rash on face and trunk.

ANSWER

b. The acute phase is characterized by fever lasting 5 days or more.

CHAPTER 38

ITEM 1 Cognitive Type: Knowledge

The major function of the epidermis is

a. temperature regulation.

b. touch sensation.

c. cold insulation.

d. barrier protection.

ANSWER

d. The epidermis provides the body with a physical protective barrier.

ITEM 2 Cognitive Type: Interpretation

A diminished subcutaneous fat layer may put the premature infant at risk for

a. infection and inflammation.

b. decreased pain sensation.

c. temperature instability.

d. increased sebaceous secretions.

ANSWER

c. The nurse recognizes that due to a lack of subcutaneous tissue, the premature infant may have difficulty with thermoregulation. The infant is at risk for cold stress.

ITEM 3 Cognitive Type: Application

A mother expresses concern about 10-year-old Timmy's dry skin. She states that he bathes daily for about 10 minutes. The nurse would instruct her to

a. limit the bath to 5 minutes every day and add oil to the bath water at the end of the bath.

b. limit bathing to once every three days and apply moisturizing cream after the skin is thoroughly dried.

c. extend bath time to 15–20 minutes and apply moisturizing cream when the skin is damp.

d. extend bath time to 20–30 minutes and add oil to the bath water before the child gets in the tub.

ANSWER

c. Extending bath time to 15–20 minutes allows skin pores to absorb water, and application of moisturizing cream before the skin dries will seal the pores.

ITEM 4 Cognitive Type: Application

The components of a diagnostic assessment of skin lesions includes a complete history and physical examination. The history should incorporate

a. symptoms, recent exposures, and medications currently being taken.

b. an examination of the lesions for size, color, and distribution.

c. collection of exudate from the lesions for laboratory testing.

d. palpation of the lesions for tenderness and texture.

ANSWER

a. The history should include a symptomatic history, exposure history, and risk factors such as medication usage and genetic predisposition.

ITEM 5 Cognitive Type: Knowledge

Impaired skin integrity related to irritation of the diaper area is a common occurrence in infancy. Diaper rashes are often related to

a. a parental lack of knowledge of prevention techniques.

b. vigorous cleansing of the diaper area.

c. exposure of the skin to air resulting in chaffing.

d. lack of use of rubber pants or disposable diapers.

ANSWER

a. Parents need to be given clear explanations about diaper area hygiene.

ITEM 6 Cognitive Type: Knowledge

Nursing history and physical examination of an infant reveals the following information: erythematous papules and vesicles, a positive history of allergy, and extreme pruritus. These are characteristics of the stage of eczema called

a. subacute dermatitis.

b. acute dermatitis.

c. chronic dermatitis.

d. seborrheic dermatitis.

ANSWER

b. Eczema has three primary stages. Acute dermatitis is characterized by intense pruritus and erythematous papules and vesicles on a background of erythema.

ITEM 7 Cognitive Type: Application

Nursing assessment of a 15-year-old girl with acne results in the following nursing diagnosis: *Knowledge deficit, related to proper skin care.* The nurse would give the adolescent instructions on the need to

a. avoid all types of cosmetics.

b. cleanse the face at least six times per day.

c. cleanse the face with lukewarm water and mild soap.

d. rigorously wash the face with a washcloth.

ANSWER

c. The nurse recognizes that acne is not a result of uncleanliness, so rigorous or frequent washing of the face will not cure acne. Water-based cosmetics can be used to promote a better self-concept in an adolescent girl.

ITEM 8 Cognitive Type: Interpretation

An adolescent female comes in for a follow-up of acne treatment. During the nursing assessment, she begins to cry and complain that nothing seems to make the acne better and that her face still looks terrible. This reaction indicates that she

a. is probably noncompliant with the treatment.

b. is concerned about her self-concept and body image.

c. understands that treatment might be lengthy.

d. has a knowledge deficit regarding acne treatment.

ANSWER

b. The nurse recognizes the impact that acne has on an adolescent's developing identity and that self-concept and body image are directly related to the adolescent's perception of how others view their appearance.

ITEM 9 Cognitive Type: Knowledge

The nurse would explain to parents that topical preparations are used in the treatment of psoriasis

a. to soften the skin for scale removal.

b. when psoriasis fails to respond to ultraviolet light.

c. to prevent infection of the skin.

d. to reduce cell division and inflammation.

ANSWER

d. Parents should understand that prescribed topical steroid and tar preparations do more than soothe the skin. They reduce rapid cell division and decrease dermal inflammation to help bring about remission.

ITEM 10 Cognitive Type: Application

A family who has an 18-month-old son is planning a family vacation at the beach in August. What anticipatory guidance would the nurse offer them about sun exposure?

a. Apply sunscreen one-half hour before sun exposure for maximum effectiveness.

b. Use a sunscreen with a sun protection factor (SPF) of less than 15 on all exposed areas of the baby's skin.

c. Plan beach or outdoor time between 10:00 a.m. and 3:00 p.m.

d. Keep the child out of direct sunlight because of his young age.

ANSWER

a. Prevention is the best therapy for sunburn. To protect skin from the sun's damaging rays, sunscreens should be applied at least 30 minutes before sun exposure.

ITEM 11 Cognitive Type: Application

The 2-year-old daughter of a vacationing family has a mild sunburn on her back and legs after her first day at the beach. The parents should

a. give the child a tepid bath and apply a water-based emollient to the sunburned areas.

b. keep the child out of the sun for the duration of this vacation.

c. apply continuous cool saline soaks to affected areas to reduce inflammation.

d. give aspirin every 4–6 hours as needed for its analgesic and anti-inflammatory effects.

ANSWER

a. For localized, first-degree sunburn, cool tap water soaks can be applied to the skin for 20 minutes. Tepid tap water baths are indicated for large sunburned areas. Water-based emollients (preferably refrigerated) have a cooling effect on the skin.

ITEM 12 Cognitive Type: Application

Nine-year-old Robby has impetigo on his leg. To prevent the spread of impetigo to other family members, the nurse would teach Robby's parents to

a. be compliant with following the schedule for oral antibiotics.

b. isolate Robby until he has had antibiotics for 48 hours.

c. cover Robby's hands with a soft cloth to scratch pruritic lesions.

d. provide Robby with his own towel and washcloth.

ANSWER

d. The infected child should not share linens with other family members.

ITEM 13 Cognitive Type: Application

Five-year-old Megan has gingivostomatitis. Her mother reports the child does not want to drink fluids because swallowing causes pain. The nurse would recommend that the mother offer Megan

a. any kind of fruit juice.

b. a glass of cold soda.

c. a bowl of beef bouillon.

d. a vanilla milkshake.

ANSWER

d. Bland fluids should be offered to the child; no fruit juices or salty liquids. Noncarbonated beverages are well tolerated.

CHAPTER 39

ITEM 1 Cognitive Type: Knowledge

The nurse can best manage common childhood communicable diseases by

a. ensuring children's current and complete immunizations.

b. teaching measures to reduce children's fever.

c. assisting children to cope with the stress of isolation.

d. helping children avoid exposure during the prodromal stage of illness.

ANSWER

a. The greatest concern for the nurse is to help parents take responsibility for preventing most childhood communicable diseases by ensuring adequate and complete immunization. Most childhood illnesses are managed at home by the parents rather than directly by the nurse.

ITEM 2 Cognitive Type: Knowledge

Body fluids of the child with cytomegalovirus that excrete the virus are

a. blood and mucous.

b. urine and stool.

c. tears and gastric contents.

d. saliva and urine.

ANSWER

d. Infants excrete the virus in saliva for approximately 6 months and in urine for 4 months or more.

ITEM 3 Cognitive Type: Knowledge

The cardinal symptoms of infectious mononucleosis include

a. difficulty swallowing and neck pain.

b. exudative pharyngitis and jaundice.

c. fever and lymphadenopathy.

d. malaise and fatigue.

ANSWER

d. The cardinal symptoms of infectious mononucleosis are fever, exudative pharyngitis, malaise, and fatigue accompanied by lymphadenopathy and hepatosplenomegaly.

ITEM 4 Cognitive Type: Application

Hepatitis A differs from hepatitis B, non-A, non-B in that

a. hepatitis A is spread primarily by fecal and oral secretions, while B, non-A, non-B are spread primarily by the parenteral route.

b. immune globulin is effective only for hepatitis B, non-A, non-B.

c. hepatitis A has a longer incubation period than B, non-A, non-B.

d. hepatitis A is the only type in which the individual is likely to remain a carrier.

ANSWER

a. The various types of hepatitis differ in their mode of transmission.

ITEM 5 Cognitive Type: Application

Clinical evidence of improvement in a child with hepatitis would be demonstrated by

a. decreasing jaundice.

b. increasing serum transaminases.

c. elevated indirect serum bilirubin.

d. increasing anorexia.

ANSWER

a. Decreasing serum transaminase and serum bilirubin levels would indicate improvement, as would decreasing jaundice and improving appetite.

ITEM 6 Cognitive Type: Interpretation

A child exposed to rabies by a bite will routinely be treated with human diploid cell vaccine (HDCV) if

a. the child does not have previous passive immunity.

b. the animal was wild and not captured.

c. the animal is domestic and healthy.

d. the skin is broken by any animal bite.

ANSWER

b. HDCV provides active immunity and would be used after exposure if the animal is wild, suspected rabid, or a domestic animal that cannot be proven nonrabid.

ITEM 7 Cognitive Type: Application

Ann is a 2-year-old child diagnosed with tuberculosis. A major impediment of proper therapeutic management of tuberculosis is the necessity for

a. 9 months of conscientious drug therapy.

b. prolonged bedrest and social isolation.

c. treatment with medications that are costly and difficult to obtain.

d. treatment in a hospital or sanitarium.

ANSWER

a. Infants and children with a positive Mantoux skin test are treated with isoniazid (INH) for 9 months.

ITEM 8 Cognitive Type: Interpretation

Tuberculosis in a child is usually first suspected when

a. symptoms of cough and fever cause family to seek health care.

b. pulmonary calcifications are visualized on an x-ray.

c. skin testing is positive.

d. there is a known exposure to someone with active tuberculosis.

ANSWER

c. Routine skin testing usually provides the first suspicion of exposure to tuberculosis and has virtually eliminated routine chest x-rays. Many children show mild or no early symptoms and may not have any known exposure to active tuberculosis.

ITEM 9 Cognitive Type: Interpretation

Toddlers and preschool children are more at risk for parasitic infections because their

a. immune systems are more immature and unable to ward off infections.

b. nutritional status is likely to be compromised because of eating habits.

c. developmental stage makes contact with parasites more common.

d. contact with other children increases communicability.

ANSWER

c. Preschoolers and toddlers engage in more outdoor barefoot activities and more hand to mouth outdoor activity and they have poorer handwashing skills than older children and adults. These developmental activities increase parasitic exposure.

ITEM 10 Cognitive Type: Knowledge

Nursing interventions in treating and preventing helminthic infections require

a. a case history of recent social contacts to locate the source of the infection.

b. teaching about handwashing and personal hygiene.

c. strict adherence to respiratory isolation techniques.

d. use of public health resources to eradicate identified vectors.

ANSWER

b. Helminthic infections are enteric. Prevention of infection and reinfection involves teaching about handwashing and hygiene as well as eradicating economic and environmental factors that contribute to the source of infection.

ITEM 11 Cognitive Type: Interpretation

The nurse who is screening school children for the presence of *Pediculus capitis* (head lice) should

a. examine the hair using a good source of artificial light.

b. use applicator sticks to systematically part hair and examine the scalp.

c. use gloved hands to separate hair in a clockwise fashion.

d. inspect and palpate each child's cervical lymph nodes.

ANSWER

b. A magnifying glass or wood light is used to inspect the scalp and hair shafts after parting the hair with applicator sticks. Lymph nodes would not be palpated on a screening unless nits or lice were found.

ITEM 12 Cognitive Type: Knowledge

Parents can be taught to help children to avoid exposure to toxoplasmosis by

a. avoiding direct contact with cat feces.

b. thoroughly cooking all fruits and vegetables.

c. teaching children to not exchange combs and headgear.

d. promptly refrigerating left-over foods.

ANSWER

a. Toxoplasmosis is spread by handling or ingestion of raw or uncooked meat and by direct contact with infected cat feces.

ITEM 13 Cognitive Type: Knowledge

Early diagnosis and treatment of Rocky Mountain spotted fever is crucial. In addition to the history of a recent tick bit, symptoms exhibited by the child will include

a. fever for 24 hours followed by headache, chills, and lymphadenopathy.

b. nausea and vomiting followed by swelling of wrists, ankles, and forearms.

c. myalgia followed in 2–4 days by a distinct, progressive rash.

d. papulovesicular rash that progresses a few millimeters each day.

ANSWER

c. Rocky Mountain spotted fever has a sudden onset with fever lasting 2–3 weeks, headaches, chills, and conjunctivitis. Myalgia is followed in 2–4 days by a rash that begins with pink and blanche macular and papular lesions. These progressively cover the palms, soles, trunk, and face within 24 hours. After 24 hours, the rash is red, palpable, and contains petechia.

ITEM 14 Cognitive Type: Application

Oral nystatin is ordered for a 2-week-old infant diagnosed with thrush (moniliasis). How would the nurse teach the infant's mother to administer this medication?

a. Apply nystatin directly to each cheek with a cotton swab.

b. Use a dropper to place nystatin in the infant's mouth before feeding.

c. Have the infant suck the medication through a nipple after feeding.

d. Insert nystatin into each cheek and rub the area with a gloved finger.

ANSWER

d. An effective method for administering nystatin is to gently rub a gloved finger inside the cheek after nystatin has been inserted. Nystatin should be applied after feeding.

ITEM 15 Cognitive Type: Knowledge

For a nurse to be effective in counseling sexually active teens, the nurse must convey that the primary responsibility for sexual decisions and behaviors belongs to the

a. individual.

b. nurse.

c. parents.

d. society.

ANSWER

a. The teen must accept responsibility for individual decisions and behaviors. The nurse must respect teens as individuals to gain their attention and cooperation in sexual counseling.

ITEM 16 Cognitive Type: Knowledge

In educating adolescents about prevention of sexually transmitted diseases, the nurse would teach them to

a. have a limited number of sexual partners.

b. cleanse the genital area thoroughly before intercourse.

c. apply a condom before vaginal penetration.

d. have regular testing for sexually transmitted diseases.

ANSWER

c. Using a condom reduces the likelihood of sexually transmitted diseases and pregnancy.

CHAPTER 40

ITEM 1 Cognitive Type: Knowledge

Which of the following statements accurately describes the differences between the nervous system of the adult and that of the child?

a. The spinal cord ends at L1–L2 in infants and at L3 in adults.

b. In children, myelination of the central and peripheral nerves is not completed until adolescence.

c. Skull ossification occurs more rapidly in adults.

d. Brain waves are more organized, rhythmic, and of increased frequency in young children.

ANSWER

b. The spinal cord terminates at L3 in newborn infants and at L1–L2 in adults. Myelination of the spinal cord is not complete until puberty.

ITEM 2 Cognitive Type: Application

A nurse who understands age-related differences in the function of the nervous system will include which of the following in her nursing assessments?

a. Obtain yearly measurements of head circumference with comparisons to baseline during the first 2 years of life.

b. Look for obvious and specific neurologic signs when a change in neurological status is suspected.

c. Obtain accurate information about when children begin to walk, talk, and attain other developmental milestones.

d. Reassure parents that the prognosis of neurological disorders is generally positive in infancy.

ANSWER

c. The nurse can best assess and identify actual or potential problems through thorough knowledge of the child's developmental history.

ITEM 3 Cognitive Type: Interpretation

When assessing the level of consciousness in an acutely ill child, the nurse should collect data on

a. the child's ability to recall and state events from the past.

b. the child's response to environmental stimuli and degree of arousal.

c. any recent changes in the child's bowel and bladder patterns.

d. the loss of any previously acquired developmental skills.

ANSWER

b. Assessment of the level of consciousness in an acute neurological check involves assessing the child's awareness of self and environment as well as the degree of arousal.

ITEM 4 Cognitive Type: Knowledge

The most sensitive behavioral indicator of a change in a child's level of consciousness is

a. low-pitched crying.

b. subtle alterations in responsiveness.

c. increased blood pressure.

d. decreased pulse.

ANSWER

b. Changes in blood pressure and pulse are late signs of altered consciousness. Decreased alertness or responsiveness is a good indicator of an altered level of consciousness.

ITEM 5 Cognitive Type: Knowledge

Which of the following diagnostic tests is a noninvasive procedure that uses radiation and a computer to provide a three-dimensional view of the density of the brain, tissue, blood vessels, and cerebral spinal fluid?

a. Brain scan

b. Echoencephalogram

c. Computerized tomography

d. Cerebral angiography

ANSWER

c. The CT scan is a noninvasive procedure that involves radiation, allows a three-dimensional look at normal and abnormal structures, and differentiates tissues by their densities.

ITEM 6 Cognitive Type: Knowledge

The parents of 2-year-old Melissa ask the nurse why their daughter needs a lumbar puncture. The nurse tells the parents its purpose is to

a. obtain a specimen of cerebrospinal fluid for laboratory analysis and to measure spinal fluid pressure.

b. visualize cerebrospinal fluid pathways and identify tumors or abscesses.

c. inject contrast media into the cerebrospinal fluid to visualize the cerebral circulation.

d. inject contrast media to visualize the structures surrounding the spinal canal and the subarachnoid space.

ANSWER

a. The lumbar puncture is done to note the cerebrospinal fluid (CSF) pressure and to obtain CSF fluid for analysis.

ITEM 7 Cognitive Type: Application

Five-year-old Mary is scheduled for an electroencephalogram (EEG). In preparing Mary for this procedure, the nurse should

a. limit verbal explanations as Mary is too old to fear noninvasive procedures.

b. draw a picture of the brain while telling Mary the purpose of the test.

c. explain in concrete terms the expected sounds, smells, and sensations that Mary will experience.

d. have Mary practice lying completely still several times before the test.

ANSWER

c. Psychological preparation for an EEG involves telling children that the smell of the EEG glue is noxious and that it will feel cold and wet.

ITEM 8 Cognitive Type: Application

Jim, a 15-year-old with a suspected arteriovenous malformation, has just returned to the adolescent unit after a cerebral angiogram. Which of the following interventions should the nurse perform to prevent potential problems?

a. Encourage immediate ambulation to facilitate excretion of the contrast media.

b. Limit oral and intravenous fluids to prevent cerebral edema.

c. Administer sedation as ordered to prevent restlessness and hyperactivity.

d. Check the procedure site every 15 minutes and note the quality and symmetry of distal pulses.

ANSWER

d. Care after an angiogram involves checking the site, monitoring vital signs and neurological status, maintaining hydration, bedrest, and observing for alterations in consciousness.

ITEM 9 Cognitive Type: Knowledge

Six-year-old Paul rode his bike into the street and was hit by a car. Upon arrival in the emergency room, he is noted to have several lacerations on his head, a temperature of 102°F, BP of 160/100, pulse 54, and sluggish pupil reactions. Paul also complains of a headache and is confused. The nurse recognizes these clinical manifestations as possible evidence of

a. elevated intracranial pressure.

b. Guillain–Barre syndrome.

c. a ruptured spleen with hemorrhage.

d. an acute anxiety attack related to the accident.

ANSWER

a. Head injury can cause increased intracranial pressure, with clinical manifestations including elevated blood pressure, headache, altered consciousness, and altered pupil reactions.

ITEM 10 Cognitive Type: Application

Medications given to a child with a head injury include the steroid dexamethasone. Nursing care relevant to this medication includes

a. asking the doctor to prescribe an antacid while she is taking the steroid.

b. checking her urine for blood.

c. giving the steroid along with her anticonvulsant to increase absorption of the anticonvulsant.

d. encouraging the child to increase her sodium intake.

ANSWER

a. When using steroids, the patient should receive antacids every 2 hours to minimize the side effect of gastrointestinal bleeding.

ITEM 11 Cognitive Type: Knowledge

Seven-year-old Becky has a craniectomy to treat a depressed skull fracture. The best position to prevent increased intracranial pressure postoperatively is

a. supine with pillows under the head.

b. prone with no pillows under the head.

c. head of the bed elevated 15° with the neck flexed slightly.

d. head of bed elevated 30° with head and neck in straight alignment.

ANSWER

d. In patients at risk for increased intracranial pressure, the head and neck position should be kept neutral with the bed elevated at 30° at all times.

ITEM 12 Cognitive Type: Knowledge

Following brain surgery for a head injury, 8-year-old James becomes irritable, has decreased urine output with increased specific gravity, and a serum sodium of 110 mmol/L. These clinical manifestations indicate the postoperative complication of

a. syndrome of inappropriate secretion of ADH.

b. diabetes insipidus.

c. hypernatremia.

d. hypokalemia.

ANSWER

a. Patients with head injuries are at increased risk for syndrome of inappropriate secretion of ADH (SIADH). Nursing care to detect this consequence includes monitoring serum electrolytes, urine specific gravity, and urine output.

ITEM 13 Cognitive Type: Application

Eight-year-old Maria had removal of a posterior fossa tumor. The position recommended for Mary in the first 24-hour postoperative period is.

a. supine.

b. side-lying.

c. prone.

d. trendelenburg.

ANSWER

b. Postoperatively, the side-lying position is preferred in the patient who has had infratentorial surgery to avoid exerting pressure on the surgical site.

ITEM 14 Cognitive Type: Knowledge

Following surgery in the cerebella-pontive angle, a patient develops dysarthria, hoarseness, and difficulty swallowing. The nurse recognizes these symptoms as manifestations of

a. early Parkinson's disease.

b. possible cranial nerve dysfunction.

c. impending electrolyte imbalance.

d. a sore throat due to intubation for anesthesia.

ANSWER

b. Dysarthria, difficulty swallowing, and hoarseness are all signs of postoperative cranial nerve dysfunction.

ITEM 15 Cognitive Type: Knowledge

Tommy, a 2-year-old toddler, starts to have a generalized tonic–clonic seizure while in his crib in the hospital. His jaws are clamped. The most important nursing activity at this time is to

a. place a padded tongue blade between Tommy's jaws.

b. prepare the suction equipment.

c. observe the seizure and protect Tommy from harm.

d. restrain Tommy to prevent injury.

ANSWER

c. The most important first-aid measures for a seizure are to remain calm, stay with the child, observe seizure patterns, and protect the child from injury.

ITEM 16 Cognitive Type: Knowledge

The most frequent cause of status epilepticus for a patient with a history of epilepsy is

a. a degenerative disease.

b. antiepileptic drug withdrawal.

c. cerebrovascular accident.

d. a head injury.

ANSWER

b. The most frequent cause of status epilepticus for a patient with a history of epilepsy is acute antiepileptic drug withdrawal.

ITEM 17 Cognitive Type: Knowledge

When charting data for the Glasgow Coma Scale, the nurse should note

a. vital signs and cranial nerve function.

b. the presence or absence of primitive reflexes.

c. eye opening and motor and verbal responses.

d. blood gas levels and electrolytes.

ANSWER

c. The Glasgow Coma Scale scores the patient's best eye opening and motor and verbalization responses.

ITEM 18 Cognitive Type: Application

An 18-month-old child has just returned from having surgery to correct plagiocephaly. The nurse should include which of the following actions in her postoperative nursing care?

a. Provide an environment with music, lots of light, and conversation to prevent sensory deprivation.

b. Force fluids to prevent dehydration.

c. Administer sedation frequently to prevent agitation and damage to sutures.

d. Monitor for the presence of periorbital edema and changes in vision.

ANSWER

d. Children recovering from surgery from craniosynostosis should be monitored for periorbital edema and vision changes. Sedatives are rarely ordered, noises are kept to a minimum, and moderate fluid restrictions are maintained.

ITEM 19 Cognitive Type: Knowledge

An infant was born with a myelomeningocele. A *myelomeningocele* is best defined as

a. the absence of meninges above a rudimentary brain stem and basal ganglia.

b. an external sac that protrudes at the base of the skull.

c. a cystlike growth that contains embryonic cells and meninges.

d. a saclike structure protruding through a spinal defect and containing meninges, spinal fluid, and neural tissue.

ANSWER

d. A myelomeningocele involves a protruding saclike structure that contains meninges, spinal fluid, and neural tissue.

ITEM 20 Cognitive Type: Knowledge

The nursing diagnosis that is most relevant in the first 12 hours of life for a baby born with myelomeningocele is

a. altered bowel elimination related to neurological deficits.

b. potential for infection related to the physical defect.

c. altered nutrition related to immobility.

d. disturbance in self-concept related to physical disability.

ANSWER

b. Care of the protruding sac is extremely important in the initial days after birth. Antibiotics and meticulous care are required to avoid contamination of the sac and to prevent meningitis.

ITEM 21 Cognitive Type: Knowledge

In helping the parents of a 12-month-old child cope with a new diagnosis of Sturge–Weber disease in their child, the nurse should

a. reassure the parents that most cases of the disease are curable.

b. encourage the parents to identify other cases of the disease in their families.

c. encourage the parents to provide as much of their child's care as they possibly can in the home.

d. refer the parents to community resources that might provide long-term care for the child.

ANSWER

d. Sturge–Weber disease does not have a recognizable hereditary pattern, it is not curable, and it often involves many hospitalizations. Parents often need help to explore long-term resources.

ITEM 22 Cognitive Type: Knowledge

A clinical manifestation commonly associated with an atonic seizure is

a. the "Jacksonian March."

b. a brief contraction of one muscle group.

c. automatic behavior.

d. loss of muscle tone.

ANSWER

d. Atonic seizures involve a sudden loss of muscle tone and consciousness. Clonic seizure activity of one muscle group, the phenomenon called "Jackson March," and automatic behaviors are manifestations of partial seizures.

ITEM 23 Cognitive Type: Application

Becca, age 3 years, is brought to the emergency room in a very drowsy but relaxed state. Her parents describe a previous seizure involving an initial upward rolling of the eyes followed by an increase in muscle tone, rigid posture, and loss of consciousness followed by bilateral rhythmic jerking of the muscles. The type of seizure Becca most likely had was

a. generalized tonic–clonic.

b. absence.

c. complex partial.

d. myoclonic.

ANSWER

a. Generalized tonic–clonic seizures involve loss of consciousness, eyes rolling upward, and muscle flexion in the flexion phase followed by a clonic phase involving rhythmic jerking of opposing muscle groups. Tonic–clonic seizures have a postictal phase in which the muscles are relaxed or flaccid and the child may be sleepy.

ITEM 24 Cognitive Type: Knowledge

Antonio, age 12 years, has had a seizure disorder for several years but is well controlled by medication. He is now complaining of "sore gums," and his doctor says he has gingival hyperplasia. This side effect is commonly caused by the anticonvulsant

a. phenobarbital.

b. phenytoin.

c. carbamazepine.

d. valproic acid.

ANSWER

b. Gingival hyperplasia is a side effect of phenytoin. It is common after chronic use of the drug.

ITEM 25 Cognitive Type: Application

Two-year-old Lindsey is brought to the hospital with a tonic–clonic seizure. If her seizure activity does not stop spontaneously, Susan will probably first be given the drug

a. clonazepam.

b. phenobarbital.

c. phenytoin.

d. diazepam.

ANSWER

d. Intravenous diazepam or lorazepam are initially given to treat status epilepticus, followed by phenytoin.

ITEM 26 Cognitive Type: Knowledge

Samantha has a genetically determined dysmyelinating disease, which will result in progressive loss of central neurological function. Such a disease is generally referred to as a

a. myeolodysplasia.

b. craniosynostosis.

c. neuromuscular disorder.

d. neurodegenerative disorder.

ANSWER

d. The large and diverse group of diseases characterized by progressive loss of central neurological function are collectively referred to as *neurodegenerative disorders.*

ITEM 27 Cognitive Type: Application

Ten-month-old Taylor is admitted to the hospital with a diagnosis of bacterial meningitis. The nurse should anticipate performing which of the following interventions?

a. Isolate Taylor once the specific organism causing the infection is identified.

b. Give him large amounts of oral fluids to prevent dehydration.

c. Administer sedatives to control irritability.

d. Administer intravenous antibiotics for at least 10 days.

ANSWER

d. Treatment of bacterial meningitis involves the administration of intravenous antibiotics. Sedatives are often withheld because they can mask neurological changes. Fluids are often restricted initially to reduce cerebral blood volume.

ITEM 28 Cognitive Type: Application

Which of the following diagnostic tests is commonly done at the time of discharge and again several weeks later to assess for potential complications in a child who has had bacterial meningitis?

a. An angiogram

b. Audiometry

c. A myelogram

d. A computerized tomography scan

ANSWER

b. Hearing loss from pressure on the eighth cranial nerve is a relatively common side effect of bacterial meningitis. Auditory testing will often be done before discharge and again a few weeks later.

ITEM 29 Cognitive Type: Application

To prevent autonomic hyperflexia in an adolescent who has a spinal cord injury the nurse should

a. check the foley catheter frequently to be sure it is not kinked and irrigate gently if plugged.

b. inspect the skin daily for signs of redness and place the adolescent on a sheepskin.

c. monitor respiration every 2 hours and encourage use of the incentive spirometer.

d. assess the adolescent's coping strategies and refer to appropriate resources if necessary.

ANSWER

a. Autonomic hyperflexia in the spinal cord injured patient is usually caused by overdistention of the bladder.

ITEM 30 Cognitive Type: Knowledge

Five-year-old Michael fell from a jungle gym and suffered a head injury 2 days ago. Michael's physical findings include "raccoon eyes" and leakage of cerebrospinal fluid from his left ear. The nurse recognizes these findings as evidence of

a. a subdural hematoma.

b. an epidural hematoma.

c. a basilar skull fracture.

d. a linear skull fracture.

ANSWER

c. A classic associated finding in basilar skull fracture is the presence of "raccoon eyes." These fractures may also present with CSF leakage from the nose or ears.

ITEM 31 Cognitive Type: Application

A nurse who monitors the vital signs (especially the blood pressure and pulse), the overall fluid status including urine output, and the hematocrit of an infant with a head injury is trying to prevent

a. the potential for infection.

b. an alteration in cerebral tissue perfusion.

c. an alteration in urinary elimination.

d. impaired tissue integrity.

ANSWER

b. Nursing care for the child with threatened cerebral tissue perfusion requires frequent and ongoing assessment of vital signs, including blood pressure and pulse. Overall perfusion status can also be assessed by monitoring fluid status and the hematocrit.

ITEM 32 Cognitive Type: Knowledge

An *epidural hematoma* is best described as a hematoma

a. in which the bleeding is usually venous and bilateral.

b. in which the bleeding is usually arterial and unilateral.

c. in which the blood accumulates between the dura and the skull.

d. that commonly occurs in infants and is usually associated with seizures.

ANSWER

b. Epidural hematomas are usually the result of a tear in an artery; they are usually unilateral, occur mostly in children over 2 years of age, and are only associated with seizures less than 25% of the time.

CHAPTER 41

ITEM 1 Cognitive Type: Interpretation

Daphne, age 7 years, has fractured her wrist and a cast is applied. The nurse performs a neurovascular assessment of her affected hand. A sign indicating a potential problem is

a. warm skin temperature.

b. rapid capillary filling of the nail beds.

c. discomfort with finger movement.

d. bluish skin coloring of the hand.

ANSWER

d. Pallor or cyanosis distal to the fracture site or terminal end of a cast may indicate interference with blood supply.

ITEM 2 Cognitive Type: Application

Nursing interventions to prevent problems associated with therapeutic immobilization should include

a. fluid restriction with strict monitoring of intake and output.

b. decreased sensory and environmental stimulation.

c. small, frequent meals that include high fiber foods.

d. limitation of active range of motion in all extremities.

ANSWER

c. Immobilization has multisystem effects that require intervention to prevent constipation, demineralization of bone, renal calculi formation, and sensory deprivation.

ITEM 3 Cognitive Type: Knowledge

When teaching to support home management of a child who has a cast, the nurse should include which instruction?

a. Wash the cast daily with warm soapy water and a scrubbing brush.

b. Gently knock on the cast at the injury site to assess for pain.

c. Use a ruler padded with gauze to scratch under the cast.

d. Check the skin at the cast edges for redness or swelling every day.

ANSWER

d. Neurovascular assessment should be taught to prevent complications associated with a cast. The presence of redness or swelling should be reported to the child's physician.

ITEM 4 Cognitive Type: Application

Which of the following would be included in the nursing care of a 10-year-old child who has just had a hip spica cast applied after completing 3 weeks of traction for a fractured femur?

a. Reposition every 4 hours to prevent skin breakdown.

b. Apply a diaper to protect the cast from urine and stool.

c. Teach the child to use the over-bed trapeze to shift position independently.

d. Arrange for hospital tutoring because of the lengthy hospital stay ahead.

ANSWER

c. An over-bed trapeze can facilitate patient positioning and foster independence if used for position changes and exercise.

ITEM 5 Cognitive Type: Knowledge

The primary purpose of instituting a schedule of active exercise in all unaffected extremities when a child is confined to bed while in traction is to prevent

a. constipation.

b. bone demineralization.

c. compartment syndrome.

d. thrombophlebitis.

ANSWER

b. The absence of normal stress on the skeletal system during immobilization produces a gradual decalcification of the bones and increased bone fragility. Active exercise against resistance (weight bearing) is of primary importance.

ITEM 6 Cognitive Type: Knowledge

Matthew, age 16 years, sustained an open fracture of his left femur after being thrown from his motor bike. A Steinmann pin is inserted and he is placed in balanced suspension traction. The nurse caring for Matthew recognizes that this was necessary to

a. protect his injury from contamination.

b. realign femoral bone fragments.

c. mobilize his fractured leg.

d. improve joint function in the unaffected leg.

ANSWER

b. Traction is the application of pull to a body part; in this instance the purpose of traction is to reduce the fracture by realigning the bone fragments.

ITEM 7 Cognitive Type: Application

The nurse checking an adolescent in balanced suspension traction would consider the apparatus intact if the

a. knots are loose enough for quick release of the weights.

b. weights are positioned on the floor.

c. mattress is gatched at the knee.

d. hanging weights are not touching the bedframe.

ANSWER

d. Traction weights should hang clear of the bed.

ITEM 8 Cognitive Type: Knowledge

A child in traction may experience a decreased appetite while confined to bed because of

a. decreased metabolic demands.

b. increased peristaltic activity.

c. dehydration.

d. postural hypotension.

ANSWER

a. When immobilized, the child's appetite decreases because the metabolic rate lowers and bodily caloric needs drop.

ITEM 9 Cognitive Type: Knowledge

Congenital hip dislocation in the infant may be recognized during physical assessment as

a. shortening of the limb on the unaffected side.

b. hyperextensibility of the tibial ligaments.

c. restricted abduction of the affected hip.

d. equalized skin folds of the thighs on abduction of the hips.

ANSWER

c. Classic signs of congenital dislocation of the hip include redundant skin folds on the inner thigh of the afflicted leg, limited abduction of the affected hip, and unequal knee length.

ITEM 10 Cognitive Type: Knowledge

The parents of 1-month-old Jasmine have just been told it is likely their daughter has bilateral congenital dislocation of the hip. The nurse is aware that treatment usually involves

a. serial application of casts over a 1-year period.

b. hospitalization for continuous Buck's traction.

c. wearing an abduction device 24 hours a day.

d. surgical correction before the child is crawling.

ANSWER

c. The most commonly used abduction device for young infants is a Pavlik harness which is worn 24 hours a day for a trial of 3–4 weeks.

ITEM 11 Cognitive Type: Interpretation

A child with Duchenne muscular dystrophy (DMD) is scheduled for surgery. When collecting the nursing history, the nurse would obtain information about the child's previous experiences with anesthesia because

a. malignant hyperthermia is a possible complication of anesthesia.

b. the child is at risk for postoperative hypothermia.

c. children with DMD require larger dosages of skeletal muscle relaxants.

d. generalized muscle paralysis generally occurs postoperatively.

ANSWER

a. Patients with DMD are at increased risk for malignant hyperthermia, a potentially fatal complication of anesthesia.

ITEM 12 Cognitive Type: Knowledge

A sign noted on musculoskeletal assessment of a child that alerts the nurse to the need for orthopedic referral is

a. mild internal femoral torsion in a 4-year-old boy.

b. knock-knees accompanied by leg asymmetry in an 11-year-old girl.

c. internal tibial torsion in an 18-month-old toddler.

d. bowlegs in a 2-year-old toddler.

ANSWER

b. Excessive knock-knees that have not corrected to a mild valgus by age 10 years require therapeutic intervention beyond the periodic follow up done to assess progressive resolution in a very young child.

ITEM 13 Cognitive Type: Application

A nursing intervention important for the child who has a slipped capital femoral epiphysis (SCFE) is

a. weight-bearing exercises for the affected extremity in the preoperative period.

b. assessment of neurovascular integrity pre- and postoperatively.

c. active range of motion exercises to the affected extremity.

d. early bilateral lower extremity weight-bearing ambulation following surgical correction.

ANSWER

b. As soon as SCFE is diagnosed, weight-bearing movements are stopped immediately. Neurovascular assessment is of primary importance in preventing complications throughout the preoperative period.

ITEM 14 Cognitive Type: Knowledge

Which of the following strategies initiated by the high school nurse would be most effective in identifying adolescents with scoliosis?

a. Encourage parents to report any changes in their teenage child's posture.

b. Educate health and physical education teachers about how to recognize the deformity.

c. Conduct a screening program that includes observation of each adolescent while walking, standing, and bending forward.

d. Interview the teenagers in the school about any deviations they may have noted in the appearance of their backs or how their clothes fit.

ANSWER

c. Early intervention for scoliosis greatly improves the prognosis and diminishes the length of time needed for treatment. Scoliosis screening programs are most effective in early identification.

ITEM 15 Cognitive Type: Application

Strategies for nursing care related to the nonsurgical management of scoliosis in an adolescent are primarily directed toward

a. promoting healthy body image and self-esteem.

b. preventing infection and immobility.

c. preserving cardiopulmonary function.

d. planning exercise and relaxation programs.

ANSWER

a. Nonsurgical interventions for scoliosis place the adolescent at risk for alterations in self-image and should be addressed.

ITEM 16 Cognitive Type: Application

The plan of care for a child with osteomyelitis should include strategies for

a. isolating the child from contact with individuals who have upper respiratory infections.

b. maintaining intravenous infusion sites.

c. performing clean dressing changes and wound irrigations.

d. promoting active range of motion, stretching, and weight-bearing exercises of the affected bone.

ANSWER

b. The child with osteomyelitis requires long-term parental antibiotic therapy to eradicate the infection completely. Maintenance of infusion sites is an important nursing responsibility.

ITEM 17 Cognitive Type: Knowledge

A common childhood fracture characterized by disruption of the periosteum on one side of the bone is called a

a. toddler's fracture.

b. greenstick fracture.

c. comminuted fracture.

d. supracondylar fracture.

ANSWER

b. A greenstick fracture is an incomplete break in the continuity of the bone. This type of fracture is common in children because their bones are more porous than an adult's.

CHAPTER 42

ITEM 1 Cognitive Type: Knowledge

When assisting with a bone marrow aspiration, the nurse should expect to

a. administer local anesthetic medication.

b. place the child in a flexed-spine position.

c. prepare the child to lie still for several hours after the procedure.

d. hold the child tightly in a prone or supine position.

ANSWER

d. The anterior or posterior iliac crest is the bone marrow site most often chosen for aspiration in children.

ITEM 2 Cognitive Type: Interpretation

Nursing interventions for the child who is receiving radiation therapy should include

a. assessing for signs of CNS hypoxia.

b. using meticulous handwashing techniques at all times.

c. administering pain medication prior to each treatment.

d. explaining immediate and long-term side effects caused by the therapy.

ANSWER

d. Immediate and long-term side effects caused by radiation treatments should be explained to parents and children.

ITEM 3 Cognitive Type: Knowledge

Which of the following statements accurately describes the action of chemotherapeutic agents used in the treatment of childhood cancer?

a. Antimetabolites interfere with the replication of DNA and are cell cycle nonspecific.

b. Treatment with combinations of antineoplastic drugs causes increased side effects.

c. All chemotherapeutic agents suppress the function of normal lymphocytes in the immune system.

d. Alkylating agents are cell cyclic specific and interfere with cell metabolism.

ANSWER

c. All chemotherapeutic agents are immunosuppressive regardless of their specific effect on cell structure or function.

ITEM 4 Cognitive Type: Application

Douglas, age 16 years, has been told that he has Hodgkin's disease. Which is the best response by the nurse when Doug asks, "Will I die?"

a. "I won't be able to answer that question until the stage of your disease has been determined."

b. "No, Douglas, you will not die. Your type of cancer is curable with chemotherapy and radiation treatments."

c. "Teenagers with cancer do die, Douglas; however, treatments available today work very well, and everyone will work together to help you to get better."

d. "Yes, Doug, you will probably die, but it will not be soon, and we'll help you to deal with death when the time comes."

ANSWER

c. When cancer is diagnosed in an adolescent, interactions and discussions should be open and honest. Direct questions should not be ignored but rather answered with gentle honesty and hope.

ITEM 5 Cognitive Type: Application

Which nursing intervention should be included in the plan of care for a child who is undergoing chemotherapy for the treatment of cancer?

a. Administer aspirin as necessary for relief of arthralgia.

b. Avoid high calorie, high protein foods to counteract nausea.

c. Offer water, tea, or coke between meals to promote fluid intake.

d. Monitor activity and playthings to decrease potential for bleeding injury.

ANSWER

d. To minimize bleeding associated with thrombocytopenia, the nurse should be aware of the need to prevent bumps, falls, and cuts. This is accomplished by monitoring activity and toys.

ITEM 6 Cognitive Type: Knowledge

Intrathecal chemotherapy may result in which of the following late effects seen in children who survive cancer?

a. Learning disabilities

b. Increased susceptibility to respiratory infections

c. Limb deformities

d. Gonadal deformities

ANSWER

a. Treatment that is directed toward the CNS, such as cranial irridation and intrathecal chemotherapy, has been shown to cause neurological and intellectual dysfunction in many children who have survived cancer.

ITEM 7 Cognitive Type: Interpretation

Alison was just diagnosed as having acute lymphoblastic leukemia (ALL). An important factor in her prognosis is that

a. she has a sibling with ALL.

b. her white blood cell count is 8000.

c. females respond better to treatment.

d. she was in good health prior to diagnosis.

ANSWER

b. Age and total white blood cell count at diagnosis seem to be most important prognostic features for children with ALL.

ITEM 8 Cognitive Type: Interpretation

It is suspected that 5-year-old Randy has acute lymphoblastic leukemia (ALL). A result from diagnostic testing that would provide a definitive diagnosis of ALL is

a. leukemic blasts seen in blood smear.

b. bone marrow contains less than 5% stem cells.

c. pancytopenia identified from complete blood count.

d. bone marrow contains 90% leukemic blasts.

ANSWER

d. A definitive diagnosis of leukemia is made from the examination of a sample of bone marrow.

ITEM 9 Cognitive Type: Application

During the induction stage of treatment for leukemia, an important nursing intervention to include in the plan of care for a child is

a. reverse isolation precautions.

b. complete bedrest.

c. high fiber, high fat diet.

d. meticulous oral hygiene.

ANSWER

d. During induction treatment, the child is at risk for bleeding and infection because of bone marrow suppression associated with antineoplastic drugs given during this stage of therapy. Careful oral hygiene is necessary to treat mouth ulceration, prevent infection, and relieve discomfort.

ITEM 10 Cognitive Type: Knowledge

The clinical manifestations commonly seen in children with medulloblastoma include

a. irritability, inability to concentrate, and visual field defects.

b. headache, early morning vomiting, and ataxia.

c. nystagmus, proptosis, and growth retardation.

d. weight loss, fatigue, and seizures.

ANSWER

b. Medulloblastoma is an infratentorial tumor that presents with signs of increased intracranial pressure.

ITEM 11 Cognitive Type: Application

Immediate postoperative care of the child who has undergone surgical resection of an infratentorial brain tumor includes

a. elevating the child's head to 30°.

b. encouraging the child to cough every 2 hours.

c. monitoring the child for cranial nerve dysfunction.

d. increasing the child's fluid intake.

ANSWER

c. Children with tumors of posterior fossa are at risk for depression of autonomic function postoperatively because edema at the operative site may cause pressure on the brain stem.

ITEM 12 Cognitive Type: Knowledge

A correct statement about rhabdomyosarcoma is that it is

a. the least common solid tumor diagnosed in children.

b. the most common soft tissue tumor diagnosed in children.

c. primarily a tumor of spinal muscle tissue.

d. the tumor is most often found in the trunk and abdomen.

ANSWER

b. Rhabdomyosarcoma is a malignancy of the skeletal muscle tissue and the most common soft tissue tumor diagnosed in children.

ITEM 13 Cognitive Type: Application

Which nursing intervention should take the highest priority in meeting the developmental needs of an adolescent who has had a lower extremity amputation for treatment of osteogenic sarcoma?

a. Encourage visits from friends.

b. Promote early ambulation.

c. Explain the phenomenon of phantom pain.

d. Teach about chemotherapeutic agents.

ANSWER

b. The primary goal for the adolescent who undergoes lower extremity amputation is early ambulation to promote independence.

ITEM 14 Cognitive Type: Application

Nursing care of the child with retinoblastoma should include strategies for

a. referring the family for genetic counseling.

b. preparing parents for the cavernous appearance of the periorbital area following enucleation.

c. teaching parents how to instill antineoplastic eye drops.

d. instituting strict isolation precautions during radiation therapy.

ANSWER

a. Once a diagnosis of retinoblastoma has been made, the risk of occurrence of the tumor in subsequent children should be discussed with parents and genetic counseling should be obtained.

ITEM 15 Cognitive Type: Knowledge

Symptoms the nurse should expect to note in a child who has a neuroblastoma are

a. anorexia, ataxia, and vomiting.

b. dysphagia, hearing loss, and cranial nerve palsy.

c. abdominal mass, irritability, and fever.

d. lymphadenopathy, malaise, and pallor.

ANSWER

c. Children with neuroblastoma may be very sick. Symptoms include abdominal mass, fever, irritability, pain, and proptosis.

ITEM 16 Cognitive Type: Knowledge

Wilm's tumor is suspected when the nurse practitioner palpates an abdominal mass in a young boy during a well child examination. When the parents are questioned about his recent health, you might expect them to report that

a. clothing are tight around his waist.

b. he has had a weight loss of 3 pounds.

c. his urination has decreased.

d. his appetite has increased.

ANSWER

a. Parents may be the first to notice increasing abdominal girth when belts or waistbands become tight.

ITEM 17 Cognitive Type: Application

Dan, age 15 years, is diagnosed with a Ewing sarcoma in his fibula. He asks the nurse how Ewing sarcoma is treated. The nurse would respond,

a. "Your leg will most likely have to be amputated below the knee."

b. "If the tumor has not spread to another site, chemotherapy is the treatment."

c. "Radiation therapy and chemotherapy are used to treat Ewing sarcoma."

d. "You will need surgery followed by chemotherapy."

ANSWER

c. Radiation therapy is important to the successful treatment of Ewing sarcoma. Multidrug chemotherapy is often used and is started at the time of primary therapy.

CHAPTER 43

ITEM 1 Cognitive Type: Knowledge

A metabolic alteration characteristic of growth hormone deficiency is

a. galactosemia.

b. hypoglycemia.

c. homocysteinuria.

d. hyperglycemia.

ANSWER

b. Growth hormone is one of the hormones responsible for maintaining normal blood sugar levels. The development of hypoglycemia is a characteristic finding related to growth hormone deficiency.

ITEM 2 Cognitive Type: Application

When providing information to support home management of the child who is receiving growth hormone replacement therapy for hypopituitary short stature, the nurse should

a. help parents to recognize the importance of interacting with the child according to age rather than size.

b. teach family members how to perform venipuncture for administration of the hormone.

c. advise parents to hold the child back in school until linear growth begins to approximate normal patterns.

d. explain to the child and family that growth in height and weight will not begin until puberty.

ANSWER

a. Recognizing potential threats to self-esteem and healthy development are important aspects of nursing care for the child with growth hormone deficiency.

ITEM 3 Cognitive Type: Knowledge

The health history of a child who has been diagnosed as having diabetes insipidus would most likely include

a. delayed closure of the fontanels, thin hair, and hypoglycemia on arising.

b. gradual onset of personality changes, irritability, and visual disturbances.

c. abrupt onset of polyuria, nocturia, and polydipsia.

d. early morning vomiting, headache, and concentrated urine.

ANSWER

c. Diabetes insipidus is characterized by deficient secretion of antidiuretic hormone leading to diuresis. Most children with this disorder experience an abrupt onset of symptoms.

ITEM 4 Cognitive Type: Application

Which instruction should be included in the home management plan for a child who is receiving DDAVP for symptomatic control of diabetes insipidus?

a. Give the DDAVP only when the urine output begins to decrease.

b. Cleanse the skin with alcohol prior to application of the DDAVP dermal patch.

c. Contact the physician for advice on altering the DDAVP dose if upper respiratory infection or allergic rhinitis occurs.

d. Increase the DDAVP dose if polyuria occurs just prior to the next scheduled dose.

ANSWER

c. Excessive nasal mucous may interfere with DDAVP absorption since it is given intranasally. Parents should be instructed to contact the physician for advice in altering the hormone dose during times when nasal mucous may be increased.

ITEM 5 Cognitive Type: Application

Nursing care of the child with precocious puberty should include strategies for

a. teaching parents to limit physical contacts with their child that may stimulate sexual arousal.

b. helping parents to understand that their child is going through a normal process earlier than other children.

c. encouraging parents to provide birth control for their child who is at greater risk for unwanted pregnancy or fatherhood.

d. fostering a child's involvement with older children whose physical maturation more closely resembles theirs.

ANSWER

b. Nursing strategies to support the child with precocious puberty include reassuring parents and the child that the puberty process is normal and that it is simply occurring earlier. The child should be treated as any other child of the same chronological age.

ITEM 6 Cognitive Type: Application

The home care plan for the parents of a child with congenital adrenal hyperplasia should include

a. teaching how to recognize signs of adrenal crisis.

b. explaining when to obtain urine specimens for glucose analysis.

c. demonstrating how to administer intranasal medication.

d. stressing that complications will not develop during periods of physical stress.

ANSWER

a. The nurse should teach parents how to take home blood pressures and interpret their readings so they can seek professional help if hypertension develops.

ITEM 7 Cognitive Type: Interpretation

Which of these should alert the nurse to a major postoperative complication in an infant following adrenalectomy?

a. A low grade fever

b. Decreased blood pressure

c. Irritability

d. A urine specific gravity of 1.010.

ANSWER

b. The major postoperative complication of adrenalectomy is shock. Increase in pulse or decrease in blood pressure are signs of acute adrenal insufficiency.

ITEM 8 Cognitive Type: Knowledge

Manifestations of thyroid hormone deficiency in infancy include

a. tachycardia, profuse perspiration, and diarrhea.

b. lethargy, feeding difficulties, and constipation.

c. dermatitis, dry skin, and round faces.

d. hypertonia, small fontanels, and moist skin.

ANSWER

b. Hypothyroidism results from inadequate thyroid production to meet an infant's needs. Clinical signs include feeding difficulties, prolonged physiologic jaundice, lethargy, and constipation.

ITEM 9 Cognitive Type: Knowledge

Which instruction should be given to the parents of an infant who is being treated with levothyroxine for congenital hypothyroidism?

a. Fussiness, sleep problems, and hunger are indications that dosage is too low.

b. Limit protein and carbohydrate intake during the first month of therapy.

c. If a dose is missed or forgotten one day, give twice the dose the following day.

d. When improvement in appetite, activity, and alertness is noted, the dosage should be decreased.

ANSWER

c. Synthetic thyroid hormone should be administered in a teaspoon or syringe, is necessary always, and forgotten doses should be given the following day.

ITEM 10 Cognitive Type: Application

Nursing care of the adolescent with Graves disease should include strategies for

a. relieving constipation.

b. promoting healthy body image.

c. minimizing radioactive iodine side effects.

d. supporting adjustment to infertility.

ANSWER

b. The physical and emotional changes associated with hypersecretion of thyroid hormone are especially disruptive to the adolescent's normal developmental struggle to establish a healthy body image.

ITEM 11 Cognitive Type: Knowledge

Therapeutic management of hypoparathyroidism is directed toward

a. preventing hypoglycemia.

b. reducing aldosterone levels.

c. reestablishing normal levels of serum cortisol.

d. maintaining normal serum calcium levels.

ANSWER

d. The goal of treatment in all forms of hypoparathyroidism is the maintenance of normal serum calcium levels.

ITEM 12 Cognitive Type: Knowledge

Which of the following is an accurate statement regarding ambiguous genitalia in the newborn infant?

a. Treatment is based on parental sexual preference.

b. It is caused by transient maternal secretion of estrogen.

c. The child will receive hormonal replacement, and surgical intervention is delayed until puberty.

d. Parents should be told that their infant's sex organs are underdeveloped.

ANSWER

d. When an infant is born with ambiguous genitalia, factual information is presented. They should be told that their infant's sex organs are underdeveloped.

ITEM 13 Cognitive Type: Knowledge

Which of the following statements accurately describes the incidence of diabetes mellitus?

a. It is the most common endocrine disease of childhood.

b. The prevalence of the disease is decreasing as a result of early detection.

c. It is an inherited disease caused by a recessive gene.

d. The asymptomatic state of the disease is more commonly seen in immune deficient children.

ANSWER

a. Diabetes mellitus is one of the most prevalent serious chronic illnesses in today's society and is the most common endocrine disease in childhood. It is not generally considered to be inherited.

ITEM 14 Cognitive Type: Knowledge

A measure of good metabolic control for the child with diabetes mellitus is

a. fewer than five episodes of severe hyperglycemia in a month.

b. hemoglobin A_{IC} values less than 12.

c. infrequent occurrence of mild hypoglycemia reactions.

d. evidence of growth proceeding in the 20th percentile range.

ANSWER

c. Criteria for good metabolic control generally include HbA_{IC} values less than 9.5, normal growth and development, and few episodes of hypoglycemia or hyperglycemia.

ITEM 15 Cognitive Type: Application

Cindy, age 10 years, has insulin-dependent diabetes mellitus. She is admitted to the hospital at the time of her diagnosis for initial management of her disease and self-care education. When teaching Cindy and her parents about insulin administration, the nurse should

a. advise the parents that Cindy should be the only one to learn about injection and site rotation techniques to foster her self-care responsibility and independence.

b. instruct Cindy to draw up the prescribed long-acting insulin prior to the short-acting type of insulin to prevent cross-contamination.

c. begin to plan demonstration, supervision, and practice time for Cindy and her parents to learn injection and site rotation techniques at the time of her admission.

d. counsel Cindy and her parents about dietary restrictions that will facilitate the use of oral hypoglycemic agents rather than insulin injections.

ANSWER

c. Children with type I diabetes mellitus require insulin injection. Both parents and children should begin to learn about insulin administration as soon as possible to allow for professional supervision, repeated practice, and positive reinforcement.

ITEM 16 Cognitive Type: Application

When discussing the effects of exercise on glucose metabolism with a school age child with insulin-dependent diabetes mellitus and his parents, the nurse should include which recommendation for preventing hypoglycemia?

a. Increase insulin dosage prior to planned strenuous exercise.

b. Carry crackers or a piece of fruit that can be eaten before or during periods of increased physical activity.

c. Perform Clinitest prior to exercising and eat a protein snack if glucose level is elevated.

d. Limit participation in planned exercise activities that involve competition to reduce physical stress.

ANSWER

b. Hypoglycemia can usually be prevented if a child with diabetes eats more food before or during exercise. Since exercise is often not planned, carrying additional carbohydrate foods is a good preventative measure.

ITEM 17 Cognitive Type: Application

How should the nurse respond when the parents of Allan, who has diabetes mellitus, ask about maintaining metabolic control during periods of minor illness because he usually loses his appetite?

a. Decrease his insulin to half the usual dose during an illness.

b. Substitute calorie-containing liquids for uneaten foods to maintain blood glucose levels.

c. Give increased amounts of diet or unsweetened clear liquids to prevent dehydration.

d. Contact Allan's physician since he will need to be hospitalized to prevent hyperglycemia.

ANSWER

b. The child with diabetes should always take at least the usual dose of insulin during an illness. Calorie-containing liquids can help to maintain more normal blood sugar levels as well as decrease the danger of dehydration in the child who is unable to eat his usual diet.

ITEM 18 Cognitive Type: Application

Which of the following should be initiated to foster adolescents' compliance with treatment for diabetes mellitus?

a. Provision for special dietary needs in the high school cafeteria

b. Education about the long-term consequences of poor metabolic control

c. Clarification of personal values to promote involvement in an acceptable schedule for management regimens

d. Identification of energy requirements for participation in sports activities

ANSWER

c. Adolescent compliance with diabetes management may be hampered by dependency versus independency conflicts and ego development. Attempts to have the adolescent clarify his or her personal values and be involved in decision making are successful strategies in fostering compliance.

ITEM 19 Cognitive Type: Application

A child with insulin-dependent diabetes mellitus tells the nurse that she feels shaky. The nurse notes the child's skin is pale and sweaty. Which of the following actions would the nurse initiate *immediately*?

a. Offer the child a complex carbohydrate snack.

b. Give a supplemental dose of regular insulin.

c. Have the child drink a glass of orange juice.

d. Administer glucagon subcutaneously.

ANSWER

c. Rapid treatment of hypoglycemia is of the utmost importance. If the child is alert, give a glucose-containing solid, semi-solid, or liquid.

CHAPTER 44

ITEM 1 Cognitive Type: Application

Which action taken by parents of a newborn who was delivered at home indicates understanding of the nurse's teaching about phenylketonuria (PKU) screening?

a. The father takes the baby to the clinic for PKU testing 24 hours after delivery.

b. The mother calls the community health nurse to arrange for a home visit on the baby's third day of life for PKU testing.

c. The mother asks the midwife to preserve a specimen of cord blood for PKU testing.

d. The parents take the baby to the pediatrician's office for PKU testing at 2 weeks of age.

ANSWER

b. Nurses are responsible for educating parents about the necessity for PKU screening, and mothers who plan to give birth at home must accept responsibility for requesting community health nursing support in performing PKU screening on the baby any time from 3 to 7 days after birth.

ITEM 2 Cognitive Type: Application

Nursing interventions to prevent neurotoxicity in the infant who has phenylketonuria include

a. instructing parents to begin feeding pureed meats, eggs, and legumes at 5 months of age.

b. supporting the mother who had planned to breast feed through the period of loss and adjustment to the bottle.

c. reassuring parents that dietary restrictions will only be necessary until the child's third birthday.

d. educating parents about the importance of measuring and calculate amounts of fruits, vegetables, cereals, and grains.

ANSWER

d. Amounts of foods are adjusted to the child's age, weight, and serum phenylalanine levels.

ITEM 3 Cognitive Type: Knowledge

The child with ornithine transcarbamylase (OTC) deficiency would receive a

a. low fat diet.

b. high protein diet.

c. high carbohydrate, high fat diet.

d. low protein diet.

ANSWER

d. Long-term management of OTC deficiency includes a low protein diet, medications to increase nitrogen removal via alternative pathways, and supplementation with arginine or citrulline.

ITEM 4 Cognitive Type: Knowledge

To prevent symptomatic episodes in the child with medium-chain acyl-CoA dehydrogenase deficiency (MCADD), the nurse would teach the parents to

a. offer frequent small meals and a bedtime snack.

b. keep the diet high in complex carbohydrates and fats.

c. limit protein intake from animal sources.

d. give regular doses of intravenous glucose.

ANSWER

a. Management of MCADD is geared toward prevention of symptomatic episodes and includes frequent feedings in infancy and frequent small meals and snacks in toddlers and small children.

ITEM 5 Cognitive Type: Knowledge

In a baby who has galactosemia, the nurse should expect to see

a. fluid retention.

b. vomiting.

c. urticaria.

d. cataracts.

ANSWER

b. Clinical manifestations of galactosemia include vomiting and diarrhea, failure to thrive, jaundice, and irritability.

ITEM 6 Cognitive Type: Interpretation

The primary purpose of genetic counseling for the family with an infant who has an inborn error of metabolism is to

a. promote coping skills for adjustment after being informed not to have more children.

b. identify health care professionals who can provide ongoing support and education.

c. provide information about the risk of recurrence of the disorder.

d. encourage questions and verbalization of understanding about the disorder.

ANSWER

c. The nurse recognizes that the purpose of genetic counseling is to provide information about the risk of recurrence of a genetic disease to help the family make their own decisions about future pregnancies.

ITEM 7 Cognitive Type: Application

When teaching about dietary management for the infant who has an inborn error of carbohydrate metabolism, the nurse should

a. stress the importance of strict adherence to offering only the prescribed amount of special formula at regular feeding times.

b. advise the parents to read product labels carefully.

c. attempt to reduce parental anxiety by providing flexible feeding guidelines that meet the baby's special nutritional needs.

d. explain to parents that dietary controls will be relaxed once the baby begins to eat solid foods.

ANSWER

c. Dietary control for the management of metabolic disorders during infancy is usually not problematic since the child quickly adjusts to the special formula. However, instructions given by health professionals may produce anxiety in a parent if they do not allow for flexibility.

ITEM 8 Cognitive Type: Knowledge

The cause of maple syrup urine disease (MSUD) can be attributed to

a. inefficient production of isoleucine and valine.

b. absence of the essential amino acids leucine and valine.

c. deficiency of the enzyme complex known as branched chain keto acid dehydrogenase (BCKD).

d. enzyme block in the first step of the metabolic pathway.

ANSWER

c. MSUD results from a deficiency of the BCKD enzyme complex.

CHAPTER 45

ITEM 1 Cognitive Type: Knowledge

A sign alerting the nurse to possible vision impairment in a child is

a. delayed language development.

b. excessive rubbing of the eyes.

c. disinterest in television viewing.

d. binocular convergence of the eyes.

ANSWER

b. The two major symptoms of refractive errors are reduced acuity and discomfort. Symptoms in children include rubbing of the eyes, tearing, and squinting.

ITEM 2 Cognitive Type: Knowledge

Screening programs to detect visual problems in children should be initiated

a. in the preschool years.

b. when puberty begins.

c. at birth.

d. during the kindergarten years.

ANSWER

c. Visual screening should begin at birth since early identification and treatment of problems can prevent serious vision loss.

ITEM 3 Cognitive Type: Knowledge

To prevent amblyopia, therapeutic management of the child with strabismus includes

a. patching of the affected eye.

b. mydriatic eyedrops.

c. patching of the unaffected eye.

d. neosynephrine eyedrops.

ANSWER

c. To encourage the child with strabismus to use the deviating eye, the good eye is patched.

ITEM 4 Cognitive Type: Knowledge

The reduction or loss of vision in an eye that is normal on ophthalmoscopic exam is called

a. myopia.

b. amblyopia.

c. hyperopia.

d. astigmatism.

ANSWER

b. A diagnostic sign of amblyopia is that visual acuity in the normal eye is at least two Snellen lines better than acuity in the affected eye.

ITEM 5 Cognitive Type: Application

Which nursing action should be included in the plan of care for a family whose child has undergone surgical removal of a cataract?

a. Explain that the child's vision will improve immediately after surgery.

b. Teach the proper administration of eyedrop medication.

c. Discuss the importance of extended activity restrictions.

d. Provide the family with developmental strategies for meeting the needs of a child with bilateral eye patches in place.

ANSWER

b. A combination of antibiotic and steroid eyedrops is given for several weeks following surgical removal of a cataract to prevent infection and minimize inflammation.

ITEM 6 Cognitive Type: Application

To prevent increased intraocular pressure in an infant following a goniotomy procedure for glaucoma, the nurse should

a. observe the infant for signs of lethargy or malaise.

b. administer miotic eyedrops as ordered.

c. maintain the infant in a flat, side-lying position, turning every 2 hours.

d. comfort the infant to prevent crying.

ANSWER

d. The nurse should institute measures to maintain low intraocular pressure in an infant following goniotomy. These include elevating the head of the bed, comforting the infant who is upset, avoiding loud noises, and treating constipation.

ITEM 7 Cognitive Type: Application

Strategies to meet the communication needs of partially sighted children should include

a. provision of additional verbal explanations to clarify exact meaning and intent during conversation.

b. use of books in Braille as the major source of learning to prevent further deterioration of sight.

c. reduction of environmental stimulation to preserve residual vision fully.

d. referral to rehabilitative services for the blind to enhance social and emotional adaptation.

ANSWER

a. Partially sighted children are often unsure of how to respond verbally to others since their perception of facial expressions and gestures used to convey messages is often distorted.

ITEM 8 Cognitive Type: Application

A play activity that would best promote socialization in the preschool age child who is blind is

a. manipulating a large geometric board puzzle.

b. exploring the facial features of an older sibling who is verbally describing each area touched.

c. holding hands with a sighted child while playing ring-around-the-rosie.

d. participating in a game of Simon Says with several other blind children.

ANSWER

b. During the preschool years when a child learns to relate to other children, the blind child must be told about an activity and must be assisted through the activity before the nature of it can be understood.

ITEM 9 Cognitive Type: Application

The Dunns' 1-month-old infant is blind. What would the nurse tell these parents about communicating with their infant?

a. Blind infants will smile in response to tactile stimuli rather than auditory stimuli.

b. Talking and singing to the infant while holding him will help the parents to get to know their infant.

c. They can expect their infant to begin smiling at 2 months of age.

d. Blind infants have very expressive facial signs.

ANSWER

b. A child's smile is important in the development of parent–infant attachment. The smile of a blind infant differs from that of a sighted child. Parents should be encouraged to talk, sing, coo to their infant to learn about the infant's responses and how to elicit smiles.

ITEM 10 Cognitive Type: Knowledge

Which of the following behaviors may suggest that a child has a hearing loss?

a. The child responds more to facial expressions than to words.

b. The infant is babbling after 7 months of age.

c. A 15-month-old toddler uses gestures and pointing more than words to express his desires.

d. A 2-year-old child has many temper tantrums.

ANSWER

a. Behaviors associated with hearing loss include more response to changes in facial expression than to words.

ITEM 11 Cognitive Type: Knowledge

The most common cause of conductive hearing loss in children is

a. ototoxic drugs.

b. serous otitis media.

c. auditory nerve damage.

d. maternal rubella.

ANSWER

b. Conductive hearing impairment accounts for most hearing loss in children and is most often caused by serous otitis media.

ITEM 12 Cognitive Type: Knowledge

Parents can facilitate their child's language development by

a. using baby talk when interacting with the child.

b. repeating mispronounced words correctly.

c. reading books with the child daily.

d. speaking slowly so the child understands the parents' words.

ANSWER

c. Reading to the child from infancy can maximize the child's language development.

ITEM 13 Cognitive Type: Interpretation

In a child who has a conductive hearing loss, the nurse should expect to see

a. poor language skills, mild behavior problems, and fluctuating attentiveness to the environment.

b. high distractibility, short attention span, and poor reading skills.

c. poor impulse control, refusal to participate in organized activity, and generalized negativity.

d. overdependence, inappropriate attachment behaviors, and reluctance to join social activity.

ANSWER

a. Hearing levels fluctuate in the child with conductive hearing loss and are usually mild to moderate losses. This accounts for the recognizable syndrome of behaviors that are usually mild and transient in such a child.

ITEM 14 Cognitive Type: Knowledge

An assessment tool useful in detecting ear pathology before significant hearing impairment has occurred is

a. audiometry.

b. a crib-o-gram.

c. tympanometry.

d. brain stem auditory evolved potential.

ANSWER

c. Impedance testing (tympanometry) measures the compliance of the tympanic membrane in response to air pressure changes in the external auditory canal. Since even mild disease can influence tympanic membrane compliance, this test is useful in detecting preimpairment hearing alterations.

ITEM 15 Cognitive Type: Interpretation

When communicating with the child who is deaf and able to speech read, the nurse should

a. maintain eye contact with the child while speaking slowly.

b. speak in a natural tone of voice using complete sentences.

c. exaggerate mouth, tongue, and lip movements when speaking.

d. use short, incomplete sentences that convey general meaning.

ANSWER

b. A deaf child's ability to speech read is improved if adequate lighting falls on the speaker's face and if natural speaking is used with normal articulation and complete sentences.

ITEM 16 Cognitive Type: Interpretation

The nurse would be concerned about a language problem in a

a. 16-month-old child who does not respond to "bye-bye" or "bottle."

b. 18-month-old girl with a vocabulary of 15 words.

c. 20-month-old boy not pointing to body parts on request.

d. 24-month-old child who speaks in two-word sentences.

ANSWER

a. If a child does not understand or respond to "no-no," "bye-bye," or "bottle" by 15 months, a language problem should be suspected.

ITEM 17 Cognitive Type: Application

Which of the following should the nurse encourage the father of a 3-year-old child to do when she stutters?

a. Supply the stuttered word for the child.

b. Practice consonant sounds with her.

c. Encourage the child to think before speaking.

d. Ignore the stuttering and maintain interest in the conversation.

ANSWER

d. Stuttering behavior during late toddlerhood is a natural manifestation of efforts to master communication skills and should be ignored. Behavioral disturbances may result if conscious controls are imposed over the involuntary act of forming words.

ITEM 18 Cognitive Type: Application

Nursing interventions for the hospitalized child who has a sensory impairment should be primarily directed toward

a. promoting optimal growth and development.

b. fostering independence in self-care skills.

c. maintaining usual methods of communication and home routines.

d. encouraging parents to room-in with the child.

ANSWER

c. Special routines of home and usual methods of communication must be maintained to provide maximum comfort to the sensory-impaired child who is hospitalized.

CHAPTER 46

ITEM 1 Cognitive Type: Knowledge

Which of the following accurately reflects developmental differences related to injuries in children?

a. Injured children should be treated as anatomically smaller adults.

b. One out of every ten pediatric deaths is due to injury.

c. Underdeveloped abdominal and chest wall muscles increase the child's risk for injury from blunt trauma.

d. Flexible neck muscles and cranial suture expandability increase the child's potential to fully recover from serious head trauma.

ANSWER

c. One out of every three pediatric deaths is due to injury. Blunt trauma is a more frequent cause of chest and abdominal injuries in children than penetrating trauma.

ITEM 2 Cognitive Type: Knowledge

Primary assessment of the injured child includes

a. weight estimation, blood pressure measurement, and body inspection.

b. allergic history, symptom analysis, and head-to-toe survey.

c. airway patency, respiratory effectiveness, and circulatory status.

d. temperature measurement, medication history, and mode of injury.

ANSWER

c. The primary survey of an injured child includes rapid assessment of the "ABCs": airway, breathing, and circulation. The secondary survey includes weight and blood pressure measurement and the head-to-toe assessment.

ITEM 3 Cognitive Type: Knowledge

Which of the following reflects recommended procedure for cardiopulmonary resuscitation (CPR) of the pediatric patient?

a. To check for a pulse in an infant under 1 year of age, the brachial artery is palpated.

b. The compression to ventilation ratio for children under the age of 8 years is 15:2.

c. If an infant is not breathing, give four quick breaths followed by a pause to allow for exhalation.

d. The cardiac compression rate for children over the age of 1 year should be 120 per minute.

ANSWER

a. The brachial pulse is palpated in CPR of infants under the age of 1 year because the chubby neck makes the carotid pulse less accessible.

ITEM 4 Cognitive Type: Application

A mother telephones the well child clinic for advice when her 9-year-old son has a tooth knocked out during soccer practice. How would the nurse advise her?

a. Clean the tooth with soap and water and come to the clinic.

b. The tooth can be kept viable for 2 hours if placed in a cup of milk; call the dentist immediately.

c. Handle the avulsed tooth carefully by the root and preserve it in 8 ounces of salt water.

d. Drop the tooth in a clean container and take it to the local emergency room.

ANSWER

b. The avulsed tooth should be gently handled by the crown and placed in a specially formulated solution marketed as "Save a Tooth" solution. If this is unavailable, the tooth can be placed in milk for 2 hours if kept at 20°C. The family should go to the local emergency room if a dentist cannot be reached.

ITEM 5 Cognitive Type: Knowledge

When conducting an educational program about first aid for common childhood injuries, the nurse should instruct parents to

a. apply warm compresses to mosquito or bee bites to reduce inflammation and discomfort.

b. obtain emergency room care for suturing of deep, gaping lacerations within 24 hours after injury to prevent scarring.

c. wash puncture wounds with soap and water and obtain a tetanus booster if signs of infection develop.

d. seek medical assistance for human bites that break the skin since prophylactic antibiotics may be necessary to prevent infection.

ANSWER

d. Human bites are highly contaminated because of the high number of organisms in saliva and are treated with debridement, irrigation, and broad spectrum antibiotics to prevent infection.

ITEM 6 Cognitive Type: Application

The Wrights are concerned about cold exposure during a skiing vacation that they are planning to take with their two young children. What information would the nurse give to the Wrights about preventing frostbite during this vacation?

a. Recommend that the Wrights arrange for indoor activities for the children.

b. Advise the Wrights to dress the children in clothing that fits snugly against the skin.

c. Teach the children to rub hands together vigorously if fingers feel cold and tingly.

d. Layer light clothing under coats and wear a hat, mittens, and two pairs of socks when outdoors.

ANSWER

d. Several layers of light clothing under outerwear provide extra warmth. Children playing outdoors should wear a hat, mittens, and two pairs of socks.

ITEM 7 Cognitive Type: Application

Home management of the child with epistaxis following the removal of a foreign object from the nose should include instructions for

a. applying nasal pressure to the septal cartilage for a full 5 minutes.

b. removing clots through gentle blowing of the nose.

c. packing the anterior nares with vaseline gauze.

d. instilling saline nose drops prior to application of warm compresses to the nasal bridge.

ANSWER

a. Home management of the child with epistaxis includes observation for repeated bleeding, correct technique for nasal pressure, and avoidance of nose blowing and picking. Nasal packing is performed by emergency room professionals.

ITEM 8 Cognitive Type: Application

Which nursing action is of *primary* importance when caring for a child after removal of a foreign object from the respiratory tract?

a. Monitor for signs and symptoms of respiratory distress.

b. Allay the child's fears and anxiety associated with emergency care treatments.

c. Facilitate resolution of parental guilt.

d. Review principles of child safety and child proofing of the home with the parents.

ANSWER

a. Monitoring the child's physical status is of utmost importance after removal of a foreign body from the respiratory tract due to laryngeal edema and/or soft tissue swelling that may cause secondary airway obstruction.

ITEM 9 Cognitive Type: Knowledge

To induce vomiting in poisoning circumstances, one should administer

a. magnesium citrate.

b. activated charcoal.

c. tannic acid.

d. syrup of ipecac.

ANSWER

d. The drug of choice for induction of vomiting to decrease absorption of ingested poisons is syrup of ipecac.

ITEM 10 Cognitive Type: Knowledge

A child has ingested an undetermined amount of 325-mg aspirin tablets. The nurse notes the child is confused and hyperventilating. These signs are related to

a. respiratory alkalosis.

b. respiratory acidosis.

c. metabolic alkalosis.

d. metabolic acidosis.

ANSWER

a. The first phase of the body's response to salicylate overdose, stimulation of the respiratory center in the medulla, causes hyperventilation, a fall in P_{CO_2} and respiratory alkalosis.

ITEM 11 Cognitive Type: Knowledge

Which of the following actions is appropriate after a child ingests liquid toilet cleaner?

a. Administer syrup of ipecac to induce vomiting.

b. Flush the mouth, lips, and face with warm water to remove the substance from these areas.

c. Offer the child a small amount of water to dilute the substance.

d. Give the child a glass of milk to coat the oral and esophageal mucosa.

ANSWER

c. Water can be given orally to dilute the corrosive substance as long as the quantity is small enough to avoid the stimulus to vomit.

ITEM 12 Cognitive Type: Knowledge

When administering *N*-acetylcysteine (Mucomyst) to a child with acetaminophen poisoning, the nurse should

a. mix the drug with a carbonated beverage.

b. give with syrup of ipecac.

c. dilute the drug in milk.

d. give the drug after administration of activated charcoal.

ANSWER

a. The nurse should recognize the offensiveness of the acetaminophen antidote (Mucomyst) and should administer it in a carbonated beverage.

ITEM 13 Cognitive Type: Application

Nursing interventions to reduce discomfort associated with chelation therapy for the child with lead poisoning include

a. use of Z-track injection technique.

b. use only the dorsogluteal sites for injections.

c. intramuscular injections of CaEDTA with procaine.

d. placement of an ice bag over the area used for injection.

ANSWER

c. Intramuscular injection of CaEDTA is extremely painful and is recommended to be given with procaine by deep injection followed by application of warm soaks to the injected area.

ITEM 14 Cognitive Type: Knowledge

The mechanism responsible for anemia in children with lead poisoning is that lead

a. prevents erythrocyte formation.

b. interferes with heme synthesis.

c. decreases the amount of free erythrocyte protoporphyrin.

d. limits iron absorption.

ANSWER

b. Lead affects heme synthesis by blocking the incorporation of iron into the protoporphyrin compound that makes up the heme portion of hemoglobin.

ITEM 15 Cognitive Type: Application

The primary purpose of performing chest physiotherapy on the child who has experienced a near drowning is to

a. facilitate gas exchange.

b. prevent hypoxia.

c. facilitate endotracheal intubation.

d. provide humidification.

ANSWER

a. Chest physiotherapy is performed to facilitate gas exchange in the lungs of a near-drowning victim by clearing the respiratory passage of excessive secretions.

CHAPTER 47

ITEM 1 Cognitive Type: Knowledge

Which of the following statements is accurate about burn injuries in children?

a. Burns are the leading cause of accidental death in children.

b. Up to 25% of pediatric burns are inflicted by adults.

c. The highest incidence of burn injuries occurs in children 3 to 5 years of age.

d. The majority of burns in children under 5 years of age are caused by house fires.

ANSWER

b. Approximately 10–25% of pediatric burn injuries are deliberately inflicted by adults.

ITEM 2 Cognitive Type: Knowledge

Tissue changes and fluid shifts that occur in the first 24 hours after a burn injury cause

a. hypernatremia.

b. hypokalemia.

c. metabolic alkalosis.

d. hypovolemia.

ANSWER

d. Fluid from injured tissues leaks out of the bloodstream and into interstitial spaces resulting in edema in the burned area and depletion of vascular volume (hypovolemia).

ITEM 3 Cognitive Type: Knowledge

Which of the following conditions would be present if a burn injury was classified as a major burn?

a. Full thickness burns have occurred that cover less than 10% of total body area.

b. Burns occur on the face, hands, feet, or perineum.

c. The child is between 5 and 10 years of age.

d. The burning agent was flames or hot liquid.

ANSWER

b. If burns are on the face, hands, feet, or perineum and/or injury is circumferential, burns are classified as major.

ITEM 4 Cognitive Type: Application

During the emergent phase of a major burn injury, a young child will require fluid therapy to prevent shock. An assessment finding indicating adequate fluid replacement is

a. increasing hematocrit values.

b. urine output of 1–2 mL/kg/hour.

c. weight gain greater than 15% of preburn weight.

d. hemomyoglobinuria.

ANSWER

b. Adequate amounts of parenteral fluids to maintain organ perfusion without overloading the circulatory system is determined by monitoring urinary output. For young children with major burn injury, outputs of 1–2 mL/kg/hour indicate appropriate fluid resuscitation.

ITEM 5 Cognitive Type: Application

A. J. is a 4-year-old boy who has full thickness circumferencial burns of the chest. Nursing actions to facilitate normal lung excursion would include

a. alternate supine and prone positions every 4 hours.

b. elevate the head of the bed 45°.

c. administer analgesics at the maximum interval tolerated by the child.

d. give mucolytic treatments followed by chest physiotherapy.

ANSWER

b. Placing the child in a semi-Fowler's position can contribute to normal lung excursion.

ITEM 6 Cognitive Type: Application

An appropriate nursing action to prevent infection in a burn wound is to

a. observe the perimeter of the burn wound for erythema.

b. culture the burn wound if purulent exudate is observed.

c. check the WBC count if granulation tissue is seen.

d. change any catheters and connecting tubing once a day.

ANSWER

a. The burn wound should be monitored for signs of infection by daily inspection for erythema, exudate, ulceration, and deterioration of granulation tissue. Often the first sign of wound infection is erythema at the burn wound perimeter.

ITEM 7 Cognitive Type: Application

Which nursing action would best promote pain relief for the child who is undergoing full thickness burn wound debridement?

a. Ensure that prescribed pain medication is given before each dressing change.

b. Use attention distraction techniques to reduce fear since full thickness injuries are not very painful.

c. Provide for active participation in wound care by allowing the child to express needs during the procedure.

d. Offer positive reinforcement for cooperation and give sedation after the procedure to provide uninterrupted rest periods.

ANSWER

a. Wound debridement for all types of burns is known to be extremely painful. Analgesia should always be given prior to wound care. Other ways to relieve pain are helpful, but they should not replace analgesia.

ITEM 8 Cognitive Type: Knowledge

The child with a major burn injury requires a high carbohydrate, high protein diet so as to

a. prevent paralytic ileus.

b. promote healing.

c. spare protein catabolism.

d. avoid anorexia and the need for hyperalimentation.

ANSWER

c. Because of increased metabolism and catabolism as a result of burn trauma, a child needs two or three times the normal amount of calories and protein. Calories should be in the form of carbohydrates to spare protein breakdown.

ITEM 9 Cognitive Type: Application

In the rehabilitative phase, how would the nurse position a child with burns of the knee and lower leg to prevent deformity?

a. Supine with a pillow supporting a flexed knee

b. Prone with a pillow under the ankles

c. Supine with the leg extended in a posterior splint

d. Side-lying with the hip and knee flexed

ANSWER

c. Extension should be maintained using a posterior splint or by suspending the heels with plastic heel protecting boots. When the child is in a supine position, no pillows should be placed under the knee. If the child is prone, there should be no pillows under the ankles.

ITEM 10 Cognitive Type: Application

Which instructions should be included in the teaching plan for parents of a child with a minor burn wound?

a. Give analgesic immediately after changing the burn wound dressing.

b. Wash the burn wound three times a day with a betadine solution and leave the wound uncovered.

c. Clean the burn wound gently with soap and water, rinse with water, and cover the area with a dressing.

d. Scrub the burn wound so partial thickness wounds are converted to full thickness for faster healing.

ANSWER

c. Minor burn wounds should be gently cleansed with soap and water and a clean dressing applied.